ADVANCE PRAISE FOR

The Best Surgeon in England: Percivall Pott, 1713–88

"Lynda Payne has achieved a remarkable reconstruction of elite hospital surgery, as it existed before the advent of anesthesia and antiseptic technique. This examination of the career of the influential surgeon Percivall Pott, 'the best surgeon in England,' explores a paradox at the heart of eighteenth-century surgical practice. Here was a highly respected and carefully cultivated form of expertise that in application proved to be fast, bloody, and all too lethal. If you would like to understand better how Mr. Pott could describe to families, teach to his many students, and walk to the table and perform a surgical procedure that might, in Pott's opinion, 'kill only 1 in 50 if done immediately,' this is your book."

—*Christopher Crenner, Robert Hudson and Ralph Major Professor of the History and Philosophy of Medicine and Chair of the Department of History and Philosophy of Medicine, The University of Kansas Medical Center*

The Best Surgeon in England

AMERICAN UNIVERSITY STUDIES

SERIES IX
HISTORY

VOL. 205

This book is a volume in a Peter Lang monograph series.
Every volume is peer reviewed and meets
the highest quality standards for content and production.

PETER LANG
New York • Bern • Frankfurt • Berlin
Brussels • Vienna • Oxford • Warsaw

Lynda Payne

The Best Surgeon in England

Percivall Pott, 1713–88

PETER LANG
New York • Bern • Frankfurt • Berlin
Brussels • Vienna • Oxford • Warsaw

Library of Congress Cataloging-in-Publication Data

Names: Payne, Lynda.
Title: The best surgeon in England: Percivall Pott, 1713–88 / Lynda Payne.
Other titles: Percivall Pott, 1713–88
Description: New York: Peter Lang.
Series: American university studies. IX, History; vol. 205 | ISSN 0740-0462
Includes bibliographical references and index.
Identifiers: LCCN 2013028628 | ISBN 978-1-4331-2319-1 (hardcover: alk. paper)
ISBN 978-1-4539-1191-4 (ebook pdf) | ISBN 978-1-4331-3727-3 (epub)
ISBN 978-1-4331-3728-0 (mobi) | DOI 10.3726/978-1-4539-1191-4
Subjects: LCSH: Pott, Percivall, 1713–1788. | Surgeons—Great Britain—Biography.
Medicine—Great Britain—History—18th century.
Classification: LCC R489.P595 P39 | DDC 617.092 [B]—dc23
LC record available at https://lccn.loc.gov/2013028628

Bibliographic information published by **Die Deutsche Nationalbibliothek**.
Die Deutsche Nationalbibliothek lists this publication in the "Deutsche Nationalbibliografie"; detailed bibliographic data are available on the Internet at http://dnb.d-nb.de/.

The paper in this book meets the guidelines for permanence and durability of the Committee on Production Guidelines for Book Longevity of the Council of Library Resources.

29 Broadway, 18th floor, New York, NY 10006
www.peterlang.com

Printed in Germany

For Bill, Beatrice and Bridget

Contents

Illustrations

Acknowledgments

I would like to thank the many institutions and people that have provided financial and professional support over the years I have been researching and writing this monograph. My colleagues and students in the History Department at the University of Missouri–Kansas City (UMKC) have remained steadfast in their interest in Pott and his world. I was fortunate to receive the support of a Women and Gender Studies Research Grant at UMKC and a University of Missouri Research Board Grant to help fund this project. Susan Sykes-Berry, a reference librarian at UMKC's Health Sciences Library, spent hundreds of hours collating primary research materials. At the University of Kansas Medical Center, Dawn McInnis at The Clendening History of Medicine Library provided invaluable help in locating surgical manuscripts and rare books. A Eugene W. J. Pearce, M. D. and Lunetta A. Pearce, M.D., Fellowship in the History of Medicine, Library and Archives at the University of Kansas enabled me to dig deeper into the wonderful collections of the Clendening Library. I also spent a summer in the Ebling Library for the Health Sciences funded by a Friends of the University of Wisconsin Libraries Research Grant-in-Aid. I wish to thank Mary E. Hitchcock and Micaela Sullivan-Fowler at the Ebling Library for their hard work in helping with my research.

Several visits to London allowed me to spend time at the Royal College of Surgeons, the Wellcome Library, Barts and The London NHS Archives, the

Royal College of Physicians, Kings College Archives, the London Metropolitan Archives, The National Archives, and the British Library. Librarians and archivists were invariably kind and knowledgeable in aiding my work. Janice O'Brien carried out an extensive enquiry into the life of Bob Pott in the British Library's India Office Records and at The National Archives. I am grateful for the primary materials she discovered and sent to me.

Finally, I would like to acknowledge the support of the late Dr. Marjorie Sirridge and her family, the wisdom and friendship of Mrs. Patricia Burton and the late Dr. Jerry Burton, and the love of my spouse, Professor William Everett and our canine companions, Beatrice and Bridget. This book is dedicated to them.

Introduction

"What Brought Each Leaden-Headed Lad to Town, What Drew Them Hither but the Name of Pott?"[1]

In 1784 there were 148 physicians, 600 apothecaries and 220 surgeons working in London. Percivall Pott (1713–1788) was one of those surgeons, and he was also the fortunate holder of one of the 62 hospital posts available in the city.[2] This book analyses the long career of Mr. Pott for what it can tell us about a period of great transition in the rank and respectability of hospital surgeons in England. Pott completed his apprenticeship with the last barber-surgeon to be elected assistant surgeon to St. Bartholomew's Hospital in 1731 and then became the first member of the new Company of Surgeons to be elected assistant surgeon to the hospital in 1745. For nearly forty years he offered a series of annual lectures on surgery to pupils, took on apprentices and trained dressers and built up a large and lucrative private practice in London and its outskirts. Pott was widely recognized for being the best practical surgeon of his generation, and his numerous publications replete with case histories were praised for the elegance of their language and clarity of approach to the bloody business of surgery. His works were avidly translated into other languages and went through many editions on the continent and in America.

Focusing on the character, pedagogy, writings and correspondence of Pott allows us to explore issues such as how did surgeons present and position themselves in a competitive world of medical men and women, what did it entail to become known as an authority in surgery, and how was knowledge structured and restructured to create a professional identity.[3] Surgery was a risky business both for patients and practitioners of the art and it aroused strong feelings of fear and hope in the minds of those who were cut upon and in those who did the cutting. Tolerance of uncertainty was required along with the ability to change a planned course of treatment based on what a surgeon discovered when he opened the body. Pott taught pupils, apprentices and dressers how to behave and think as surgeons through narratives composed of words, emotions, and actions. He sought to construct certain patterns of behavior and inculcate reserve in how his young charges acted when making a diagnosis, carrying out a treatment, or offering a prognosis. Surgery for Pott was an intellectual and sensory experience, where emotional engagement with the patient was a necessity and honesty was the best policy. Long before amphitheatres became common in London hospitals, Pott opposed heroic measures, theatrical performances, and displays of temper by surgeons.[4] He instructed his pupils to maintain an unruffled composure and to have the fortitude to cut as deep and wide as needed to allow a surgeon to effectively treat the patient.

At the age of forty-three Pott had a horse accident that badly injured his leg. During several months of enforced rest, he wrote *A Treatise on Ruptures*. It was published in 1756 and discussed one of the most common ailments a surgeon treated, namely hernias. It was to be the first in a prolific stream of books and treatises. A cursory glance at the titles of some of Pott's books provides a view into the workaday existence of a London hospital surgeon in the eighteenth century and the sorts of conditions he would encounter: *An Account of a Particular Kind of Rupture, Frequently Attendant upon New-Children; and Sometimes Met with in Adult; viz. that in which the intestine, or omentum, is found in the same cavity, and in contact with the testicle*, 1757; *Observations on that disorder of the corner of the eye, commonly called fistula lachrymalis*, 1758; *Observations on the nature and consequences of those injuries to which the head is liable from external violence*, 1760; *Practical Remarks on the Hydrocele or Watery Rupture, and Some Other Diseases of the Testicle* 1762; *Remarks on the disease, commonly called a fistula in ano*, 1765; *Some few general remarks on fractures and dislocations*, 1773; *Chirurgical Observations relative to the Cataract, the polypus of the nose, the cancer of the scrotum, and the mortification of the toes*, 1775; *Remarks on Curvature of the Spine*, 1779; *Observations on the necessity and propriety of amputation, in certain case and under certain circumstances*, 1779; and *Farther Remarks on the useless state of the lower limbs in consequence of a Curvature of the Spine*, 1782.

Along with the production of books on various conditions, a significant part of Pott's life was spent teaching surgery. Notes from his apprentices and pupils survive in surprising numbers in manuscript form, some anonymous and some not, some as fair copies and some as scribbles. As Susan Lawrence has posited, lecture notes reflect an interaction between the instructor and the student, rather than a verbatim account of what an instructor said and the student understood.[5] Read in this way, the surviving manuscripts of Pott's lectures, often completed by boys between the ages of fourteen and seventeen, offer glimpses into how knowledge and practice was passed on from teacher to student. The gentlemanly virtues Pott considered requisite for a successful surgeon are constantly stressed: courage, a cool head, a steady hand, a keen eye, and the ability to gain and keep the trust of patients upon whom you were going to generally inflict great pain. The notes also reveal how Pott trained and influenced other surgeons, ways in which surgical knowledge was produced and transmitted, and how surgeons learned to judge what to treat and what to leave alone. Case histories included in the lectures and Pott's many publications establish that certain conditions and parts of the body were viewed as being so closely linked with particular operative surgeons that they became part of that surgeon's professional identity. Pott had several conditions named for him, and the terms were in use soon after his death if not just before. They were "Pott's puffy tumor" (periosteal abscess formation in the brain that is often recurrent[6]), "Pott's disease of the spine" (tuberculous spondylitis[7]), and "Pott's dislocated fracture of the ankle" (a complicated break). Pott was the first medical man to argue that an external agent could cause cancer, namely that soot trapped in the skin folds of young chimney sweeps could lead to scrotal cancer in adulthood.[8] Cancer Scroti was often referred to as "Pott's disease" in the twentieth century. Not for nothing did Sir D'Arcy Power dub Pott the "Prince of Eponyms."[9] Such labeling of disorders in the late eighteenth century reveals the importance and power of rhetoric in crafting the increasingly rigid definition of medicine as a sophisticated scientific activity rather than a mundane lay experience of treating sickness. It also helps lay bare the power of surgeons to classify and essentially come to own certain disorders in the body.

The appearance, the smell, and the feel of infected body parts are vividly recorded in Pott's lectures and books. Surgeons saw patients in acute crises and in chronic disorder and pain. Networks of care and neglect, conditions for living and working, and the dangers of child play and innocent games are revealed through case histories of accidents, violence, paralysis and deformity. Questions of power and control in the history of medicine arose when surgeons sought to coerce patients into revealing information about their illnesses and to get them to agree to an operation. Equally such questions arose when patients insisted on surgery or a more forceful therapy. Surgery before the availability of general anesthesia has been viewed as brutal for the patient and potentially brutalizing to the surgeon. An analysis of Pott's and his patients' rhetoric helps reveal when surgery was resorted to and when it was not. Piecing together some of the details of the lives and deaths of men, women, and children Pott encountered and contextualizing their experiences results in a rich social history of events generally neither shared nor captured in non-medical sources.

The scholarship on early modern English surgeons is limited, and consideration of the social and cultural history of surgery has largely been overshadowed by studies on the lives of physicians and medicine in general. Where surgery and surgeons are addressed, it has been largely in terms of technology (the development of instruments, anesthesia, asepsis) and innovation (new techniques in operating).[10] Notable exceptions include Wendy Moore's *The Knife Man: The Extraordinary Life and Times of John Hunter, Father of Modern Surgery* and Peter Stanley's *For Fear of Pain: British Surgery, 1790–1850*. Andrew Wear and Roy Porter have considered connections between early modern surgery and pain, as have I within my study of the development of dispassion.[11] The rise of general anesthetics, not surprisingly, has received considerable attention from historians. Only recently, however, has its transformative effects on surgery been problematized. Stephanie J. Snow has discussed the social, economic, and political aspects of anesthesia, noting that its genesis has been celebrated and treated as a watershed moment in medical history, for this was when pain was banished from operative practice and surgery became modern, meaning painless.[12] But much remains to be written about the history of surgery. Thomas Schlich has noted that we are especially lacking histories that tackle "What surgeons actually did in their jobs …"[13] Pott's training in surgery began when he was 15, and he treated his last patient at age 73. Examining and contextualizing what Pott did over the course of his life to earn the epithet of being the best surgeon in England is one of the principal goals of this book.

The first chapter examines how Pott successfully clambered up the ladder of surgery and business over a half century to become a gentleman of means and respectability. Pott's origins, apprenticeship, patrons, marriage and the lives of his eight children are explored to establish the social, cultural and economic contexts within which Pott found fame as a hospital surgeon. He achieved a high degree of respect through producing well-trained apprentices and dressers, holding authoritative roles in the new Company of Surgeons, obtaining a senior post at a major hospital, demonstrating calm dexterity in operating, treating well-known patients, and writing praiseworthy books. A biography written by Pott's son-in-law, the surgeon James Earle has achieved canonical status among scholars as the source on Pott's life. It is analyzed for what it reveals of sentiments toward the barber-surgeons of Pott's youth and the characterization of Pott as the epitome of the new professional surgeon.

The next chapter analyzes how Pott visualized the doing of surgery. It was a risky occupation that required physical strength, dexterity, and a strong amount of authority. Pott's words and deeds as captured in his pupils' lecture notes signify changing professional and cultural ideologies. They allow us to examine the interplay of forces and structures in shaping surgical aspiration and status. Pott's life both impacted on and reflected broader historical changes in what it meant to be considered skilled in surgery. His systematic and focused approach to carrying out surgery, which he both practiced and taught, reveals the physical and sensory experiences of pre-modern surgeons and their patients. Pott advised his pupils to cultivate certain comportments, values, and traits in order to become successful and authoritative surgeons that point to the ambitions and anxieties of medical men in the mid to late eighteenth century.

The third chapter focuses on acute injuries, especially ones to the head, and those to the limbs that meant amputation was recommended. Pott published a seminal text on wounds to the head that includes many case histories which vividly depict the dangers and violence of daily life in Georgian England. Case histories were key components in the education of pupils and fellow medical men in the art of surgery, and Pott's are quite numerous and lengthy in comparison to other hospital surgeons of the era. They typically contained information on the context for the injury, the appearance of the injured body part, and the treatment and outcome of the intervention; however, they were far from being just accounts of diagnosis, treatment and prognosis. Pott constructed his narratives to warn of common mistakes in surgery, criticize quackery and mediocre surgeons, explain women's bodies, and teach the correct way to interact with other medical men and patients. Over decades of lectures he used his vast store of case histories to educate, persuade and occasionally amuse his pupils. Finally Pott expressed strong views in person and in print on the need to amputate when a wound was fresh. He entered into debates with medical men in Europe that show what a surgeon did well was promoted as evidence of the superiority of their physical approach to operating and of being bred in a country with higher morals.

The fourth chapter continues the analysis of Pott's case histories for what they reveal of chronic conditions such as hernias, cancers and venereal swellings of the genitals. The economic and social fears of patients can be glimpsed in the conversations, letters and case notes that surrounded such diagnoses. Pott followed some patients for years, and their situations could raise pity, amusement, and derision in him. In particular he experimented with different treatments on children with spinal deformity and paralysis of the legs from tuberculosis and published his findings to mixed reviews. The relation of practicing surgery to morality is further examined through a public dispute Pott had with William and John Hunter over the discovery of the formation of congenital hernia in infants. Both sides attempted to create a negative association of values around the other. Pott drew attention to the unsavory and vindictive nature of those who taught anatomy in private schools, while William Hunter attacked Pott for his willingness to steal and plagiarize findings from the hard work of those who possessed knowledge from dissecting hundreds of bodies.

The epilogue considers how Pott's legacy was shaped soon after his death and what has happened to it since. Pott is first viewed through the eyes of the generation of surgeons who came after him and reinforced his title of being the best surgeon in England. The comments of his contemporaries and successors, however, were not uniformly positive or hagiographic. Over time his reputation was twinned with that of John Hunter, with Pott being characterized as a doer and Hunter as a thinker. Finally in the twentieth and twenty-first centuries, Pott was lauded as the founder of preventive oncology and environmental epidemiology based on a brief essay he published on the development of cancer of the scrotum in chimney sweeps who survived to adulthood.

CHAPTER ONE

"Climbing the Ladder"

Business and Surgery

In 1777, a seventeen-year-old Irish boy named Ludford Harvey began a five-year apprenticeship with Mr. Percivall Pott, a person he described as "certainly the finest surgeon in the world."[1] Harvey had wanted to join the army, but his mother and brother overruled him, "and much to my regret, the Truncheon & the Mitre gave way to the Probe, & the Lancet … and frequent scenes of distress." In his "Diary Containing Memorandums relating to avocation, Accounts, Correspondances [*sic*], Anecdotes, &tc. Which may serve as a reference on my private concerns,"[2] Harvey describes the shock of suddenly being transplanted from a quiet home in rural Ireland to Pott's mansion off Hanover Square, London, where "Routes, Balls, Lords, Ladies, Opera Singers, and all other fashionable Topics were eternally agitated." Harvey bemoaned that he could only witness these events as an outsider in the Pott household, consigned as he was "to a Solitary Corner in this Temple of Mirth."[3]

Eventually Harvey had learned enough of the business of surgery to become invaluable to Pott. He assisted at capital (major) operations, took sole care of patients at St. Bartholomew's Hospital, and attended private fee-paying ones in their homes. Harvey also answered Pott's letters and collected money for surgical services. Buoyed with hope that he could rise from Pott's indispensable assistant to become a member of the family, Harvey fixed his sights on Pott's third eldest daughter, Mary, but found he had left it too late. Harvey recorded that "a

Courtship of one fortnight terminated the [indecipherable word] virginity of Miss Pott, now become Mrs Earle, & gave my Patron an Aspiring Surgeon for his Son in Law, whom for the past 10 years the whole Family had most cordially ridiculed & abused."[4] Harvey realized that all hope of succeeding Pott in his practice was now lost.[5] For the time being his climb up the ladder of surgical business was arrested.

In 1782, the same year that Harvey's apprenticeship came to an end, James Earle married Mary Pott and solidified his position as the surgeon who would take over his father-in-law's patients as needed. Earle also became Pott's first and only biographer: his 46-page memoir of Pott, which appeared just two years after the death of its subject, was subsequently published as the introductory piece to all the editions of Pott's complete works after 1790.[6] Earle's biography has achieved canonical status as the source on Pott's life and work.[7] This unquestioning acceptance appears to have occurred not just from the author's close relationship to the subject but because the biography was framed as a satisfying rags-to-riches romance. At the center of the tale is a saint-like Pott surrounded by admiring colleagues and grateful patients. Above all Earle stresses the humanity of Pott and contrasts it with the barbarity of previous surgeons.

Formative Years: St. Bartholomew's Hospital, and the Company of Surgeons

Earle begins his tale with the birth of Percivall Pott on December 26, 1713[8], in his parents' home on Threadneedle Street, London, adding that the Potts' home stood where the Bank of England is now located. The Bank moved to Threadneedle Street in 1734, but Pott's family home was probably demolished sometime between 1766 and 1788 when the great east and west wings were added. Percivall Pott's grandfather was John Pott (1642–1705), a grocer and oilman who made a good second marriage to the daughter of a pot maker.[9] Pott's father, also named Percivall (1681–1717), was the second of twelve children and worked as a scrivener and notary.[10] In 1712 he married Elizabeth Houblon (neeé Symonds), a widow with one daughter.[11] Her first husband, Lieutenant Benjamin Houblon, had died in Lisbon in 1708, probably while on business for his father, Sir John Houblon (Earle refers to him as Jacob), Governor of the Bank of England.[12] The Houblons were Huguenots, as were many subscribers when the bank was set up in 1694.[13] The elder Percivall Pott died at age 36, and his son Percivall, the future surgeon, was likely his only child, since the younger Pott in his writings only mentions the existence of one sibling, a stepsister named Elizabeth.

The younger Percivall Pott was only three-years-old when his father passed away, and according to Earle, the family was poor. No firm evidence suggests, however, that Elizabeth Houblon Pott and her children were left in dire circumstances after the death of her second husband. Earle bases his claim on the fact that after Percivall Pott's death in 1788, a £5 note was found in a box among his papers, and that this supposedly constituted his entire inheritance from his father. Earle mentions that Pott's mother received help after her second husband's death from Dr. Joseph Wilcox, a relative of her first husband. Wilcox (1673–1756) was a Chaplain to the English Factory in Lisbon and successively bishop of Gloucester (1721) and Rochester (1731). The English Factory was a trading station for those carrying out business as foreigners in Portugal from the 1650s.[14]

Earle's biography continues with the assertion that at age seven young Percivall was sent to a private school at Darenth, Kent, under Wilcox's protection. Just as evidence is lacking about the financial situation of Pott's family in 1717, no records survive for a school in Darenth that existed for boys such as Pott.[15] Nonetheless, at age 15, Pott was apprenticed to Edward Nourse (1701–61), a surgeon at St. Bartholomew's Hospital.[16] This cost his widowed mother the considerable sum of 200 guineas. A surgical apprenticeship may seem a surprising choice for a young man educated in the classics at a good country school with an extended family that had done well in selling dry and wet goods for at least two generations.[17] Surgery, however, was rising in status in the eighteenth century, especially in London. Christopher Lawrence lists three factors that enabled this: a "positive valuation of practical arts by Enlightenment thinkers and the attempt to base those arts on rational principles," "the rise of a medicine of populations, to which surgical-like models of specific disease were applied," and most relevant to Pott, "the increasingly successful employment of hospitals by surgeons as their institutional base."[18]

Fortunately the apprenticeship indenture for Percival Pott has survived.[19] An indenture was a legal document that defined the mutual obligations of master and apprentice. In London it was a particularly prized item for a seven-year apprenticeship "offered a path to gaining a freedom of the City." As Drew Gray notes, the gentry were willing to pay high prices to get life-long skills.[20] Pott would have had to pass an examination in Latin at the Barber-Surgeon's Hall before he could be bound to Nourse as his Master.[21]

Once an apprentice, Pott appears to have spent much of his time dissecting, prosecting, and preparing specimens for Nourse to use in his lectures on anatomy and surgery. These took place at Nourse's home in Aldersgate Street, close to St. Bartholomew's Hospital. Earle gives a damning summary of the theory and practice of surgery at the time Pott was laboring as an apprentice under Nourse:

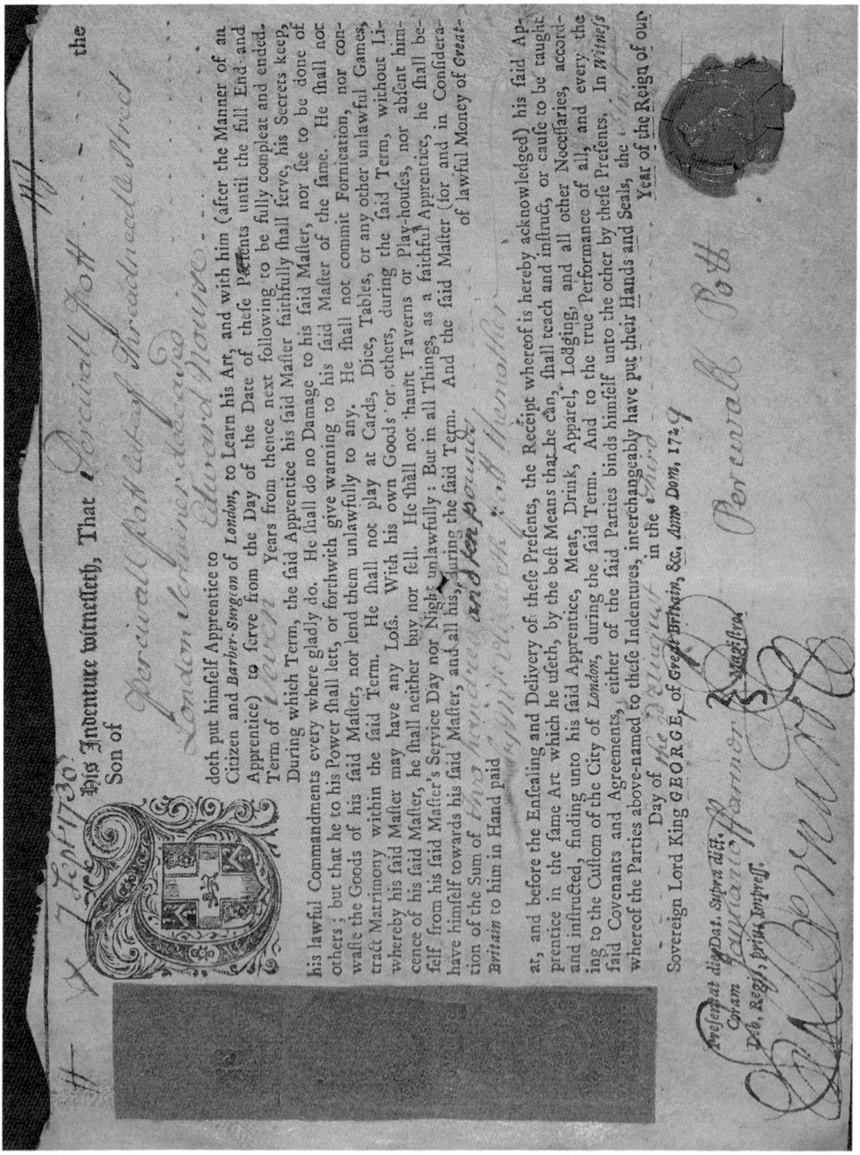

7 Sept 1730

This Indenture witnesseth, That Percivall Pott the Son of Percivall Pott late of Threadneedle Street London Scrivener deceased doth put himself Apprentice to Edward Nourse Citizen and *Barber-Surgeon* of *London*, to Learn his Art, and with him (after the Manner of an Apprentice) to serve from the Day of the Date of these Presents until the full End and Term of Seven Years from thence next following to be fully compleat and ended. During which Term, the said Apprentice his said Master faithfully shall serve, his Secrets keep, his lawful Commandments every where gladly do. He shall do no Damage to his said Master, nor see to be done of others; but that he to his Power shall lett, or forthwith give warning to his said Master of the same. He shall not waste the Goods of his said Master, nor lend them unlawfully to any. He shall not commit Fornication, nor contract Matrimony within the said Term. He shall not play at Cards, Dice, Tables, or any other unlawful Games, whereby his said Master may have any Loss. With his own Goods or others, during the said Term, without Licence of his said Master, he shall neither buy nor sell. He shall not haunt Taverns or Play-houses, nor absent himself from his said Master's Service Day nor Night unlawfully: But in all Things, as a faithful Apprentice, he shall behave himself towards his said Master, and all his, during the said Term. And the said Master (for and in Consideration of the Sum of two hundred and ten pounds of lawful Money of *Great-Britain* to him in Hand paid by Elizabeth Pott the mother at, and before the Ensealing and Delivery of these Presents, the Receipt whereof is hereby acknowledged) his said Apprentice in the same Art which he useth, by the best Means that he can, shall teach and instruct, or cause to be taught and instructed, finding unto his said Apprentice, Meat, Drink, Apparel, Lodging, and all other Necessaries, according to the Custom of the City of *London*, during the said Term. And to the true Performance of all, and every the said Covenants and Agreements, either of the said Parties binds himself unto the other by these Presents. In *Witness* whereof the Parties above-named to these Indentures, interchangeably have put their Hands and Seals, the first Day of the August in the Third Year of the Reign of our Sovereign Lord King GEORGE, of *Great-Britain*, &c. *Anno Dom.* 1729

Presentat die Dat. Supra dict. Coram [illegible] *Magistro* [illegible]

Percivall Pott

Figure 1. Entry from the Freedom Admission register for Edward Nourse, September 1730, Indenture signed by Edward

> At that time the art was miserably defective; the instruments were clumsy and unmanageable; the operations unscientific, and unnecessarily painful: the established mode of practice, incumbered with a farrago of useless medicines and applications, tended rather to mislead than direct the inquirer; prescription too frequently held the place of reason; and want of real knowledge was concealed under a pompous garb and specious demeanour.[22]

Although all of these vices would be ones that Pott would address in his lifetime, Earle specifically draws attention to Pott's rejection of the cautery, or the use of hot irons, to seal wounds. Each of the surgical wards at St. Bartholomew's Hospital had a fire where the irons were "regularly heated and prepared whenever the surgeons visited the hospital."[23] According to Earle, the old-fashioned Nourse contemptuously opposed Pott's rejection of the cautery in favor of milder measures. Truth won out, and "Mr. Pott lived to see the remains of barbarism set aside, and a more humane and rational plan, of which he was the chief author universally adopted."[24] Earle loftily concludes that surgery, having shaken off the great part of its horror thanks to the courage of Pott, became "comparatively, a pleasing study."[25] By this Earle meant that the ends of surgery, if not the means, are pleasing—to relieve distress, to soften anguish, and to aid in the treatment of accidents and misfortunes.

Earle had no doubt taken into consideration the differing status of the master and the apprentice in his account of ancient versus modern surgery. Nourse was the last barber-surgeon to be elected assistant surgeon to St. Bartholomew's Hospital in 1731, while Pott was the first member of the new Company of Surgeons to be elected assistant surgeon in 1745.[26] In *Desire and Disorder: Fevers, Fictions, and Feelings in English Georgian Culture*, Candace Ward specifically cites Earle's biography of Pott as proof of a "sympathetic disposition" that was beginning "to replace class affiliation, as the hallmark of the successful practitioner."[27] Various attempts were being made to draw a firm line between the supposedly lamentable brutality of the old barber-surgeons and the praiseworthy gentlemanly demeanor of the new surgeons. That Pott was conscious of the fact that he straddled the supposed change from barbery to surgery is shown in occasional teasing remarks he made to his pupils.[28] For example, Pott "used sometimes pleasantly to say to his pupils that they might remember they had been dressers to a barber-surgeon."[29]

Having completed his apprenticeship at the age of 22, Pott presented himself before the Court of Examiners of the Company of Barber Surgeons with the intent of proving himself qualified as a surgeon. In the Minutes of the Court for 7 September 1736, the following is recorded concerning the unusual circumstances under which Pott was examined:

> the question being put whether Mr. Percivall Pott should be examined by this Court, he not having waited on all the Governors and Examiners to desire the favour of their presence at his examination, and it appearing to the Court that Mr. Pott had been sent for out of town to attend Sir Robert Goodesall's lady, where he was detained so long as not to be able to return within the time limited for his attendance on the Governors and Examiners, and Mr. Warden Petty having been pleased to say that he would make his excuse to the Court: It was resolved that the Court would proceed to the Examination of the said Mr. Pott notwithstanding his default in attending Examiners: But this is not to be a precedent in time to come to any other person.[30]

Sir Robert Goodesall was in all probability Sir Robert Godschall (1692–1742), a wine merchant, master of an ironmonger company, alderman, ardent Tory, and in 1736, a city sheriff. He later became the lord mayor of London and president of St. Bartholomew's Hospital in 1741. Lady Godschall (née Catherine Tryon) came from a Huguenot family in Kent. She died in 1755. The Goodschalls lived at Weston House in Albury, Surrey, about 33 miles from London. All in all she was an important patient for Pott (or any surgeon), and the examiners took this into consideration. They passed Pott, and following his admission into the Company, he proceeded a few hours later to be examined for the more prestigious Grand (or Great) Diploma to practice, a rarely offered option. Pott succeeded in passing this examination as well and paid six guineas for the pleasure of doing so. He was also required to pay each member of the Court of Examiners a fee and to put 5 shillings in the poor box.[31]

In 1739 Pott applied for the post of assistant surgeon at St. Bartholomew's Hospital but was rejected, a decision that was not unusual for a young and largely unknown surgeon.[32] Medical positions at hospitals were secured by election and depended upon courting, flattering, and bribing either the voting members of the board of governors or those who already held medical appointments at the hospitals to which the applications were made. Ludford Harvey, Pott's former apprentice who we met at the beginning of the chapter, refers bitterly to the election he lost in 1784 to become an assistant surgeon at St. Bartholomew's Hospital. Things had not changed much in the forty-five years since Pott's unsuccessful application. Harvey writes candidly about the amount of money the endeavor cost him:

> The beginning of this year a vacancy of Surgeon to St. Bartholomews Hospital occurred by the death of Mr Young, and I became a Candidate for the office of Assistant Surgeon in opposition to Mr Long. The contest was very severe; as the Event was long expected my letters from Mr Pott had been in preparation—my Friends were anxious in my support—but Mr Heavyside became also a Candidate which divided My Interest, and above 15 friends of Mr Long on one day having made themselves

> generous in his behalf gave him on the day of Election a decided majority—. This event I had Endeavour'd to parry by also *making* governors (presents) Gentlemen were nominated who were so *generous* as to permit *me* to pay their fine of £50 each—which I verily believe exhausted the last penny I was master of.[33]

When Nourse, Pott's former master, was made senior surgeon at the hospital in 1745, Pott easily won election for the post Nourse had just vacated and hence became an assistant surgeon. Pott was promoted (elected) to the rank of full surgeon in 1749 and remained at the hospital for the next 38 years. Although hospital surgical appointments were largely honorary and paid little, they allowed for two lucrative activities that hopefully would lead to money, fame, and the attraction of students and private patients. First Pott could start lecturing on-site at the hospital.[34] Fees were not charged for lectures, but pupils generally attended the lectures as part and parcel of having paid to follow a particular surgeon. All fees paid by pupils were shared amongst the surgeons at the hospital. This was not the case with monies paid by dressers, for like apprentices, they contracted with an individual surgeon for a set period. Permission to take on dressers was the second privilege that Pott gained from becoming a senior surgeon. Dressers were young men who typically paid twice what a pupil or "walker" did to gain experience in operating and treating more serious conditions.[35] Pott's dressers paid him 50 guineas per year while his pupils paid 25. The more poverty-stricken dressers generally lodged with their surgeon and his family and essentially paid for this privilege through helping take care of the private patients. Pott had several live-in dressers, the best-known being John Heaviside (1748–1828)[36] and Robert Rainey Pennington (1766–1849).[37] John Abernethy (1764–1831) and James Hutchinson (1752–93) were dressers who lived out and paid for boarding at the hospital.[38] Some idea of what dressers did can be gleaned from their letters to family and court records in which they appear as witnesses to describe fatal injuries and the findings at postmortem. Hutchinson described his duties in a letter to his uncle:

> I dress daily at the Hospital, and am often permitted to perform some of the less Capital operations myself, and generally assist in the performing of the more Capital ones; this distinction I owe in a great degree to the kindness of Surgeon Pott ...[39]

Only rarely do the feelings of dressers towards each other emerge. Rivalry between Pennington and Abernethy for the attention of Pott appears to have been fierce. The two nearly came to blows when Abernethy shoved Pennington out of the way when they spotted Pott crossing the quadrangle at the hospital, surrounded by apprentices, pupils, and dressers. Pott was busy giving a summary of a case in which Pennington was particularly interested. But then,

> Abernethy came up and absolutely (pushed) me out of my position. I then found it was time to put a stop to his impertinence, particularly as the insult was given in the presence of so many of our fellows. I took no notice of it at the moment, though the circumstances did not escape the observation of Mr. Pott. Immediately on the conclusion of 'the round,' I made up my mind to act, and accordingly, in the presence of a number of students, I addressed Abernethy—'Jack, this won't do; I have given way to you too long, and for the future you must be content to play second fiddle.' Abernethy began to bluster, and said—'I'll be d—d if I do.' At that time disputes of the kind were settled in a summary way, and I immediately prepared to assert my right by an appeal to the fist. The place of combat was in the corner of the ground which is near to the anatomical theatre, and thither we repaired followed by our anxious and admiring *confrères*. I took off my coat and prepared for action. Jack did not follow suit, and began, like Bob Acres,[40] to show unmistakable symptoms of not coming up to scratch. In fact, he declined the ordeal of battle, and I was for the future first.[41]

The total number of pupils Pott taught during his lifetime is unknown, as it is impossible to document such activity.[42] This is partly due to the circumstances under which pupils (as opposed to dressers and apprentices) were accepted as students by surgeons. Often from rural areas, pupils came to study with Pott for varying lengths of time, although usually it was for just one winter, which allowed them to attend Pott's course of surgical lectures and perhaps observe a few operations.[43] Some pupils were already apprenticed to other surgeons at St. Bartholomew's Hospital but worked with Pott, such as Charles Blicke (1745–1815). Blicke became a senior surgeon at the hospital in 1787 and is famously satirized as toothless and senile in George Cruikshank's 1811 print *The Examination, of a Young Surgeon*. Henry Park (1745–1831) of Liverpool, the American John Jones (1729–91), and William Pryce (1735–90) from Cornwall also registered as Pott's pupils.[44] Others briefly attended lectures or observed operations. John Hunter (1728–1793) did the former and may have gone on hospital rounds with Pott. There is also evidence that William Bayly[45] and Bradford Wilmer (1737–1813)[46] trained at some point with Pott. Solomon Wadd is described as being Pott's pupil in 1767.[47] John Howard, a surgeon to the Middlesex Hospital who established the first ward specializing in the treatment of cancer at the hospital in 1791–2, was also a pupil of Pott's.[48]

In 1761 the governors of the Middlesex Hospital in London read and handed rules to each pupil and dresser. Along with requirements not to go to the female wards except at times of "dressing" or treatment of a patient by a surgeon or his deputy, they were to swiftly leave the hospital each day when their duties were over. Furthermore,

> That during the time they are in the hospital, there be no swearing or noise made, or any kind of indecency committed, nor the medicines, &c., of the hospital wasted or embezzled, and that every offender in these particulars be reported to the weekly

> board by the house pupil, and be liable to be suspended, or even expelled from the hospital, at their discretion.[49]

The similarity to the language in Pott's indenture of 1729 and the twin concerns of manners and money are striking but unsurprising. Pupils and dressers were treated like apprentices and vice versa. Behavioral expectations may have been interchangeable, but it often proved difficult to control a group of adolescent boys in a bustling hospital. As will be discussed in chapter two, Pott would both comment on and increasingly include instructions in his lectures on the ideal deportment of pupils at Saint Bartholomew's Hospital.

Pott practiced at a time of flux in how young men were being trained in the art of surgery. Part of this can be seen in the fact that he had not only dressers and pupils but also apprentices.[50] Pott started taking apprentices in 1743.[51] The first three we know of, Richard Powney (1743), Julian Herring of Jamaica (1747), and William Atkinson (1749), paid £262, £350, and £367 respectively for a "Company of India" seven-year apprenticeship.[52]

Many of Pott's apprentices were candidates for the Honourable East India Company, or HEIC, which, along with the army and navy, required large numbers of surgeons. From 1629 the Barber-Surgeons Company was responsible for examining anyone who hoped to become a surgeon's mate in the navy. In the early to mid-eighteenth century the examination before the Court of Examiners may have only lasted fifteen minutes, but that did not mean that candidates did not need instruction in anatomy and surgery in order to pass it.[53] As outlined in the following chapter, it is probable that Nourse's and Pott's joint private lecture courses were created for and sustained by this need for military and naval surgeons. After 1745 and the separation of the barbers and surgeons, the new Company of Surgeons was made responsible for examining both navy and army candidates.[54] Besides the HEIC candidates, Pott's other apprentices that we know of (and their fees) were Thomas (Peter) Clare (1752), £420; James Gordon (1757), £105; John Ravell (1760), £315; James Earle (1762), £420; Henry Thornhill (1769), £315; Thomas Pemberton (1770), £420; Samuel Rayley (1773), £210; and Ludford Harvey (1777), fee unknown[55] The higher fees probably reflect who lived in the Potts' home versus those who boarded at the hospital.

In January 1745 several London-based surgeons petitioned Parliament for separation from the Barber Surgeons Company. In spite of strong opposition from leading barbers, the surgeons were successful. The "Company of Surgeons for the promotion of the Science as well as the Art of Surgery" received the Royal Assent and met for the first time on July 1, 1745, in Stationers' Hall.[56] It is likely that Pott supported the splitting of the barber and surgeons into separate entities, given the eager interest he showed in obtaining leadership positions in the new organization.

The causes and effects of this split have been much argued, especially in terms of the impact on the professionalization of surgeons.[57] Margaret Pelling concluded from a close analysis of the Journals of the House of Commons that when it came to causes, the "primary concern (of the surgeons) was with licensing and control, and that they wanted a full share of company property."[58] The effects of the split, according to Bernice Hamilton, were twofold: 1) a premium was put on pure surgery, and 2) the hospital surgeons gained control of the Company.[59] Her primary evidence for this assertion is the wording of the new by-laws:

> no person practising pharmacy or following any other trade or occupation than that of a surgeon was to be chosen as Examiner or for the Court of Assistants *on any pretext*. The Company insisted on 'being now of no trade but of the profession of Surgery only.' This placed the entire control of the corporation in the hands of the hospital surgeons, since all other members were compelled to practise midwifery and pharmacy in order to get a living.[60]

Pelling disagrees with Hamilton that the split occurred due to the desires of a group of "progressive" surgeons. She makes the interesting point that the dissolution of the barber-surgeons can be read as the triumph of old élite surgeons who commanded high fees from patients and apprentices than new forward-looking surgeons.[61] Pelling also questions the role of the development of London hospitals as teaching institutions in redefining surgeons in terms of their professional and corporate identity. This relates to arguments made by historians such as Susan C. Lawrence that hospital surgeons were able "to flourish individualistically in a new institutional framework which was only loosely connected with any form of civic responsibility."[62] Pelling concludes that it was not élite surgeons nor medically minded MPs who were behind the desire to separate the Barber-Surgeons Company, but instead a network of politicians eager to reform the navy and ensure the provision of adequate surgical services. Parliament and the navy were not interested in creating a profession of surgeons but in winning the war at sea.[63]

Pott's old master Nourse was among the surgeons who provided bonds to finance the Company of Surgeons, and Pott himself held several posts in the new organization. In 1753 he and William Hunter were elected the first masters of, or lecturers on, anatomy. One of Pott's tasks was to serve on a committee that considered new supplies and security for the anatomy lectures. On 12 July 1753, Pott met with several other surgeons, including Nourse and Hunter. Among their recommendations was one that a new table for the body be bought and iron spikes be installed in the theatre "to prevent the mob getting over the outer rail."[64] Three years later Pott became a member of the Court of Assistants, and in 1761 he was elected to the Court of Examiners. By 1763 Pott was an under warden and the following year he became the upper (or first) warden. Finally in 1765 Pott became the master of the company.[65] Evidence gleaned of what Pott actually did in any of these roles is largely anecdotal. For example, Forbes Winslow in *Physic and Physicians: A Medical Sketch Book, exhibiting, The Public and Private Life of the Most Celebrated Medical Men of Former Days* (1839) reported that John Abernethy, a dresser to Pott and later a surgeon at St. Bartholomew's Hospital, recalled the types of questions Pott would ask when examining candidates at the company:

> Abernethy related in his lectures that Pott would frequently question the treatment of a compound oblique fracture of (the) Tibia. And such was the question that he put to his pupil: "What would you do, sir, in such a case—would you enlarge the wound or saw off the bone? And knowing the desired answer, Abernethy replied: "I would rather enlarge the wound than saw off the bone." Another favourite question for his candidate would be: "What would you do, sir, in such a case of retention of urine?" "Sir, I would bleed and bathe with tepid water and so on to allay irritation." But would you introduce a catheter?" "No sir, I would rely on other measures," was deemed a good answer by Pott.[66]

The first question on the fracture of the tibia was one based on personal experience, for at age 43 Pott fell from his horse and only escaped amputation of his leg through the caution of other surgeons. The case of catheterization for urinary retention, however, shows Pott's own caution. He viewed it as an intrusive measure and recommended it only as a last resort to his pupils in lectures. It was also a procedure Pott associated with quacks, a group toward whom he kept an ambivalent attitude.

As one of the ten members of the Court of Examiners in 1769, Pott took part in what became the controversial questioning of the surgeon John Foot on evidence he gave at the Old Bailey regarding the fatal injuries George Clarke sustained at the Brentfield Election Riot in December 1768. Clarke was bludgeoned on the head during the melee that followed radical journalist John Wilkes's (1725–1797) election to parliament[67] and died five days later. Foot was called to carry out a postmortem at a public house in front of the coroner's jury.[68] The surgeon later gave evidence of his findings at the trial of the two men charged with Clarke's murder and categorically stated that the blow to the head had killed Clarke. The defendants, two Irish chairmen, Edward Quirk, Kirk, or McQuirk and Lawrence Balf, or Balfe, were found guilty and sentenced to death.[69] It is probable that the government employed the two men charged with Clarke's murder to start the riot in the hope that it would prevent Wilkes being elected for Middlesex. After the guilty verdict, a royal pardon was sought for the men, and Foot was "encouraged" to change his opinion.

Yet there was much more to this appeal than simply saving the lives of Quirk and Balf, for it also concerned saving the reputation of one of Pott's close colleagues, William Bromfeild (1712–1792), surgeon to the Princess of Wales.[70] Bromfeild had treated Clarke for the blow to his head but had refused to carry out, attend, or even send one of his assistants to observe the postmortem. Most likely Bromfeild feared that he would be dragged into the court case. Bromfeild had directed an apothecary, Solomon Starling, to treat Clarke for the fever that developed after the blow to his head.[71]

Bromfeild pressured Foot into signing a statement before three other leading surgeons of the company that it was the fever that killed Clarke and not the injury to the head. This was of crucial importance to Bromfeild, since a patient dying of fever was not unexpected, but one dying from the neglect of a head wound was a different matter. Foot's statement was then leaked to the appropriate governmental authorities, and they, in turn, directed the Court of Examiners at the Surgeon's Hall to call Foot before them and interrogate the evidence he gave at the trial.[72] Unlike other inquisitions, the court met in camera (secret). As a member of the court, Pott was, along with Bromfeild, one of Foot's questioners. By 1769 Pott's expertise and publication on head wounds was well-known, and he naturally took the lead in asking about the appearance and extent of the injury. Foot described his interrogation:

> The secretary read over my evidence as given at the Old Baily [*sic*]; I was desired to be attentive to it … I then was interrogated;
> Q Mr Pott. On what part of the head was the wound?
> A On the crown of the head.
> Q What do you mean by the crown of the head?
> A On the right parietal bone, by the sagittal structure.
> Q In what manner did you take off the scalp?
> A By a circular incision.
> Q In what state was the pericranium?
> A Much inflamed, it was almost separated from the cranium for about two inches in circumference under the wound.[73]

After a few brief questions from other members of the Court of Examiners, Pott spoke again: "I would ask you two questions as a man of experience and an artist"[74] (craftsman). Pott wanted to know the condition of Clarke's dura mater and cranium, since this information would provide crucial information as to the cause of death. At the end of his interrogation Foot once again agreed that the blow to the head was not the likely cause of Clarke's death and that the fever was a more reasonable explanation. Quirk and Bafe could not therefore be held responsible for the death of Clarke and more importantly, neither could Bromfeild. The Court of

Examiners wrote up their findings and sent them to the government. Quirk and Balf received a royal pardon a few days later. Foot was highly embarrassed by the whole event and engaged in a long war of pamphlets on the matter with Bromfeild but to no avail.[75] Press reactions were vociferous. Among these was a print called "A Consultation of Surgeons" that showed the ten surgeons of the Court of Examiners, including Pott, being influenced in rendering their verdict that fever killed Clarke through the liberal gift of bags of money.[76]

Eleven years later, in March 1780, Pott became embroiled in another legal matter at the Company. He volunteered to write a letter to Joseph Cruttenden, the long-serving clerk, asking about reparations for irregularities that the finance committee of the Court of Examiners had discovered in the accounts.[77] Cruttenden had already resigned from his post and although neither Pott's letter nor Cruttenden's reply have survived, the minutes of the Court of Assistants to which the finance committee reported do exist. They reveal that the Company's assets in early 1780 should have been £837 7s. 5d., but in fact only £74 8s. 0d. was in the coffers. The Company owed £285 16s. 4d. Cruttenden's resignation was accepted, but he was not prosecuted nor made to pay back any of the missing monies.[78] Wall speculates that this may have been due to 35 years of service and the "selection as an envoy of Percival [*sic*] Pott, who had married a Miss Cruttenden in 1746, (this) suggests an additional incentive to leniency though the similarity of name is the only clue to relationship."[79] Research reveals that Joseph Cruttenden was in fact Pott's brother-in-law. Wall adds that Pott only appears to have attended the last session of the finance committee, unlike the other members who attended regularly. Pott's lack of attendance was perhaps due to family embarrassment. Okey Belfour (1752–1811) was elected the next clerk and would in time take on one of Pott's sons as a legal apprentice.

Pott was also part of a specially formed committee in 1786 that considered the legal right, under an Act of 1784, of retired army and navy surgeons to practice in London and Westminster without the permission of the Company of Surgeons (i.e. without having passed and paid for the examinations at the Hall). In the end the committee decided not to oppose this action.[80] Pott's role in all three of these cases—Foot, Cruttenden, and the military surgeons—suggests that he was not one to rock the boat.

Friends and Family

In his biography of Pott, Earle stresses that his father-in-law was not just a hospital surgeon but someone who also kept a large practice of private patients. These included the writer Samuel Johnson (1709–1784), the actor David Garrick

(1717–1779), and the painter Thomas Gainsborough (1727–1788). Pott treated Johnson for testicular swelling, as will be discussed in chapter four. The case of the diseased prostate of the "late David Garrick Esq." is included in "Lecture 40th On Complaints of the Urinary Passage" from c. 1780. In spite of taking a lot of laudanum, Garrick still had times when his pain was excessive.[81] A letter from Pott to Garrick in June 1776 suggests that a friendship had developed between surgeon and patient:

> My Dear Sir,
> I love and esteem you more than most other people, and therefore feel all your obligations more powerfully. This morning I gave away my dear Bessy [probably Pott's daughter Elizabeth] (a very sincere admirer of you): the whole family are gone to Mr. Pott's uncle, Mr. Hindley, at Twickenham; I follow to dinner, and the pair will stay there a few days.
> You are sure in your retirement to enjoy the otium cum dignitate, [Cicero, retirement from public life with dignity] and I hope to God it will always be cum salute. Believe me always and truly yours. P. Pott[82]

Pott's role in caring for Thomas Gainsborough was limited. Pott was called in along with Dr. Richard Warren (1731–1797) when John Hunter (1728–1793) and Dr. William Heberden (1710–1801) could do no more for the artist. Gainsborough had developed a wen (cyst) on his neck that had slowly "grown inwards" and then suppurated. Hunter had diagnosed it as a "swelling on his glands," but when it began to drain, he stated it was cancer. The growth was so large that it made it difficult for Gainsborough to breathe and swallow. Pott, sadly, was unable to help.[83]

A great deal of effort and money was needed to secure private patients. Ludford Harvey records that in his own attempt to obtain referrals, he subscribed to assemblies that helped fund social events, entered any gentleman's club that would take his money, and even resorted to holding dances at his home.[84] As David Cannadine describes in *Class in Britain*, the eighteenth century had several ways of ranking people in society: first by their prestige (hierarchic), second by their place in the range of poorest sort, middle sort or better sort (triadic), and third as high or low (dichotomous).[85] This was the world that surgeons such Pott had to negotiate if they were to ever gain a foothold on the ladder of fee-paying patients. Negotiations became far easier if one could marry well and secure powerful patrons.

Pott's devotion to his mother is a recurring theme in Earle's narrative. Before his apprenticeship, Pott was no wild youth and led a quiet life at home with his mother and stepsister, deliberately choosing (according to Earle) not to look for a wife until after his mother's death in 1744.[86] Given the meager income of an assistant hospital surgeon and the time-consuming need to be always on the prowl for private fee-paying patients, Pott's decision to wait to marry may not have been entirely based on devotion to his mother but rather was a circumstance forced upon him. Nevertheless when Pott finally did wed in 1746, he married up. His bride, Sarah Cruttenden (1723–1811), was the daughter of Robert Cruttenden (1694–1763) and Elizabeth (née Holden) (1701–?). Pott's biographers have often identified Sarah's father as a director of the HEIC, but this is not the case. Robert Cruttenden was the son of Joseph (c. 1658–after 1731), a wealthy wholesale apothecary in London.[87] Robert was bred to become a Congregational minister like his uncle Robert Bragge (1665–1738) but could not reconcile himself with some of the religious views Congregationalists held, especially their belief in the Trinity. So Cruttenden became a bookseller instead and then unwisely followed the investment advice of his brother-in-law, Robert Surman (1696–1759), assistant to the Chief Cashier of the South Sea Company. By 1723 Cruttenden was bankrupt from the South Sea Bubble.[88] He then, somehow, obtained the office of *Common Hunt*, an ancient position that originally involved caring for the hounds of the lord mayor and citizens but was now one that simply paid a sinecure. This gave Cruttenden good connections, and he also became an accountant in the Penny-Post–Office, where he earned £70 to £90 a year.[89] Cruttenden underwent a conversion in 1742 and became an enthusiastic follower of the evangelists George Whitefield (1714–1770) and Philip Doddridge (1702–1751).[90] He married Sarah Cliff in 1716, and they had three children: Edward Holden (1717–1771), Joseph (the aforementioned disgraced clerk to the Surgeons' Company), and Sarah, the future wife of Percivall Pott. Sarah's connection to the HEIC was through her brother Edward. This is why Pott's family would receive notice and consideration from the HEIC.

Edward was first employed by the HEIC in 1737 as a writer in Calcutta on a salary of £5 per annum.[91] This low paying but coveted position opened up other possibilities to make a fortune in India. Within a year Edward had moved on from keeping the accounts and copying the company's letters in triplicate to working in the Export Warehouse and collecting consulage, a duty paid by merchants to protect their goods and trade. By 1748 Edward was a senior merchant with an annual salary of £40. In 1755, however, he was dismissed from the HEIC for using fraudulent means to obtain a contract to supply the marine stores. Edward remained in India and worked as a merchant until he returned to the HEIC in 1757. The same year his wife, Elizabeth, died on board one of the ships that fled Calcutta when Fort William was besieged.[92] Edward returned to London in 1759–60 and eventually rose to become a director of the HEIC, a position he kept from 1765 until his death in 1771. During this period he solidified his large Bengal fortune (reportedly £50,000) and became the principal owner of several Indiamen (ships).[93] These included the *Cruttenden*, on which his nephew, Robert Pott, would sail as an employee of the HEIC to China and India.

Percivall Pott and Sarah Cruttenden were married at St. Augustine's Church in London on 27 June 1746.[94] They then moved into a house on Watling Street, and Pott started to give private classes in surgery and bandaging from home. The classes appear to have been largely for his pupils and dressers. Earle recounts that Pott spoke at first with hesitation and reserve and struggled to come up with a system for teaching surgery. Pott eventually decided to first discuss general disorders of the body and then diseases affecting each part of the body, starting with the head and moving down. An examination of the lecture notes that survive shows that he kept refining this system throughout his life.[95] Pott also developed an easy and eloquent style of speaking. Ludford Harvey praised Pott for his easy manner but criticized what this talent led to, namely an ability to take advantage of others in order to "push his Fortunes" and the vanity that came from hobnobbing with the nobility:

> He was universally acknowledged to be the first in his Profession; a Rank which he obtained, not merely on account of his Chirurgical Knowledge & Ability; but also for his address, which was exactly callculated [*sic*] to bring him forward in the publick Estimation. Lively in conversation, full of anecdotes, with an Excellent memory his Company was always desirable; as an Observer of mankind, he had an advantage, which careless People of Equal Ability do not possess of knowing how & when to push his Fortunes, & the quickness of his parts never sufferd him to let slip any opportunity of doing so.[96]

It is difficult to determine how much patronage Pott secured in order to "push his Fortunes" throughout the course of his life. A "Eulogium on Percival Pott" in the February 1789 edition of *The European Magazine* states that "Pott arrived at the summit of his profession alone by superior excellence without any particular patronage."[97] This assertion is not true, for Lord Thurlow (1731–1806), a supporter of the Duke of Bedford[98] and of Warren Hastings, was in fact also Pott's patron.[99] This firmly fixes Pott as a Tory and a supporter of George III rather than of the Prince Regent. Edward Thurlow was a MP (Tamworth, 1765), a judge, and from 1778, the lord high chancellor and a baron. In 1788, the year of Pott's death, Thurlow lost favor due to the Regency crisis and the impeachment of Warren Hastings.[100] Thurlow's control of vast lay and ecclesiastical patronage (his younger brother Thomas was Bishop of Lincoln and Durham) was instrumental in helping Pott and especially his sons succeed in life.

How far Pott's connection to Thurlow goes back is a matter of conjecture. Thurlow attended Westminster School in the 1740s, where his schoolmates included the poet William Cowper and two leading members of the HEIC, Warren Hastings and Elijah Impey.[101] (Impey was to play a considerable role in the fortunes of Pott's youngest son, Robert.) Thurlow was a member of the Inner Temple and spent many hours in Nando's coffeehouse on Fleet Street, close to Temple Bar and where Pott also appears to have gone on occasion.[102] Real evidence for a close connection between Thurlow and Pott, however, emerges sometime in the early 1770s. Pott and his family moved to Lincoln's Inn Fields, where Thurlow lived, in 1769. The second volume of the *Recollections* of R. J. S. Stevens (1757–1827), an organist at Charterhouse and professor of music at Gresham College who taught Thurlow's daughter music, begins,

> When a Barrister, Lord Thurlow was very intimate with Mr. Pott the Surgeon, who then lived in Lincoln's Inn Fields. It so happened that when he was dining with Mr. Pott, a Bricklayer's labourer had fell from a scaffold, and alighting upon his feet, both the Ancle [*sic*] bones were broken, and his feet beat to pieces. This poor man was brought to Mr. Pott in the greatest agony. Amputation was absolutely necessary. Mr. Pott took off both his feet, and the man was put to bed in his house. Mr. Thurlow attended the operation, and was astonished at the accuracy of the Surgeon upon the occasion.[103]

Stevens gave tangible evidence of the importance and necessity of surgery and the radical relief it could provide. Watching Pott operate caused a reaction in Thurlow that included self-reflection and admiration for the mechanical and aesthetic skills of Pott. Thurlow would remain Pott's patient and patron for many years.[104] On another note, Stevens's recollection reveals that capital operations were carried out in Pott's home where no doubt they would have been heard if not seen by family members and servants. It is likely that another duty of Pott's live in dressers and apprentices was to attend to such patients.

Some flimsy evidence suggests that late in life Pott may have been a surgeon at some point to the first Royal Dragoons, a regiment of mounted infantrymen. In 1786 Pott cared for Lord George Augustus Herbert (1759–1827), the son of the tenth Earl of Pembroke, and on October 25 of that year, his father's chaplain sent him the following letter:

> So you have not done with that Butcher Pott, as I hear he is termed by the Royals, who have discarded him from their service for cutting and slashing too deep. I agree with him that you ought to be possessed of a full quota of patience, & no bad constitution to stand up agst his operations & those of a Medicinal Doctor for 12 months together. Get rid of your Pethrox, & never for God's sake see a d—d D—ct-r again as long as you live. Upon your account I abhor the idea of medicines, & wish all the faculty at the Devil.[105]

Lord Herbert's father was colonel of the first Royal Dragoons from 1764–94, and in all likelihood these are the "Royals" mentioned in the account. In a letter to his father in December of the same year, Lord Herbert reported that he had received extensive surgical treatment for a wound in his groin that resulted from drunken revelry at a military dinner:

> My health has been tolerablly [*sic*] well lately, but I have a wound in my groin, which nobody can perswade [*sic*] to heal; it looks better now however than it has done some time, & I have been cut five times owing to Sinum [sinus or cavity] forming under the flesh; I believe I shall be under the necessity of submitting to one more cut, but it will be a very slight one in comparison to what have been. ... Now for some account of my own proceedings lately with respect to your affairs. I was stopped short here by the entrance of Butcher Pott ...[106]

How much Pott's appointment to the Royals as surgeon came from the patronage of the Pembroke family is unclear, but it is apparent from these letters that he had lost the position by 1786. Pott would be far more successful in obtaining and keeping Lord Thurlow as a family patron, which was fortunate as he and his wife would eventually have eight children to support.

By the time of Pott's election to joint master in anatomy with William Hunter at the Company of Surgeons in 1753, Sarah Pott had already given birth to four babies. The first, a son called Percivall, sadly died at just five months and was buried at the church of St. Mary Aldermary on 24 February 1747. The other three children, Percivall (1749–1833), Sarah (1751–1791), and Elizabeth (1752–?) survived and would in time be joined by five other siblings, Mary (1754–1831), Robert or Bob (1756–1795), Joseph Holden (1758–1847), Anna (1760-?), and Edward Holden (1766–98). Not surprisingly Ludford Harvey described Percivall Pott as a family man and damned him with faint praise, "In his Family, he was most Amiable for as a Husband, & a father he was faulty only, in being too indulgent, for his Childrens sake he was inconsistent, could be insincere."[107] The eight children who grew to adulthood put considerable strain on the household budget. Fortunately all the daughters married well.

The Daughters

Sarah (1751–1791), the eldest daughter, married John Ravel Frye of Montserrat (1743–1799) in 1771[108] and gave birth to two daughters and three sons. Susan Burney (1755–1800) described the daughters, Sarah and Mary, rather unkindly: "plain, inelegant looking Girls I think."[109] She added that Mrs. Frye was a great favorite with her mother, Esther. The family lived on Wimpole Street, and Frye was listed as a member of the Corporation of Surgeons in the Medical Register of 1783.[110] Whether he ever practiced as a surgeon is unknown, but evidence confirms that the previously mentioned John Ravell who apprenticed to Pott in 1760 was in fact his future son-in-law John Ravel Frye. He came from a wealthy family who owned sugar plantations on Montserrat and were prominent in governmental affairs.[111] We do not know Pott's views on slavery, but the fact that Sarah married John Ravel Frye suggests he was not concerned about the source of his son-in-law's fortune.[112]

In May 1771, Pott visited John Baker (1712–1779) who was a lawyer, brother to two surgeons, and close friends with Julian Herring, one of Pott's former apprentices. Baker, like Frye, had family connections in the Caribbean. He recorded in his diary that Mr. Pott the surgeon had visited him on the 18th and 19th of May. This was probably to examine and then drain an infected wound. During the second visit Pott told Baker a convoluted story of a girl who had been caught lying about having sex for money with a Lord G ** r.[113] Pott also mentioned the news of his eldest daughter's engagement to a gentleman from Montserrat, and Baker was interested in finding out more. Ten days later he was successful:

> May 29. Dined below Mrs Ann [once Gordon] Smith, Mr. Shephard a very sensible man and a scholar—has 3 pupils under his care. The gentleman she [Miss Pott] is engaged to is John Frye of Montserrat (son to Edward Frye), he having been bred under (apprenticed to) Mr. Potts, that the family had notion his estate was £2000 a year.[114]

John Baker gives us a glimpse of Pott's home in 1771 in which he concurs with Ludford Harvey that it was a happy family:

> June 7. … Mr. Banister set me down at Mr. Potts [*sic*]—I dined there. After dinner played Miss [Sally] Potts [*sic*] and sister, Eliza and Mary (which last 17 years old today), a younger sister Ann, about 11 or 12, and son Holden (so named from Uncle Cruttenden, I suppose), a sweet boy about 5—all these dined—a lovely and amiable family indeed—while young ladies playing, about 6 came in another son, a grown-up young gentleman.[115]

Pott had proudly told Baker on his first visit that his wife was formerly a Cruttenden. The last mention of Pott in Baker's diary is on 13 June when Baker recorded, "Mr. Pott afraid now (that there is) swelling under the old wound."[116]

Pott's second daughter, Elizabeth, married a Mr. Samuel Potts (1735–1792) in June 1776. He was the nephew of Henry Potts, and when his uncle was promoted to Secretary of the Post Office in 1760, Samuel became Comptroller of the Inland. Both Potts were dismissed in 1762 but restored to office in 1765. This mirrored the fortunes of their patron, Thomas Pelham-Holles, the first Duke of Newcastle upon Tyne and the first Duke of Newcastle-under-Lyne (1693–1768).[117] Samuel Potts was forcibly retired in 1768 when the General Post Office was established. He was then on a salary of £200 a year.

Horace Walpole (1717–1797), author of *The Castle of Otranto*, wrote from his villa Strawberry Hill in Twickenham to the Earl of Strafford in August 1782, "Here we cannot stir, but armed for battle. Mr. Pott who lives at Mr. Hindley's, was attacked and robbed last week at the end of Gunnersbury-lane, by five footpads who had two blunderbusses."[118] Mr. Pott was in fact Samuel Potts, who at the time was living in a mansion called Radnor House. The bachelor Lord Radnor had left the furnished home to his steward, Frederick Atherton Hindley (c. 1710–1781) in 1757. Percivall Pott wrote to Thomas Gainsborough in 1776 that Elizabeth and Samuel had gone to stay with "Uncle Hindley" after their marriage. Potts and his family lived in Radnor House on and off between 1779 and 1785, and besides being his nephew, Samuel was also Hindley's heir-at-law. Unfortunately Hindley was a poor manager of finances, and a series of disputes over ownership of Radnor House drained his income.[119]

Samuel and Elizabeth had two daughters, Frances and Elizabeth, and a son, William Percival. William entered the service of the HEIC as a writer in 1798 and rose to the level of a factor in Bengal before dying in Furruckabad in 1806.[120]

Mary, who we met at the beginning of this chapter as the object of Ludford Harvey's hopes, married James Earle, a former apprentice of her father and his early biographer. In 1782 John Opie was commissioned to paint portraits of the newly married couple.[121] The couple had three girls and six boys. Like Pott's other sons-in-law, he did well professionally. He was elected assistant surgeon at St. Bartholomew's Hospital in 1770 and senior surgeon in 1784. Earle was knighted in 1807.

Pott's youngest daughter, Anna, married Samuel Compton Cox of Lincoln's Inn in 1787. Cox became a judge, was appointed master of the High Court of Chancery and was elected treasurer of the Foundling Hospital, a post he held for 33 years.[122] Anna and Samuel had five daughters, Anna, Mary, Sarah, Eliza, and Charlotte.

The Sons

Percivall and Sarah Pott had four sons who grew to adulthood. The eldest, Percivall, attended Eton College and in 1785 was listed as a partner in the banking company of Walpole, Clarke, and Pott, located at 28 Lombard Street. Richard Walpole, whose name appears first in the partnership, was a former captain of an East-Indiaman and as a banker acted as an agent for the East India Company. No doubt Sarah Pott's connections to the HEIC through her brother Edward Holden Cruttenden helped her son gain this position. Percivall appears to have married for the first time at the age of 75.[123]

Robert, the second son, died penniless in India in 1795, leaving behind a wife and two natural daughters. Pott had intended his son to be a Charterhouse Scholar and solicited and gained the patronage of the Duke of Newcastle to fulfill this wish, since the Duke and his wife were his occasional patients.[124] Robert, however, had other ideas, and in a letter from his father dated 18 July 1765, Percivall withdraws his request for aid from the Duke to have his son nominated for Charterhouse.[125]

> My Boy, whom his Grace, the Duke of Newcastle, at your request, was so kind to intend to make a Charter house Scholar, has taken such a dislike to letters, and such a liking to be a Sailor, that I think I ought not to resist him. The Charter house education not being calculated for a Seaman, I would by no means be the occasion of it being thrown away; and therefore must beg the favor of you to present my most humble, and most grateful Compliments to his Grace, with all possible thanks to his intended kindness, and to assure him that I shall allways retain a just sense of it.[126]

At age 14 Bob (as he was now called) realized his wish to be a sailor and was apprenticed on a ship of the HEIC through Cruttenden family contacts since in 1770, Edward Holden Cruttenden, his mother's brother, was a director of the HEIC. It is possible to follow the rise and fall of Bob Pott through HEIC documents, family letters, and the lurid memoirs of his close friend William Hickey.[127] Such an analysis also reveals how closely Percivall Pott's reputation was tied to the fortunes of Lord Thurlow and his patrons.

William Hickey (1749–1830) was articled in 1766 as a clerk to Mr. Bayley, a partner in his father's law firm. There he ran errands for an up-and-coming lawyer, Edward Thurlow.[128] Three years later Mr. Hickey discovered that his son had embezzled £500 from the firm, and William was forcibly enrolled in the HEIC as a lawyer and sent to China aboard the *Plassey*. In Canton "one of the most lovely boys I ever beheld" greeted William Hickey. This was the 14-year-old Bob Pott, who Captain William Baker of the *Cruttenden* described as "a boy of uncommon talents, but volatile to excess."[129] Baker told Hickey that,

> Pott was the son of the surgeon so well known for superior abilities in his profession, who having a numerous family of children, was compelled to put them into different lines of life. Robert was intended for the sea, this being his own choice, and was accordingly shipped as a Guinea pig [the name given to boys on their first voyage] on board the Cruttenden, so called after a brother of Mrs. Pott's, who was in the India Direction, and principal owner of that and other vessels of the Company, of one of which he (Robert) was to have the command when competent to assume it.[130]

In 1769 Robert went back to London, and after his friend William Hickey returned a few months later from India, they frequently dined with Pott's father in Lincoln's Inn Fields. Hickey already knew Robert's younger brother, Joseph Holden. The two had been together at Eton College where Joseph had "tipped" for William, meaning the younger boy had acted as his servant.[131]

Percivall Pott meanwhile was receiving reports from Captain Baker that his son had behaved poorly on board the ship and also in Canton.[132] In 1770, however, Baker reluctantly agreed to take Robert to India again on board the *Cruttenden* as his fifth mate.

After another visit to Canton, Robert returned to his family in early 1772. Hickey recalled dining with the Pott family that spring and noted the tension between father and son:

> the father complained to me in strong terms of Robert's conduct, observing that what might have been forgiven in him a mere boy became inexcusable at a more mature age. He said he had scrupulously enquired into all the circumstances of his last voyage, in every point of which he found Robert in the wrong, and that his behaviour to his commander had been most improper and disrespectful, in some instances scarcely short of mutiny.[133]

Some background to Hickey's remarks is in order, for it illustrates aspects of not only the conflict between Bob and his father but also the personality of Percivall Pott. Pott had spoken earlier with Captain Baker of the *Cruttenden*, who had promised to "bury in oblivion" Bob's outrageous behavior as mate of an Indiaman on the voyage to Canton and back to England; Bob apparently had even spat in Baker's face at one point.

Bob responded to his father's complaints to Hickey by laughing, which (not surprisingly) further enraged his father. After only one more voyage, Bob could have been promoted to command of a ship, but Pott stated, "the bastard has the impudence to tell me he will not upon any terms go (on such a) voyage!"[134] Bob then interrupted his father's conversation with Hickey, saying he would not go back to serve on any ship because the commanders were not gentlemen. Pott responded that this was a very proud position to take but wasn't realistic as far as Bob's financial future was concerned, for "By God, that fortune will not come from me. Already more than your just proportion has, I am sorry to say, been wasted upon you, and certainly I shall not stint the rest of my children to support you in extravagance and folly."[135] Pott was probably further aggravated from the fact that Hickey, being a close friend of his son, had a reputation as a troublemaker within the family. Around 1757, for example, Hickey feigned drowning from Uncle Hindley's canoe, which "caused consternation."[136]

With the plan of Robert becoming a ship's captain now in ruin, Pott once again turned to his wife's relatives for aid. In 1772 Robert Pott was appointed a writer to the HEIC, following the path of his uncle Edward Holden in 1737.[137] Despite threats to cut Robert off, once he returned to Bengal, his father continued to send him money. For example, in December 1774 Pott sent his son the equivalent of 960 rupees (£100).[138] Three years later Robert asked permission to resign from the civil service in Bengal and return home after a company surgeon had certified him as suffering from a chronic disorder of the liver.[139] He did so, though in 1779/80 he sailed back to India on the *Hillsborough* and with the permission of the Governor-General of the HEIC, Warren Hastings, Robert was reinstated without prejudice. During the journey, Spanish pirates attacked Robert's ship. Robert was held prisoner for several weeks before being released to return to London and ship out again.[140]

Money and manners were not the only bones of contention in Percivall Pott's dealings with his son—there was also the question of morals. For several years, Bob Pott maintained a relationship with the courtesan Emily Warren. In 1779 he set her up in a "handsome well furnished house in Cork Street" stocked with "all sorts of Wines, Coals, Candles."[141] As Karen Harvey writes,

> sex was not simply regarded as an act—whether of reproduction, desire or violence; sex was a place for men to visit. Rendering the act of sex spatial enabled it to be contained and firmly situated.[142]

Cork Street, where Emily was installed, was just southeast of Hanover Square, where Bob's parents resided. As a courtesan, Emily led a public and ostentatious life. Hickey described being met by Emily in a

> dashing bright yellow Vis a Vis having Pott's arms emblazoned thereon, an Elegant pair of bay horses, The Coachman and footman in smart frocks of blue faced with yellow and trimmed with a broad silver lace but what was all *this* outside shew, compared to the lovely creature within looking more than mortal.[143]

Indeed much of what we know about Emily comes from Hickey's memoirs, including the oft-quoted description of the night in 1780 that he spent in her bed:

> Where I past a night that many would have given thousands to do: I however that night experienced the truth of what I had heard said, That she was as cold as ice, seemingly totally void of feeling.[144]

This incident took place at the house in Cork Street (Pott was travelling to India on board the *Hillsborough* at the time). Indeed Pott had tried to smuggle Emily on board the *Hillsborough* but the Captain had seen through the deception of dressing Emily as a boy, and Pott was forced to sail alone.

Hickey also provided the origin story for Emily that has been accepted, largely without question, by scholars ever since:

> Charlotte Hays [a well-known brothel owner] met her in the streets of London, when not quite twelve years of age, leading her father, a blind beggar about, soliciting charity

> from every person that passed. Struck with the uncommon beauty of the Child's countenance she set her myrmidons [hired ruffians] to work and without difficulty soon got her into her clutches, the young scholar proved an apt scholar so far as walking, and common address, the more substantial points being totally neglected. She could neither read nor write.[145]

In *London's Sinful Secret: The Bawdy House and Very Public Passions of London's Georgian Age*, Dan Cruickshank questions the validity of this account. He suggests that the story of Emily and her blind father borrows from the popular poem of the time "The Blind Beggar of Bethnal Green." In 1765 a version of the poem was included in Thomas Percy's *Reliques of Ancient English Poetry*, and Charlotte perhaps used the story of a "blinded rebel knight led through London by his beautiful young daughter as a romantic background for Emily."[146]

Emily initially worked for Charlotte Hayes in her brothel. Once groomed to be a courtesan, Emily was kept by a series of men, the last of whom was Bob Pott. Leading artists of the day painted her, including George Romney (1734–1802) and Joshua Reynolds (1723–1792). Reynolds probably met Emily in the late 1770s when she was being kept by Charles Greville (1749–1809), the second son of the Earl of Warwick. It was Greville who commissioned the Thäis portrait.[147] (Thäis was a legendary courtesan of Alexander the Great who had supposedly persuaded him to burn Persepolis in 330 BCE after its capture from the Persians.) By the time the Thäis portrait was completed, however, Greville had finished with Emily, and it was several years before he paid Reynolds for the painting.[148] When Thäis was unveiled in 1781 at the Royal Academy, it created a sensation.[149] Just three years earlier, Reynolds's dignified three-quarter length portrait of Percivall Pott had been exhibited in the same room.[150]

Still distraught about his son, in 1782, Percivall Pott sent a letter to Hickey asking to meet at Pott's new home in Hanover Square. He described Pott as "almost in tears," and he begged Hickey to use his influence to persuade Bob to return home from Portsmouth, where he was already on board the *Lord Musgrave* preparing to cross to India. With him was "that infamous and notoriously abandoned woman, Emily," who had already spent most of Robert's money. Pott lamented that once it got out that she had been smuggled on board the ship disguised as a cabin boy, Bob would be shut out of all proper society and would never again hold a respectable and well-paying position in the HEIC.[151] Hickey also received a long letter from Bob in which he wrote that the ship was marooned off Portsmouth due to lack of wind, and he was uneasy that "the old buck" (his father) would persuade the Court of Directors of the HEIC to intervene and take his "dear woman" off the ship. Percivall Pott indeed had already sent a letter to the Court and another to the ship's captain, Urmston, "admonishing him against so unpardonable a fault

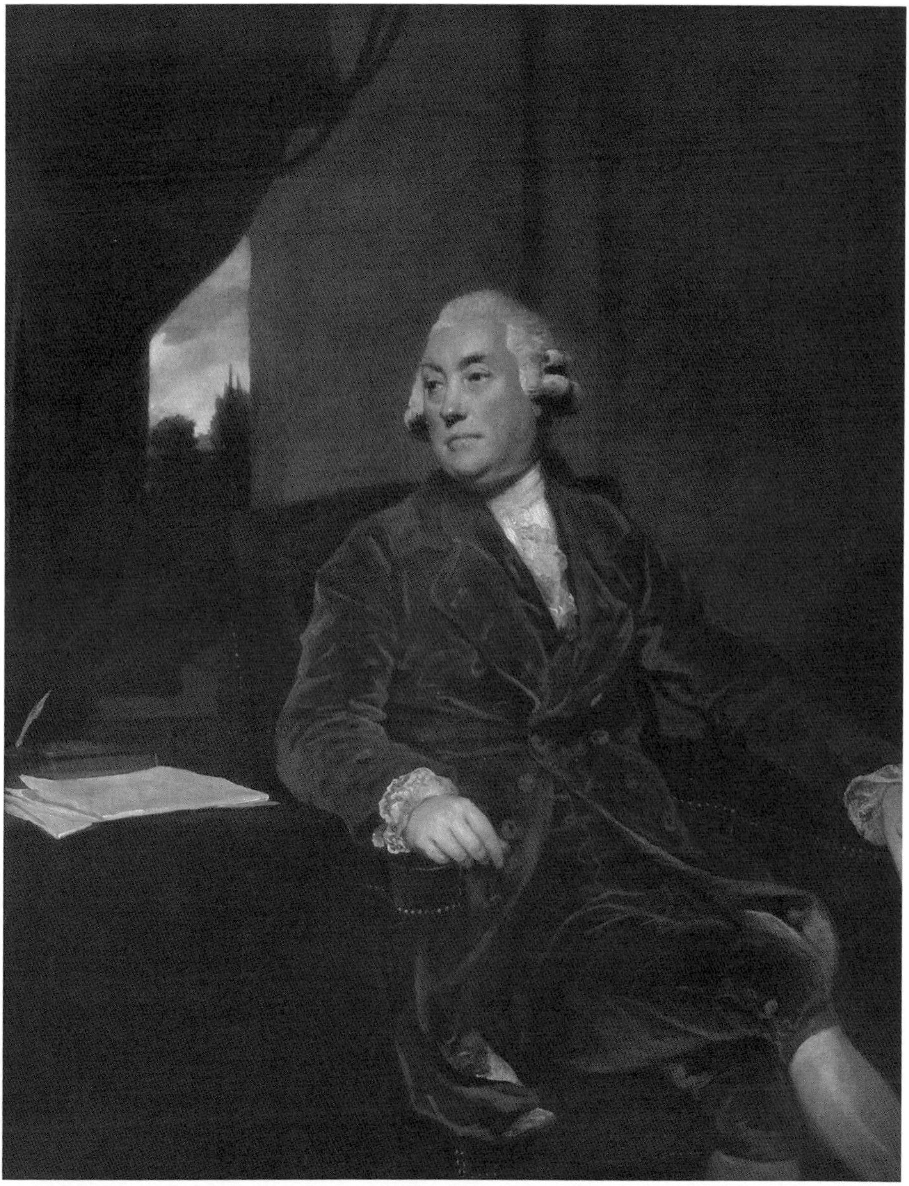

Figure 2. Portrait of Percivall Pott by Joshua Reynolds, 1784, SBHX7/16. Courtesy of St. Bartholomew's Hospital Archives.

as permitting a common prostitute to find her way to India on board his ship."[152] Captain Urmston was now in a panic as he feared losing his command, but Bob wrote Hickey that he simply planned to pay the few hundreds pounds he suspected

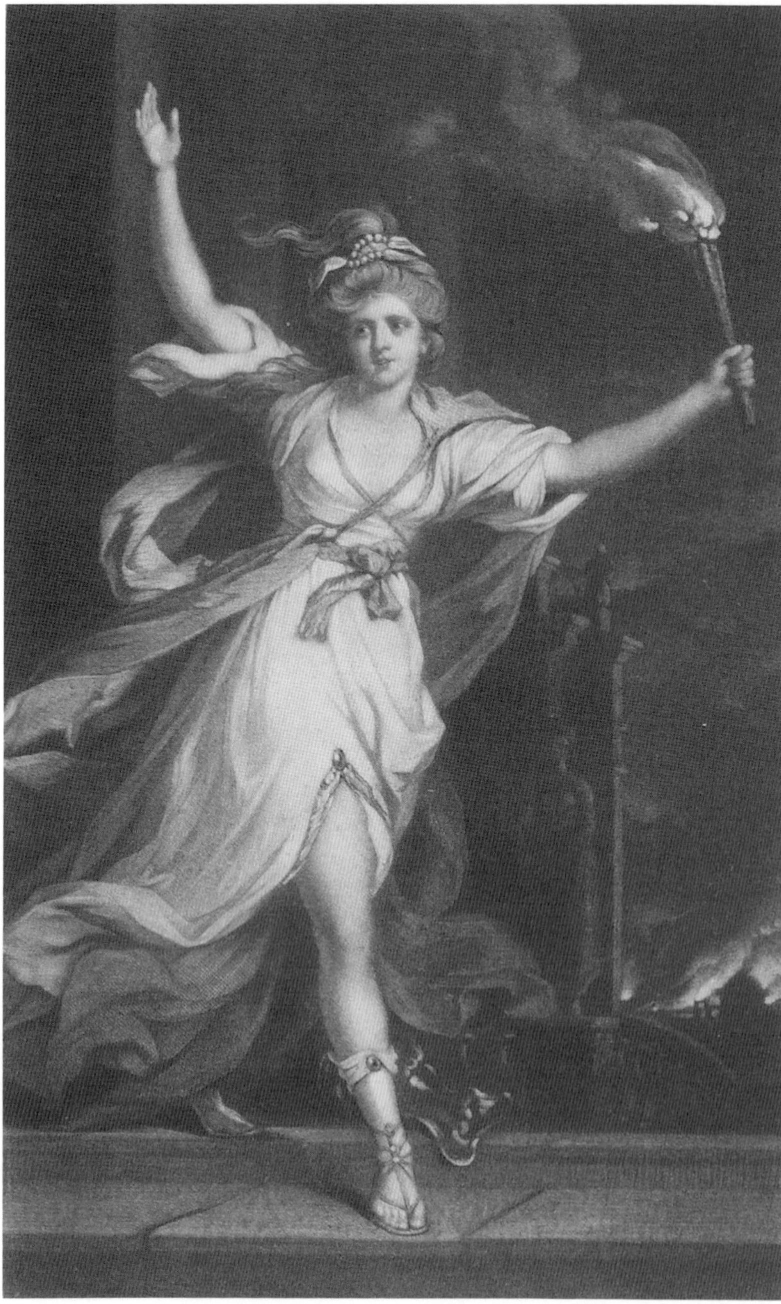

Figure 3. Emily Warren (Emily Pott) Thäis by Sir Joshua Reynolds, D14709, Mezzotint, 1837. Copyright of National Portrait Gallery, London.

the directors, or as he described them, "the cheese-mongering varlets of Leadenhall Street," would "mulct" (milk) out of Urmston.[153] Bob had already paid a large sum of money to Urmston to reserve the whole of the Round house and "half the Great Cabin of the Ship *Lord Mulgrave*" for Emily and himself.[154]

The passenger list of the *Lord Mulgrave*'s 1781 voyage indicates that Robert Percival Pott and his servant, William Bodifield, would be sharing a berth. Bodifield was no doubt Emily Warren.[155] The couple reached India but a few months later, in May 1782, Emily died while traveling with Pott by ship from Madras (Chennai) to Calcutta (Kolkata). Hickey wrote that Emily died from the consequences of drinking a cold substance when she had prickly heat. Following her death, Bob Pott was initially:

> inconsolable and outrageous in his grief; For several hours he would not be persuaded that she ceased to exist. He however but too soon has unanswerable evidence such way the fact, from the body becoming black and putrid, emitting the most offensive smell, a Coffin therefore being prepared with the utmost dispatch, the Corpse was finally enclosed therin, placed in a boat, astern of the vessel, with a very long painter, or head fast, and thus was towed up to Calcutta, where it was interred in the burial ground of the town.[156]

No information about exactly where Emily was buried in Calcutta has been found, despite Hickey claiming that Pott paid nearly £3000 for a magnificent mausoleum and a further £1000 to build a column in Culpee (Kalpi) close to where Emily breathed her last.

Hickey relates that Pott soon recovered from his grief and eventually landed a fine post in India. The diarist recorded that, in July 1784:

> my friend Robert Pott accomplished his great object by obtaining the Appointment of President at the Durbar of the Nabob of Bengal, at the City of Moorshedabad, which was at that time considered as the most lucrative office in the Company's service, the whole stipend or salary allowed by Government to the Nabob passing through such President's hands in which channel a considerable portion of it always stuck to his fingers ...[157]

Hickey, Bob Pott, and Percivall Pott all acknowledged that Bob's position in Moorshedabad (Murshidabad) was awarded through the influence of Lord Thurlow, a supporter of Warren Hastings.[158] Percivall Pott counted the Hastings family among his patients and in early August 1784 had written to Warren Hastings, reassuring him that he had examined his wife, who had been sent home from India to recuperate from a debilitating illness, and found her better. Pott included his best thanks "for your kindness to my son Robert" in the letter.[159]

Percivall Pott's relief at having his son finally settle down was soon gone, for two years later Robert Pott was unemployed and living in disgrace on a small pension. Robert appealed directly to Earl Cornwallis for relief in a series of letters over the course of several years.[160] In May 1789 Robert sent Cornwallis a description of his extensive work experience in India, and in June wrote him a forlorn letter:

> My Lord. The affection I know that parts of your lordships family held my father in induces me to think that your lordship may have received some certain intelligence relative to him. Perhaps contradicting of the newspaper report.[161]

Bob Pott had obviously read, or been told of, a newspaper report concerning the death of his father. A month later a letter was recorded from Cornwallis' clerk to Pott stating, "that he had no intelligence whatsoever of the melancholy circumstances mentioned in your letter of this 17th. last."[162] The news of his father's death had taken nearly five months to reach Bob in India.

At the time of his father's death Bob Pott had fallen on very hard times and no relief would be forthcoming in the shape of an inheritance. In 1786 John Addison, Pott's chief assistant, appealed to Cornwallis for Pott to be dismissed from his position in Moorshedabad on the basis of a new Act passed about the holding of multiple offices in the HEIC.[163] More lurked behind Addison's appeal than a new law being passed, for Addison had been the natural successor to the post Pott received, and the two were bitter enemies. They accused one another publicly of fraud and theft so extensively that the company was forced to dismiss both of them from their positions.[164]

Pott was a broken man. In December 1787 he wrote to Cornwallis to document his misery and once again to ask for aid from the company:

> I have my Lord now lived near three years in a state of anxiety of mind, which is intollerable [*sic*]. My health is destroyed by it, and I feel my situation so degrading, and unmanly, that any alteration is infinitely preferable. In an unfortunate hour did the patron of my family Lord Thurlow solicit my succession to the Durbar of the Director. Retrenchments, and reductions immediately followed, my obtaining it.[165]

Bob Pott died in Calcutta in late 1794. He left behind a wife, and two illegitimate daughters. Pott's wife was his cousin Sarah Cruttenden, who he married in India in 1788. Sarah had been baptized in Calcutta on 9 April 1754 and was probably the sister of George Cruttenden, who had been on board ship with Bob when Emily Warren died.[166] Hickey described Sarah as "a very charming woman who was universally admired and respected and who proved an exemplary wife."[167] In 1797 the HEIC finally granted her a widow's pension of £100 a year if she went to live in England.[168] If Sarah did go, we have no record of her journey. The *Calcutta*

Gazette reported that she died somewhere near Dacca in November 1807.[169] Of Pott's daughters (and their mothers) little to nothing is known. Anna Hiatur Pott was baptized in Burrampore in 1789, and Bertha Sarah Russell Pott was baptized in May 1798, when she was seven years old, in Bhagalpur. Nothing else is known of Anna, but Bertha married a British Army Ensign in 1809 and died in 1836.[170]

Joseph Holden Pott (1758–1857), called the "exemplary Archdeacon of St. Alban'd," was Percivall Pott's third living son and the longest-lived of all the children. He was educated at Eton College and St. John's College, Cambridge, where he obtained a B.A. and then proceeded to a M.A. in 1783. He was ordained in 1781 and rapidly rose through the ranks of the Anglican Church. A Thurlow connection is again evident, as Joseph Holden's patron was Lord Thurlow's brother, the Bishop of Lincoln and Durham. Between 1783 and 1790 Pott was the priest for several parishes in Lincolnshire, including Beesby-le-Marsh and Bratoft.

A short letter dated 1783 from a Reverend Robert Percival Pott to Sir Elijah Impey of the HEIC concerned "the happy news that Lord Thurlow has presented a living to the Reverend's younger brother."[171] It ends with the writer revealing that he is not in a fact a real parson but only a mendicant. The letter's author, Reverend Robert Percival Pott, was of course in reality Bob Pott.

In 1784 Joseph Holden was appointed as Chaplain to Lord Thurlow, and in 1787 he became vicar of St. Olave Jewry, with St. Martin's, Ironmonger Lane, London. Two years later Pott was made archdeacon of St. Albans, the position he was holding at the time of his brother Edward Holden's death. Joseph Holden then served as a rector in Essex and Middlesex and became vicar of St. Martin-in-the-Fields in London. He was made archdeacon of London in 1813, Canon of St. Paul's Cathedral in 1822, Vicar of Kensington in 1824, and Canon and Chancellor of Exeter Cathedral in 1826. Joseph Holden resigned his archdeaconry and vicarage in 1842 but held both canonries until his death.

Joseph Holden was part of the Hackney Phalanx, an influential group of Anglican high churchmen who often came from banking and mercantile backgrounds. He was a governor of the Society for Promoting Christian Knowledge and later became its treasurer. At the time of his death in 1847, Joseph Holden was the last survivor of the Hackney Phalanx. Throughout his life he wrote poems and essays on religion and painting.[172] He also took care of his mother from the time of his father's death in 1788 to her death in 1811. Two years before Sarah Pott passed away Joseph Holden had a letter published in *The Gentleman's Magazine* in response to a letter from "Clericus" who:

> professes to have some Letters written by Mr. Robert Cruttenden to Dr. Doddridge, which he is willing to communicate to any survivors of Mr. Cruttenden's family. It would very much satisfy me to see these Letters of my grandfather: my mother, the only

> surviving daughter of Mr. Cruttenden, unites with me in requesting your offices on this occasion with your Correspondent. Mr. Cruttenden possessed considerable talents as a Writer, and was connected with many distinguished persons in the Literary world. My mother is now in her 86th year, and has survived all the children of Mr. Cruttenden.[173]

Joseph Holden Pott died in February 1847, at Woburn Place, London. He was buried with his parents at St. Mary Aldermary and left an estate of £20,000.[174]

Comparatively little is known about Percivall Pott's youngest son, Edward Holden Pott (1766–1798). He married a woman called Sarah (1775–1865), and they had one daughter, Mary Ann (1796–?). Some information on Edward Holden's life appears in an obituary published in *The Gentleman's Magazine and Historical Chronicle*:

> Found dead in his bed at Liverpool, *Edward Holden Pott*, esq. major in the Westminster regiment of the Middlesex militia. Major P. was in his 33rd or 34th year. He was the youngest son of the late Percival P. esq. the celebrated surgeon, whose abilities as a professional man stand not in need of any encomium. He … went to Eton … [and] was placed by his father under Mr. Balfour [Belfour], a solicitor, and clerk to the Surgeons Company. After remaining the usual time with that gentleman, he practiced in one of the Inns of Court, where his business soon increase[d] in such a manner as would probably have placed him at the head of his profession, had not his inclination for arms led him to embrace a military life.[175]

Evidence supporting the article of clerkship (5 years) made between Okey Belfour and Edward Holden in 1782 survives in a statement of one of its witnesses, the surgeon Thomas Warrell. Ludford Harvey also served as a witness. According to the document, Percivall Pott paid Belfour £400 to:

> accept and take the said Edward Holden Pott to be the Clerk of him … and should use his best and utmost endeavors to procure the said Edward Holden Pott to be admitted and sworn an Attorney of his Majestys Court of Kings Bench and also a solicitor of his Majestys High Court of Chancery.[176]

On 14 December 1791, Edward Holden Pott of 9 Gray's Inn, witnessed the will of Mrs. Philadelphia Hancock (1730–1792).[177] She was the sister of the Reverend George Austen and aunt to Jane Austen. She also had strong associations with the HEIC, particularly with Warren Hastings. Scholars have indeed speculated whether Hastings was the father of Philadelphia's child, Eliza (1761–1813), rather than just the godfather.[178] All we know of Edward Holden Pott's life after he witnessed Philadelphia Hancock's will is that in 1793 he was made Captain of a Company in the Westminster Regiment and four years later was promoted to

Major of the Regiment.[179] Edward Holden is buried in Henry Park's family grave at St. James Toxteth Park, Liverpool.[180] Henry Park had been one of Percivall Pott's pupils, and a close friendship had obviously developed between the Pott and Park families.

Edward Holden Pott's obituary ended with the comment that though his situation in life was highly respectable, "as his father lived in an elegant and liberal manner, and had eight children, it was impossible for him to have been in the enjoyment of a very ample fortune."[181] Edward Holden Pott's survivors were listed as his mother and two brothers:

> the eldest formerly in the banking-house of the Hon. Richard Walpole; the second the learned, pious, and exemplary Archdeacon of St. Alban'd; and three sisters, all married; the eldest to Samule [*sic*] Potts, esq. late of the General Post-office; the second to Mr. Earle, the surgeon; and the youngest to Samuel Compton Cox, esq. lately, from his abilities, appointed to the situation of a Welsh judge. Robert Pott, esq. the Major's eldest brother, died lately in the East Indies; and his eldest sister who was married to Mr. Frye is likewise dead since her father's decease.[182]

The Deaths of Percivall and Sarah Pott

Percivall Pott became ill after he returned wet and exhausted from visiting a patient on horseback on 11 December 1788. Earle, as Pott's assistant, rode out three days later to see the patient on the understanding that Pott would stay home and recuperate. Pott instead went on a round of his patients in London. He became progressively ill, with shivering, fever, and finally delirium. The best doctors were brought in, but on 22 December, Pott died. His last coherent words, according to Earle, were "My lamp is almost extinguished. I hope it has burned for the benefit of others."[183]

Pott was buried a few days later near his mother at St. Mary Aldermary Church, close to where he had been born 74 years earlier. In his will Pott left his wife, Sarah, £3000 and all his household goods, furniture and silver. She also received a house that was rented out in Charlotte Street, Bloomsbury with the instructions that it should go to their son, Edward Holden, on her death.[184] Percivall, the eldest son, was left £500 and his father's gold watch chain and seals, while Edward Holden and Joseph Holden were left £1000 each. Joseph also received all of Pott's manuscripts and books, except the ones on surgery. They went to Pott's son-in-law James Earle, a surgeon. Bob Pott fared poorly. As his father had told him when they argued many years earlier, Bob had already received more than his fair share of monies:

> and wheras my son Robert Pott when he wanted my assistance had it Therefore and because he is in a Situation to do much better for himself than I can do for his Brothers

> and Sisters I desire him to accept of one hundred guineas for a Ring in memory of a parent who loved him tenderly.[185]

In 1811 Joseph Holden Pott commissioned Law and Gilbert of St. John's Square, Clerkenwell, to print *An Address to Her Beloved Children*, which Sarah Pott had written in 1808. In a brief six pages in a formulaic fashion, she covers her long life and commands her children to obey God. With pathos Sarah writes:

> Your honoured Father left me an ample and noble income; but circumstances, public and private, have for some years past reduced it full half, leaving barely sufficient to bring the balance of my annual expences even. In consequence of which, I am deprived of the pleasure of bequeathing to my dear Children any lucrative token of my affection and regard, though fully and always possessed with the opinion, that, happier is the giver that the receiver. I must submit to this inability.[186]

Sarah Pott's probate shows that she was living with Joseph Holden in the Rectory at Little Burstead, Essex, when she composed her will.[187] Her wish was to have as plain a funeral as possible, to avoid all unnecessary expenditure, and to be "buried in the vault with the remains of my most dear and honoured husband and my beloved daughter Sarah Frye." Sarah Pott left instructions for mourning rings of 2–3 guineas in value to be distributed to "her 5 children and 4 children in law, 16 grandchildren, 2 grandchildren in law, my niece Sarah Cruttenden, [and] my nephew George Cruttenden."[188] The gold repeating watch given to her by her husband was to go to Anna Potts, her granddaughter, with the command that she was never to part with it, and she left £50 to her granddaughter Sarah Frye. Any remaining monies were to be divided equally between her two living sons, Percival and Joseph Holden, as was the furniture and portraits.

In print and in person, Pott was key in promoting attributes that were associated with being an eighteenth-century leading professional surgeon in London. These included producing well-trained apprentices and dressers, holding authoritative roles in the Company of Surgeons, obtaining a senior post at a major hospital, demonstrating great skill in operating, treating famous patients, and writing praiseworthy books. It was also important to cultivate politeness, be a patron of the arts, have sons that were well-educated and daughters that married well, and reside in the more fashionable areas of the city.[189]

Pott's training in surgery began when he was 15, and he treated his last patient at age 73. For nearly half a century Pott successfully clambered up the ladder of business and surgery to become a gentleman of means and respectability.[190] The next chapter analyzes how Pott achieved eminence in the profession of surgery. It was a risky business that required physical strength, dexterity, and a strong amount of authority.

CHAPTER TWO

"Be Firm Without Appearance of Brutality"

Authority and Surgery

> Another thing which I will observe to you is the pretty manner of expressing yourself as in taking of a Limb or the like, I will affirm there are more people afraid by the different terms used as to call them operations amputating breasts & going on with so formal a way with their damnable long Gowns and dress than by removing the cancer which are things abominable.[1]

> I have often told you Gentlemen that forming true Prognostics was what constituted the great difference between Practitioners, and that there is no other part of our profession in which a Man gives a more conspicuous proof of his abilities than in this.[2]

Pott practiced and published during a time of fluidity in the status of medical men, especially that of surgeons. His own life bridged one of the biggest changes, for Pott held the title of barber-surgeon from 1736 to 1745 and then that of surgeon from 1745 until his retirement in 1787 from St. Bartholomew's Hospital. This chapter examines Pott's influence on the shaping of the embryonic profession of surgery through a two-prong analysis of his lectures and published works. First, Pott's systematic and focused approach to carrying out surgery, which he both practiced and taught, reveals the physical and sensory experiences of pre-modern surgeons and their patients. Second, Pott advised his pupils to cultivate certain comportments, values, and traits in order to become successful and authoritative surgeons. This points to the ambitions and anxieties of medical men in the mid to late eighteenth-century.

The Teaching of Surgery

As Roy Porter, Susan Lawrence, and Toby Gelfand have demonstrated, offering a course of lectures could be a source of consistent income for surgeons in eighteenth-century London.[3] In 1719 John Douglas (d. 1743) added a section on chirurgical operations and bandages to his syllabus of anatomical lectures to the Company of Barber Surgeons. In the preface Douglas explained that the course was:

> entirely calculated for the Students of Surgery; and the main Design of it, is to shew them a shorter and more direct Way of acquiring that excellent and useful Art, than any has hitherto been propos'd.[4]

After an anatomical overview of the body, including three demonstrations of the bones, Douglas turned to the "scarf-skin" and two demonstrations of fat and membranes. He then outlined demonstrations of adenology (glands), angieology (arteries), the genital parts, and myology (muscles). Douglas gave a total of twelve anatomical demonstrations prior to the actual Operationum Chirurgicarum Syllabus.

The Operationum Chirurgicarum began with a discussion of "punctions," from bloodletting to tapping water to opening abscesses. This was followed by advice on sutures and hernias, then fistulas[5], sounding with a probe or fingers, and cutting on the body in a variety of operations. In each case, Douglas chose to first demonstrate the instruments that had been, and in his opinion, should still be used in a particular operation. For example, when discussing "Errors committed in cutting Breasts," Douglas wrote:

> The forks and needles that are pas'd thro these Tumours, to hold them by, cruel and inconvenient. The Purse and Forceps, used by others, troublesome and uncertain. An easy and certain Way of holding them. The great, long or crooked Knives used to cut them with, frightful and very inconvenient. A proper Knife.[6]

Douglas pointed out the anatomy of the part to be operated on, and finally, showed what dressings should be used and how they should be applied. He did this with recourse to a corpse and defended what students could learn from the dead versus the living:

> Some are apt to fancy that the seeing Operations made on dead Bodies is of little if any Use. I own, that the bleeding, crying and struggling of the Patients, and the preternatural Structure of the Parts in some Cases, are wanting here: But then Operations on dead Bodies have all the other Advantages, which those on living ones have, and besides, a great many peculiar to themselves, which will more than Compensate abovemention'd.[7]

The peculiar advantages that came from working on the dead were to do with being able to demonstrate a large variety of operations on one body and the factor of time. Douglas explained that a living patient would not allow a surgeon "full leisure" to explain instruments, operative techniques, or dressings to pupils. In particular, "doubts and objections" could not be raised and answered in front of a patient.

D'Arcy Power speculated that Edward Nourse (1701–1761) at the Barber Surgeon's Hall and Samuel Sharp (ca. 1700–1788) at Guy's Hospital both copied the format of Douglas's lecture series. Certainly the title of Nourse's single publication, *Syllabus totam rem Anatomicam humanam complectens et praelectionibus aptatus habendis Authore E. Nourse, huic accredit syllabus chirurgicus quo exhibentur operations quarum modus peragendarum demonstrandus. Londini* (1729) suggests this.[8] Sharp's *A treatise on the operations of surgery, with a description and representation of the instruments used in performing them: To which is Prefix'd an Introduction on the Nature and Treatment of Wounds, Abscesses and Ulcers* (1739), which went through multiple editions, also reflects Douglas's influence.[9] Sharp provided lectures for the edification of future naval surgeons (see chapter 1), and Nourse and Pott would follow suit.[10] Exactly when Nourse first began to offer an extended course on anatomy and some surgery from his home in Aldersgate Street is unclear. Pott probably assisted him in this enterprise as an apprentice and then as a qualified surgeon.

In 1734 the Governors of St. Bartholomew's Hospital decided to allow their surgeons and assistant surgeons to give lectures on anatomy in the dissecting room.[11] Nourse immediately took advantage of this opportunity and Pott joined him. They developed two courses a year, one beginning in February and the other in November. Their series, advertised in London newspapers as "a Course of Anatomy to which will be added, the Method of performing all the *Operations* in *Surgery*, with their proper Bandages by E. Nourse, F.R.S. *Assistant Surgeon, and Lithotomist to St. Bartholomew's Hospital* and P. Pott, *Surgeon in Bow Lane*," was offered for the last time in November 1741. Pott's income from lecturing with Nourse is unknown, but Bow Lane was a respectable address.[12] A year later, a report in the *Daily Advertiser* indicated that Pott was able to afford clothes of good quality and employ a manservant:

> Lost on Tuesday last, from a Washer-woman in White's Alley, Little Moorfields, six fine Holland Shirts, ruffled, mark'd P, and number'd 1, 3, 7, 9, 15, and one the Mark unknown. Whoever will bring them to Mr. Pott, Surgeon, in Bow-Lane, Cheapside, shall receive Two Guineas Reward, and no Questions ask'd; if offer'd to pawn or sell, pray stop them, and give Notice as above, and you shall have the same Reward.
>
> Lost at the same Time, three Shirts belonging to a Servant, mark'd R. J. tied up in a red and white spotted Handkerchief. Whoever will bring them to Richard Jones, at Mr. Pott's as above, shall have Half a Guinea Reward, and no Questions ask'd.[13]

It is not clear why Pott and Nourse stopped offering their course of surgical lectures. Until his death in 1761 Nourse worked alongside Pott at St. Bartholomew's Hospital, and Pott became Nourse's most famous apprentice.

A somewhat mysterious and anonymous essay satirizing Pott and Nourse, among other medical men, was published in 1748, by which time their joint lectures had ended. *Egregious quackery display'd. Or, a narrative of the late memorable case of Seignor Capitano Masseo/Written in Spanish … And translated into English by a faithful hand (Sarificato Sangresugeo)*[14] strongly attacks the physicians, quacks, and surgeons who treated and by implication murdered Captain Robert Massey.[15] Characters include Don Ricardo de Prato (based on Richard Mead, a well-known London physician), Guardo (inspired by Joshua "Spot" Ward, a rich purveyor of medications), Antihectico Poterio (Percivall Pott), and Cavaliero Norsario (Edward Nourse). The close business relationship of Nourse and Pott forms part of the narrative, for Poterio is described as Norsario's "Creature," to whom he had for some time "consecrated" himself.[16] Pott's satirical nickname of Antihectico Poterio refers to the surgeon's belief in the theory of inflammation in the body as the cause and complicating factor in many illnesses—Pott believed that air entering a wound was invariably fatal. Nourse's Cavaliero title mockingly draws attention to the myriad of instruments, or the armory, that operative surgeons would need to carry with them.

For sixpence you could purchase and read the sad story of "Seignor Masseo," aged 48, who had been "seized with a *Spina Ventosa*, or White Swelling in his Elbow" [probably a skeletal manifestation of tuberculosis].[17] Prato sees the patient, then Guardo, and finally, Norasio and Poterio:

> At this Juncture an officious Visit was made him by *Antihectico Poterio*: who, assisted by *Cavaliero Norsario*, had, to his immortal Honour, the Courage, even in this deplored Condition of *Masseo*, to make an Amputation.[18]

The chief accusation made in the satire is that Pott amputated the patient's arm when Masseo became too ill to bear the pain. The writer also notes that a senior surgeon should have carried out the procedure, which did not happen, and Massey died two days later. On the final page Norsario is attacked as uncouth and uneducated, not a gentleman.[19] This certainly coincided with Pott's view of his former master and his criticism of Nourse's eagerness to operate, even in the most hopeless of situations. As Pott became more gentrified he sought to distance himself from the barber-surgeon who trained him.

In 1745, as a member of the Company of Surgeons and a newly appointed assistant hospital surgeon, Pott began to offer his own winter lecture course for the price of five guineas.[20] The timing was good for Pott since he had just moved to new and expensive lodgings in Watling Street with his bride, Sarah Cruttenden, where he could lecture and dissect, board pupils, and see private patients.

Sometime between the death of Edward Nourse in 1761 and the designation of a dedicated lecture space at Saint Bartholomew's in 1765, Pott stopped offering private lectures from home and began to offer them publicly at the hospital. Earle writes that this move was due to the large number of students Pott was attracting from Edinburgh, Dublin, and abroad. While this was probably true, a more compelling reason was that the governors of the hospital had finally responded to calls to provide a new space for physicians and surgeons to read their lectures rather than in the old and dark dissecting room. Medical men were given permission to now "make use of the Theatre for operations and also of the Room adjoining."[21] Pott did not charge a fee to those attending his lectures at the hospital, but this does not mean that his income was not increased from offering them there.[22] The fact that Pott attracted so many pupils to the hospital would have led to considerable income for, as previously noted, all pupils' fees were shared amongst the hospital surgeons. In 1775 James Hutchinson, one of Pott's dressers, lamented in a letter to his uncle Israel Pemberton in Philadelphia: "My giving fifty Guineas to the Hospital, besides paying for all the different lectures, Cloaths and board, has left but a very small sum, & I know not how much it may cost me to come back to America."[23]

Pott offered his course in surgery at St. Bartholomew's Hospital twice a year from spring 1765 until autumn 1787. As the lectures were only open to pupils who had paid a fee to one of the medical men at St. Bartholomew's, only one advertisement for the lectures seems to have appeared in London newspapers between 1765 and 1787. The advertisement for what would be his final course before retiring suggests that perhaps there had been speculation as to whether Pott would be willing to offer it:

> London, St. Bartholomew's Hospital, Sept. 1, 1787.
> Chirurgical Lectures.
> Mr. Pott intends to continue his Lectures as usual at this Hospital.[24]

In his usual grandiose fashion James Earle describes his father-in-law as envisioning the lecture series as an index to the great book of disorders that his students would have to learn to read when taking care of patients at St. Bartholomew's Hospital.[25] Earle claimed that Pott struggled at first to organize his thoughts:

> He had not then digested and arranged his ideas, but spoke, as I well remember, with hesitation and reserve … In a few courses he overcame all obstacles, and communicated his thoughts with eloquence and ease. He was not satisfied with following any system which had been laid down by others, as he thought they in general dwelt too

> much on the operative part, which, though very important, is by no means the most difficult part of surgery, nor the most worthy of attention.[26]

Pott was forthright about the importance of the physical location of the lecture series as a place where information could be best imparted by a surgeon to his pupils:

> The great Benefit of Hospitals is not confined to the Poor only, but indeed extends to all Ranks of Mankind, such Variety of Cases affording much information & Practice in the Arts of Physic & Surgery. Surgeons & Physicians who have the Care of Hospitals, & to whom the medical Care of others is entrusted should be particularly circumspect with regard to their Practice, & should be perfectly communicative to their Pupils: for these reasons & that the Pupils might not be necessitated to ask many questions at Times when perhaps neither convenient nor Opportunity would admit a proper discussion of them, the following lectures were intended, & from these Circumstances I have purposely omitted descending into systems, physiological or Anatomical disquisitions, my sole aim being to give Descriptive signs & symptoms of Diseases as they have appeared to me many years.[27]

This statement includes several aspects that warrant closer examination. First it shows that it was not necessarily when walking the wards with medical men that pupils learnt about surgical procedures or diseases. Pott was conscious of the need to be "circumspect" when treating patients in the crowded, bustling halls of St. Bartholomew's hospital.[28] Second, legal cases reveal all too clearly that whatever a surgeon would say to a patient, pupil, or nurse would be overheard by many others in the ward. Third was the issue of "convenience." This term can be read in many ways—Pott was in a hurry, the patient was in pain or needed immediate attention that precluded lengthy discourse on his or her condition, or Pott needed to focus on doing or ordering things to be done to his patients, rather than instructing the pupils that trailed behind him. In any event, the lectures are indicative of Pott's desire to impart surgical knowledge in a setting where only future surgeons are present. Lectures were meant to supplement bedside teaching and sometimes to replace it.

Based on evidence from rewritten student notes that survive of Pott's lectures at St. Bartholomew's Hospital, the earliest of which dates from 1767,[29] the full course in surgery consisted of sixty-four lectures. Pott divided it into two parts, with the first beginning in early November and the second in early February. This was in line with other lecturers' courses in the capital, such as those of William Hunter.[30] The syllabus changed little over Pott's lifetime.

In the introductory lecture, Pott would simply state that if his pupils wanted to know about bandages they could consult Joahnnes Scultetus and if they wanted to know about instruments, they could read Lorenz Heister.[31] Early on in the course he would also tell his students that traditional methods of teaching surgery were unsatisfactory and particularly singled out the plan recommended by Johannes van Horne (1621–1670):

> One great author whose Plan has been generally followed has divided Surgery into several parts each of which has a Greek derivation from the manner of operating, as Synthesis, Diaresis, Pharesis, Aphaeresis, Prosthesis, & Diarthrosis—It is a pretty good plan as far as it goes, & for the Time it was written in, but whoever thinks of studying the art of surgery from it will be misled, & at last find himself entangled in many gross errors.[32]

Van Horne was a professor of anatomy and surgery at Leiden University.[33] In 1717 and again in 1730 an English translation of his *Micro-Techne; or, a methodical introduction to the art of chirurgery* was published in London.[34] The work included an introduction to the antiquity and usefulness of surgery, followed by a section on instruments, bandages, and compresses, then:

> Of Syntheis, or a Conjunction of what is disjoin'd. Of Fractures … Of Luxations, Of Wounds and Ulcers, Of Dislocation of the soft Parts, as Ruptures, Of Diaresis, or a Division of entire Parts, Of the soft parts. Of Exaresis, or an Extraction of noxious Substances sticking in our Bodies, such are generated there … as come from without. Apharesis, or an Ablation of what's superfluous, which is either occultly … or manifestly. Of prosthesis, or a supplying by Art what is deficient. Of Diorthosis, or rectifying what is crooked.[35]

Pott would sometimes briefly explain what each of van Horne's six divisions covered, such as "Prosthetic, as the Putting in of artificial teeth, Eyes and Wooden legs …"[36] But he always ended the discussion of van Horne's plan with condemnation, remarking that it was superficial and narrow since it only covered operations and:

> it leads not to the knowledge of Diseases. A Young Man by studying this Plan would become an Imposter, without knowing why to perform the Operation. He may perhaps doe it [but] not perhaps Dexteriously.[37]

For Pott, knowing the nature of the patient's disease was the first step in mastering the art of surgery, for from that knowledge came the ability to observe the symptoms that would indicate whether an operation was even necessary.

The second step was learning how to perform the operation in "the best safest and easiest Manner as Possible."[38] Pott lectured his pupils that:

> In order to render you capable to accomplish this, my intention in the following Course of Lectures, and which I shall endeavor to lay before you … My Plan is to

> make my five or six first sections general, and to speak of those diseases which are Confin'd to particular Parts but are liable to happen in all Parts of the Body, and having finished these begin Scalp; and so end regularly at the Extremities.[39]

Pott followed his introductory lecture on the nature of surgery with two lectures on the different varieties of tumors that could be found in the body. He then discussed different types of wounds, starting with those that could occur to the head and moving down the body. He then considered specific disorders of various parts of the body, usually beginning with the fistula lachrymalis (obstruction and infection of the tear ducts), cataracts, polypus (nasal tumors), the "hare lip" and extirpation of the tonsils. The lectures continued with diseases of the breast, including empyema and cancer, and then those of the abdomen, such as ascites. Pott spent considerable time on hernias, diseases of the testicle, bladder, and urethra, gonorrhea, and diseases of the anus and, very occasionally, of the uterus and vagina (Pott remarked that these latter topics were best left to lecturers on midwifery[40]). He completed the course with an explanation of aneurisms and the operation of amputation, both of which affected the limbs, or inferior members.

Pott wove stories of the beliefs of the ancient authorities and of patients and medical men about the nature of the body in sickness and in health into his lectures. He wryly told his audience that while

> Hypocrates thought wounds of the Bladder mortal, & therefore made an Oath never to cut for the stone, If Every Body had trod in his Steps to this time, There would many have died in great Misery, who have been brought to lead very happy lives from the Operation.[41]

Pott's lectures and publications reveal the surgeon's own assumptions about what were thought to be spurious conditions, the workings of women's bodies, and how surgeons attempted to negotiate authority to treat, or sometimes, to refuse to treat, patients. At times Pott questioned whether certain medical conditions even existed. In lectures given in the 1770s, he spoke of a condition where water accumulated between the heart and the pericardium, or the sac in which the heart is encased. Pott told his audience that it caused a "total incapacity of breathing and they all die." The name *angina pectoris* had been proposed for the condition, and Dr. William Heberden (1710–1801), according to Pott, "has taken considerable Pains to discover the Cause of this Disease, but has not succeeded."[42] Heberden proposed that excess fat around the heart led to the swelling, but Pott dismissed his idea, stating that, "on Dissections we find Hearts abundantly loaded with Fat, with out [*sic*] having a single Symptom of the Disease." Pott then told a story of a patient he knew, "one Jones" who had the mysterious condition of angina pectoris for seven years and when it struck, "whither he was on Foot, Horseback or in a Coach, he was oblig'd immediately to stop and take a Spoonful of Brandy." Pott added that he has not been able to determine whether this helped him or not, but at least the man died quickly, for Jones dropped dead in mid sentence, apparently in "perfect Health."[43]

Pott dismissed some conditions and surgical claims out of hand because of their nation of origin. For example, "some french writers have mention'd a disease term'd a dropsy of the Periteneum, which I never saw nor do I believe it to exist."[44] France and Britain were on different sides at many times during Pott's life; this remark, however, was not just a matter of patriotism. What particularly aroused Pott to a state of righteous indignation was the French claim of having superior skills in performing operations. In the first few minutes of his introductory lecture, he generally included references to the cruel and irrational nature of French surgeons:

> [The surgeon's] resolution should by no means lead him to barbarity, he should make a distinction between the dead senseless and the sensible extreme irritable part of a miserable, unhappy, but feeling patient, you find the French us'd to cruelty in their operations, you read of their tracing the Spermatic Chord 4 or 5 inches in the Abdomen, for the removal of a Schirrous Testicle & Chord, could we ever suppose they did it but in an inaminate body, or if otherwise they were mere brutes for the attempt, how they do this cannot be envi'd by a rational Surg.n, yet if they lay this down as authenticat'd or as a matter of fact & the cures have been perform'd. I can't [for my own part] believe they ever have been perform'd on a dead body.[45]

Here Pott shared his doubts that a living patient could tolerate the pain of this procedure and his suspicions that the French must have done it on a corpse. In another introductory lecture around 1775 he concluded his presentation of the case with the comment that if the French had operated on a patient in this fashion, "they are madmen."[46]

Pott also refers to the rivalry between French and English surgeons in his lectures on hernias when discussing the case of a child who had a large swelling between its legs. Five surgeons in Bath all diagnosed the swelling as a *hernia congenita* and recommended that the child be sent to Paris for surgery.[47] Instead, the child was first sent to London and brought to Pott for his expert opinion on whether the hernia could be surgically removed or if the child should be left to die. Pott recounts that on unwrapping the swelling, which was encased in "some hundred yards of filleting" (linen) to try and keep it pressed up against the body, he found that this was not in fact a case of hernia congenita. Rather, "the Testicle not yet come down into the Scrotum but lying in the Groin which by their bandage it was Enlarg'd to thrise [three times] its natural Size." Essentially the supposed large hernia was in fact a small testicle wrapped in many layers of linen. Pott concludes that, "if I had not discovr'd it the Child would have been sent forwith to Paris to serve the french a laugh upon our profession."[48]

Another theme that emerges from an examination of Pott's lectures over several decades is a certain characterization of the bodies and emotions of women. While he did not address childbirth, except for brief comments on the urgency of seeking aid when confronted with the "Prolapsus Vagina, Uteri; & Inversis Uterus," Pott did have strong views on how women should be cared for once they had given birth. He particularly disliked the practice of providing copious amounts of caudle or alcoholic tonics, since this not only made the woman drunk but also overheated her and caused breast inflammation:

> Bothe [*sic*] the rich and Poor after Parturition are almost always wrong treated; instead of being kept cool, quiet, & free from everything which could occasion their being heated, or Irritation; till lately & still too often, every means to inflame the Blood is us'd, by drinking Caudle of different kinds, so that a woman who usually does not drink but moderately, shall drink sometimes a Pint of Brandy, or a Quart of Wine, strong Beer be made into Caudle every day, by which they are sometimes little better than drunk for the whole Month ...[49]

Among the topics regarding women on which Pott lectured were dropsy of the ovary and diseases of the female breast, such as abscesses and cancer. Dropsy or swelling of the ovary could be due to a cyst, but if seen in older women, it generally meant they had cancer. Why cancer occurred in females was something Pott addressed cautiously. Bruising from falling or being hit in the breast was often given as the cause of cancer, but Pott was unsure as to whether this was the most common cause. He added that a melancholy habit of the body (prone to disease and chronic ailments) also appeared to play some role[50] and suspected that cancer of the breast was similar to cancer of the testicle in that it progressed slowly and remained hidden until like yeast it fermented and caused a rising in the body.

In lectures on menstruation Pott stated that it was well-known that women were more liable to cancers after their menses ceased.[51] Similarly if their menses started late, they were also more susceptible. He gave the case of a 25-year-old woman who died of unknown causes and was opened after death. Pott referred to the patient as a girl, presumably because of her lack of menses (and implied virgin status):

> Blood if kept from the Air (contrary to the received opinion) will not form matter as for—instance A Girl having an imperforated Vagina & not her menstruations until twenty five if opened after death the Blood is always pure nor would it ever have come to matter.[52]

This remark fit with Pott's views on the causes and consequences of inflammation in the body (see chapter three).

Pott's ideas about cancer being found more often in the female body after the cessation of menses were in line with those of other surgical authors. Among these was Lorenz Heister (1683–1758) whose *A General System of Surgery in Three Parts* (1739) was the most comprehensive work on surgery available in the eighteenth century and went through many editions. Pott and William Hunter both recommended the book to their pupils. Heister wrote,

> It is observable that old Maids and even married Women that do not breed, are very subject to Cancers in the Breast; this generally happens to them when they are turned of forty Years of Age, at the Time when the menstrual or haemorrhoidal Discharge begins to decrease or disappear; though I have frequently known this Case happen to Persons not so far advanced in Years, even between twenty and thirty.[53]

Heister noted that "tumours in the Breasts of Child-bed and Suckling women sometimes cannot be dispersed for years" but continued that this was not cause for alarm as: "The Surgeon's Business here is to take care to keep the afflicted Patient in good Heart by his Persuasions: and to the Tumor itself is to be applied Emp. De Spermate Ceti," (a wax found in the head of sperm whales). Heister reported that the tumors often shrank and even disappeared with the constant use of this wax. The cessation of menses, though, changed the odds:

> But the Case is usually otherwise in Women who are advanced in Years, and of a melancholy or sorrowful Disposition; for in such there is great Danger of the inveterate Tumor turning to a *schirrhus* or Cancer.[54]

Although medical practitioners and patients claimed external violence as the most common explanation for cancer of the breast, other theories existed as to how one developed the disease.[55] In 1758 Benjamin Gooch, a well-respected Norfolk surgeon, published *Cases and Remarks in Surgery. With Sketches of Machines, of Simple Construction, Easy Application and Approved Use*. One of the cases he included was of a gentlewoman who had a "cancerous disease which arose from drinking some liquor impregnated with the matter that issued from an ulcerated cancer."[56] Gooch added that the patient was "of great virtue and veracity,"[57] which suggests that he had trouble reconciling the patient's narrative of her disease with his surgical knowledge and perhaps suspected that his readers might have the same dilemma. The gentlewoman's story, "confirmed by relatives," was that when:

> she was a child about three years old, she went with her mother to visit a friend, who had an ulcerated cancer upon her breast, which had just been dressed, and some of

> the liquor with which it had been washed, standing in a tea-cup upon the table, she drank a little of it.[58]

A large ulcerated tumor grew within weeks on the girl's tongue and eventually spread to the inside and outside of her cheek. Surgeons were consulted in London, and eventually one managed to stop the growth of the tumor. Twenty or so years later, "the leaven (tumor) shewed itself upon her thigh, where she had received a contusion some years before."[59] The two theories about the cause of cancer come together here: first that cancer was contagious and hid in the body, rising up much like leavened bread, and second that it was caused by external violence, a contusion or bruise. For the next fifteen years the woman enjoyed tolerable health until she "discovered a small scirrhous[60] knot in her breast."[61] It grew slowly until her menses ceased and "began then to increase very considerably, and in a few years occupied the whole breast, with all the glands in the Axilla at last."[62] The woman died shortly after Gooch saw her. As Pott warned, it was after menses ceased that cancers would grow and take hold of the body.

But there is another issue here too. Cancer in the living could only be diagnosed if it surfaced and could be felt and then seen. In essence this meant that breast tumors were the most common cancer treated by surgeons, and the fact they occurred in middle-age women reinforced the link of menstrual flow to the formation of schirrous tumors.[63] Heister referred to a hard painless tumor "entirely covered with Skin" as an "*occult Can*cer." Once it broke through the skin it was called an "*ulcerated Cancer*"[64] and was exquisitely painful. His description of the intolerable stench of an ulcerated cancer, the increasing pain from the discharge, anorexia, and insomnia, "till at last Death delivers them from a miserable stinking Carcase,"[65] captures all too well the fear filled end of a patient with breast cancer.[66]

Pott told his pupils that getting women to submit to the knife was difficult and often impossible. Marjo Kaartinen surmises that women who hid their breast problems from eighteenth-century surgeons until the tumor became too large to conceal were in fact not just being modest or fearing the pain and disfigurement left by the knife, but were living in hope that the lump would disappear.[67] In the cases given by Gooch and Pott, it appears that women approached surgeons when a tumor had ulcerated and become painful and/or so large that it made life in general unbearable. In *Female Patients in Early Modern Britain: Gender, Diagnosis, and Treatment*, Wendy D. Churchill adds the interesting point that women probably knew someone who had died from breast cancer, and surgery may have appeared worse than any death.[68] Some women chose the use of caustics, such as paste made up with arsenic, instead of surgery. Pott opposed this method because it was more painful to the patient than being cut, and furthermore, it took longer to work, was often applied by a quack, and left a large scar. Cutting off a cancerous breast was much quicker than burning it off. But "patients would sooner suffer the Caustic [applied by some quack] than submit to the knife."[69] The words Pott chose to contrast the procedures, namely *suffer* and *submit*, perhaps reflect another factor that caused women to reject having their breast tumors amputated with a knife as opposed to having them burnt off with a chemical. Suffering when the caustic was applied implied some measure of control, as opposed to submitting to cutting, which did not. Suffering could also be done in private while submitting involved the public event of having an operation. Finally one further reason for the choice of caustic over the knife is hinted at in a note taken by Richard Whitfield when attending Pott's lectures on cancer of the breast. He wrote "such is the horror of the Knife in many people, that they will submit to endure ten times the pain by any other method, rather than undergo a sanguinary operation."[70] Sanguinary is the keyword here for, as eighteenth-century surgeons recorded, amputation of the breast was a bloody affair.[71]

Why women might fear and avoid an operation for cancer of the breast becomes crystal clear in Pott's description of the instruments and procedures that older surgeons had used to amputate a breast. They included "a large knife something like a common carving knife & a fork to be stuck in the Breast to hold it by, & from a foolish fear of Haemorrhage, they added to the horridness of the operation by making the knife red hot …" Pott considered this to be barbaric as well as unnecessary because, as he informed his pupils, amputations of the breast were straightforward procedures that simply involved two deep semicircular cuts, removal of the muscles, and careful scraping of the ribs. Once the surgery was over a *pledgit*, or a wad of lint, should be applied to the wound and changed daily for a week.

Henry Fearon (d. 1803), a surgeon to the Surrey Dispensary, reported that Mrs. Elizabeth Ellis of Camberwell had been dissuaded from being operated on for breast cancer by a neighbor's account of her excruciating ordeal. In *A Treatise on Cancers, with a New and Successful Method of Operating, Particularly in Cancers of the Breast and Testis* (1784), Fearon describes how Ellis finally changed her mind on hearing of the success of a breast amputation performed by Fearon, and that he was then able to successfully operate on her cancerous right breast.[72]

Pott considered the operation to remove cancer of the breast to be relatively painless, except for the initial phase. He stated that "The only pain of any Consequence in this Operation is in the Division of the Skin," and therefore, it should be done with *celerity* or quickness.[73] This operative technique was recommended not only to minimize pain for the patient but to also prevent the development of possibly fatal inflammation. Pain was a shock to the body that led to overheating, which in turn created the ideal environment for inflammation. Pott therefore counseled his pupils to cut fast and especially to cut deep. This must be done in spite of the feelings it could arouse:

> of whatever size the Breast may be, it is always best to divide the skin by two semi-circular Incisions, which should be deep enough; All the operating Part is done anterior to the pectoral Muscles & Ribs. Young surgeons are sometimes embarrass'd from the great depth they appear to cut this, but it is nothing but skin, teat & cellular membrane.[74]

Henry Fearon's account of his operative technique echoes that of Pott in many ways. Fearon relates the necessity to cut quickly and not being hurried by embarrassment from the depth of tissue to be cut through and the heavy bleeding that could ensue. In particular, he agreed that the most painful part of the operation was the first incision. Fearon studied with John Hunter in 1780 and may have availed himself of the opportunity to attend Pott's series of lectures on surgery.[75]

Certainly the letters of two patients to family members confirm the agonizing pain of the first cut in a breast amputation. Fanny Burney's well-known account written in 1811 recounts how she began to scream when "the dreadful steel was plunged into the breast—cutting through veins—arteries—flesh—nerves …"[76] A lesser known letter of October 1855 from a mother to her daughter describes the procedure: "Then came a gash long and deep, first on one side of my breast, then on the other. Deep sickness seized me, and deprived me of my breakfast. This was followed by extreme faintness. My sufferings were no longer local. There was a general feeling of agony throughout the whole system. I felt, every inch of me, as though flesh was failing …"[77]

Given the fear of being cut, however, Pott recognized that women often chose caustics and reluctantly counseled his pupils to be prepared to use them when the knife was refused. In doing so he also managed to attack quackery again and mock the old idea of cancer being like a crab in how it attached itself to the body. In 1767 John Heaviside recorded that in a lecture on cancer of the breast, Mr. Pott stated:

> I cannot see a reason why the Surgeons should be afraid to do it by Caustic as well as the Quacks. The Caustic is tedious in its Operation, inefficacious, & horridly painful but set from a dread of the Knife (Which in fact is not half so painful as the Caustic) … From this Quackery Destruction has happened to thousands, & probably will to many more; besides the Caustic hardens the surrounding Parts & it was this that gave origin to the ridiculous absurd Idea of the Schirrus [a cancerous tumour] having Claws, Roots & so on. However if Caustic are us'd, which I would by no Means advise, the more active ones are the best. [78]

A decade later Pott attacked quacks for marketing their recipes for caustics as secret and efficacious. To probably a great deal of laughter from his audience of pupils, Pott described the "Boasted Secret—brought from Stephens hospital, Dublin" as consisting of "The Meadow crow-foot, Dogfennel, Sulph. Vivum & Arsenic made into a paste with a yoke of Egg."[79] This paste supposedly would find and burn out the roots of the cancer. What Pott did advise his pupils to use as a caustic, though, is not recorded.

A milder complaint that occurred in the breast concerned milk abscesses. Pott asserted that these frequently developed because women were not willing to breastfeed as "it causes them trouble or to keep the shape of their breasts." He explained that the abscesses form "from the milk being driven back from the breasts to the uterus and a resultant high fever."[80] In another course of lectures Pott again commented on this style of rearing infants and told his pupils that "There is a very odd way now prevailing amongst the folks of fashion all over Europe and that of not suckling their Children." Pott described this as "contrary to Nature" as it "drives back the milk, and causes fever," and the mother's milk is needed to purge "the Meconium in the infant."[81] Physicians and surgeons recognized the mother's first milk or colostrum as what rid the child of its earliest stools of meconium in the first few days after birth. These statements by Pott reflect the concern of surgeons following William Cadogan and others to promote suckling or breast-feeding rather than the use of wet-nurses, who became identified with infant mortality.[82] No evidence suggests whether Mrs. Pott suckled all nine of her infants or resorted to wet-nurses.

Pott's first concern in counseling suckling was a medical one. He remarked, "you will find much in the Conexion [*sic*] between the breast and Uterus." Pott was alluding to the ancient and common knowledge that breast-feeding possessed some contraceptive properties, and if a woman chose not to breast-feed, "the uterus being again impregnated so soon after delivery it must Certainly be prejudicial to the health of the woman."[83] Although Pott did not address the issue of a woman having too much milk in her breasts, advice on this topic was certainly available in surgical texts:

> But if the Breasts are internally very much distended with Milk, it will be proper to discharge it by the Sucking either of an Infant, an old Woman, or a Puppy, or else by the Application of a Glass Instrument which we shall hereafter describe.[84]

Pott did not teach midwifery per se but made passing references to the difficult business of diagnosing pregnancy.[85] He cautioned that women and their friends often mistook dropsy (swelling) of the ovaries for pregnancy and that surgeons needed to be careful to not make the same assumption. They should attend to the signs of the body and note that if the swelling is only on one side of the body, then it is probably not due to pregnancy but rather dropsy. The only way to cure dropsy of the ovary was to pierce the ovary with a trocar, but surgeons should be prepared for the significant amount of lumpy stinking drainage. In the case of one patient Pott treated:

> as soon as the incision was made there gush'd out a deal of very offensive matter mix'd with Hydaties some as large as turky [*sic*] Eggs, and to Spake within Bounds it was a full gallon, the Lady rcover'd after sometimes.[86]

Female bodies could be tricky to diagnose. The reproductive parts were occult or hidden from view, and many mistakes were made because of this. Pott related the case of a nineteen-year-old virgin diagnosed with a bladder stone by hospital physicians, who "desired she might be searched."[87] Pott was called in and felt the stone with his catheter, but her pain was excessive and so he stopped. Two months later, Dr. William Pitcairne Senior, one of the physicians at the hospital, called Pott back to search again. "I searched again, & kept the instum.t so as to touch every mathematical point in the bladder, but could find no stone." The woman was put on opium, and died suddenly "in a fit." On opening her body, Pott found "a schirrus of the neck of the womb."[88] There was no stone.

The Comportment of Surgeons

Pott's training in surgery began in 1729 when at age 15, he was apprenticed to Edward Nourse, a senior surgeon at St. Bartholomew's Hospital. There is no doubt that the theory and practice of surgery at the time left a poor impression on the young Pott, for he was frequently damning in his summary of it. In his first book, *A Treatise on Ruptures* (1756), written after a narrow escape from having his leg amputated, Pott began with a description of the "antient surgery" as coarse, horridly painful from the use of caustics, and "encumbered with a multitude of awkward, unmanageable instruments, and pieces of machinery."[89] Operations as a result were complex, messy and longer than need be. Pott contrasted this ancient surgery to the modern one, where practitioners were concerned to lessen pains, to preserve the elegance of the figure (through fewer scars), and to strive for a shorter confinement period following operations and treatments.

The charges of old surgeons having used too many instruments, caustics, and burning irons were always part of Pott's first lecture to his pupils. In practice it was more difficult to operate when surrounded with a large choice of instruments, some of which would have required two people to use them. An anonymous student laconically—and succinctly—recorded in notes from autumn 1767, "Lect. 1st Was an introductory lecture, As to the use of surgery, & to lessen the Bandages to no more than usefull; with an abhorrence of that cursed instrument Probe Scissards."[90] Pott castigated surgeons who used probe scissors in several of his printed works, including *A Treatise on the Fistula in Ano*. He disliked that they pinched as they cut and so did further damage when dividing the skin. Pott wrote that "they may assist an awkward or an unsteady hand, but are more fit for a farrier, that for a surgeon."[91]

Pott followed his criticism of crude instruments that could not be directed by the finger of the surgeon with an attack on medications:

> Another Circumstance which you will find in your Researches is a prodigious barrage of Medicamenta, such as Epithems, Embrocations, Plaisters, Balsams, Ointments black, yellow, red & green, which they [old surgeons] dignified with the epithets of digestive, detersive, mundicative, incarnative & so on. I remember forty years ago when the [Surgeons'] Boxes of this Hospital had forty different colored Ointments & Balsams at one time, all for various kinds & states of Wounds & Ulcers, which were seldom made better but often worse thereby.[92]

Jargon also came under attack. Pott used this term on several occasions in his writings to mean a collection of unintelligible terms relating to a diseased condition that surgeons had developed over time so "that it is next to impossible to understand often what they really mean."[93]

Pott continued throughout his life to bring his pupils up-to-date in how to treat patients. Such advice was generally offered in a rapid-fire manner in lectures. John Heaviside recorded the following from having attended Pott's lectures in 1777. First, do not be seduced by symptoms into operating on patients who have convulsions but try opium and warm baths instead, and use "woollen Night Caps" rather than a myriad of bandages to avoid putting pressure on a wounded skull. Second, a "Formidable collection of bandages" may look "extremely neat on Paper, but [is] troublesome to apply."[94] Pott also informed his young charges, somewhat sarcastically, that if they wanted a list of bandages, "you may furnish yourselves with much better notion of from reading in your closets, if the diversions of this City will allow you ever to spend an evening at home."[95]

In his final years of lecturing Pott often included the following case history as an example of the changes he had made to the practice of surgery at the hospital and in private practice. Fifty years ago, he told his pupils, when he first came to St. Bartholomew's, they had been using medicated bougies, but Pott had "done away with them and sees them as quackery and roguery."[96] To drive this point home, he first caught the audience's interest with a story about a patient:

> I remember a waiter at a coffee house, had a very bad disease of the neck of the bladder, and was on a sudden seized with an impossibility of making water, I found him in

> the greatest agonies I ever saw any body in my life, I endeavored to introduce a bougie but found it impossible, I made use immediately of warm emollient formentations, & the warm bath, injected glisters of warm water, oil and opium, by which means the urine began to come away by drops, I found it was now impossible to pass the smallest bougie. By attending to the rigor, symptomatic fever, giving the bark freely for 14, or 20 days, he got well without the use of any bougie, or any other application to the urethra.[97]

Throughout his lectures Pott updated his pupils on the theory of diseases as well as the practice of surgeons. In the 1770s as part of lecture 29 on diseases of the urethra, he commented, "The virulent Gonorrhae is a desease which has exeris'd the Wit & imagination of almost al [*sic*] Writers in all Ages, as well in regard to the Origin of it as cure." Pott continued that the old theory of gonorrhea being a poison "now appears very stupid."[98] He was careful to point out throughout the forty or so years he lectured that his pupils must not regard the advancement of surgery "with vanity but ambition to accomplish more"[99] and "no doubt some years hence our Successors will be as much astonished at our ignorance as we are of our Predecessors."[100] Pott also drew attention to the fact that "Many useful improvements come from fools—Frère Jacques and the lateral operation. Smallpox treatment is widely different now," but cautioned pupils to not listen "too greedily to a sudden new puffing Practice, before you have thoroughly consider'd it."[101] The rhetoric of persuasive strategies was something to consciously develop but not to unconsciously consume.[102]

It is difficult to untangle how much of this criticism and advice on practice and theory reflects Pott's actual early experiences as an apprentice to a barber-surgeon and as an assistant surgeon at a large hospital versus coming from a desire to bolster the aspirations of his pupils to become gentlemen-surgeons. As Michael Stolberg has noted, "Medicine shapes perceptions, creates meanings, and provides practical guidance and implicitly or explicitly imparts a specific world view rooted in the power structure of the day."[103]

The precise image of surgery that Pott held and desired his pupils to attain—as a profession, occupation, trade, and/or livelihood—is difficult to puzzle out. Traditionally the three professions were the law, the church and medicine. These were occupations that required lengthy training and the acquisition of learning, resulted in a formal qualification, and dealt primarily with human beings rather than material objects. Profession was also used in the eighteenth century to mean a body of people engaged in an occupation. Anne Digby has asserted that medical men were members of an occupation who were also engaged in a trade and a profession. She sees professionalization as "a drive towards an ideal rather than a static attainment of a set of essential criteria."[104] Much appears to hang on this distinction between the promotion of professional values and the process of professionalization. Pott certainly promoted values that he considered to be professional; he refers to fellow surgeons throughout lectures as "members of a profession" and his "brethren." Andrew Edgar's work is useful to note here as well, for he views professionalism to a significant degree as an historical process of gentrification. By this Edgar means that etiquette and social skills are as important as any distinctive form of skill or value.[105] What makes a profession different to a craft or a trade is that:

> the values of a profession are articulated intrinsically to the profession, in terms of the contested understanding that the professionals themselves have of the meaning of the profession and the narratives within which its history is to be told.[106]

If professionalization can be defined as collective action by members of a particular occupation to protect its interests, Pott certainly participated in this process as a member of the Company of Surgeons. He told his pupils stories of the barbarous nature of surgery in the old days and urged them to mind their manners. Yet, is this evidence of a self-conscious desire to raise the low status of surgery and, as Julie Doyle puts it, "to resignify surgery as a scientific practice, and anatomy as exemplary of scientific knowledge"?[107] Certainly Pott viewed surgery in its highest form as a "great and noble science" rather than merely a way of making a living. Science was knowledge acquired through sustained study with someone who had mastered the theory of a branch of learning. This fitted with the aspirations and rising status of those who chose to be apprenticed or become pupils to surgeons in the great hospitals of London. There they could learn the theory of surgery from leading men in the field and obtain the discipline to systematically apply the principles in practice.

The power structure in relation to medical men was in flux throughout Pott's life and is reflected in surviving copies of notes taken during Pott's courses. Specifically, the introductory lecture always addressed the mixed image of "that useful and importance [*sic*] Science Surgery" in Georgian England.[108] Pott would tell his pupils that:

> I am sorry to say that many people consider Surgery in two different lights, if its in practical for the sake of getting a livelihood very little art and ability are requir'd, but if consider'd a great and noble science, it requires a steady application, ability, integrity, and as you acquire these you will despise and abominate the other.[109]

Here Pott was directly addressing not only historical changes in the ways in which surgery was being practiced as a trade or as a profession but also changes in the places surgeons were being trained, namely hospitals. The latter issue resulted in straightforward advice; pupils who didn't take full advantage of their time at St. Bartholomew's would learn to regret it:

> In an hospital you will have frequent opportunitys [*sic*] of this kind of knowledge [of symptoms and causes of diseases] & if you omit it, the faults will be yours & you will have a great deal to answer for.[110]

During Pott's lifetime, there was a great expansion of beds in the capital as new hospitals were built and old ones expanded. Pott was conscious of what such large institutions could provide in terms of material for teaching:

> The great Benefit of Hospitals is not confined to the Poor only, but indeed extends to all Ranks of Mankind, such Variety of Cases affording much information & Practice in the Arts of Physic & Surgery.[111]

St. Bartholomew's hospital was partially rebuilt and expanded in the 1730s. The governors commissioned one of their own, the architect James Gibbs, to design a grandiose symmetrical quadrangle of buildings to replace the higgledy-piggledy structures that had grown up since the twelfth century and were full of vendors of food and beggars.[112] The North Wing was completed in 1732, the South in 1740, the West in 1752 (women's wards), and the East in 1769. Pott was a barber-surgeon when the first two wings were built and a senior surgeon when the latter two were constructed. As Pott was planning a rational and informative series of lectures of surgery, architects and builders were streamlining the structure of hospital life itself for patients and those who cared for them. Gibbs's choice of a quadrangle of similar buildings echoed the new fashionable squares of gentlepersons' homes that were starting to populate the western edges of London, including Hanover Square, where Pott and other wealthy surgeons would choose to live.[113]

Pott was quick to tell his pupils that if they wished to succeed in earning the accolades of their peers and the fees of their patients, they must cultivate certain character traits along with their clinical skills. His advice changed little over several decades of lecturing but it did get longer. He remarked in the late 1770s, after many decades of experience:

> Anatomy and Physiology are absolutely necessary to make the surgeon: to these should be added natural Philosophy to form part of the studies, as that will point out to you the various beauties attending this noble Science; greatly assist the natural genius, and explain to us the many deviations nature sometimes puts on: to these must be added a temper steady & Resolute, patient in Enquiry & not biased by prejudice; nor to be led by the first appearance as that is unmanly. His resolution should by no means lead him to Barbarity, he should make a difference between the senseless dead, & the Sensible & Extream [*sic*] irritable, parts of a miserable unhappy but *feeling* patient.[114]

As Roy and Dorothy Porter have argued, "Georgian patients had little conception of the medical profession as a comprehensive entity, a collective abstraction. It

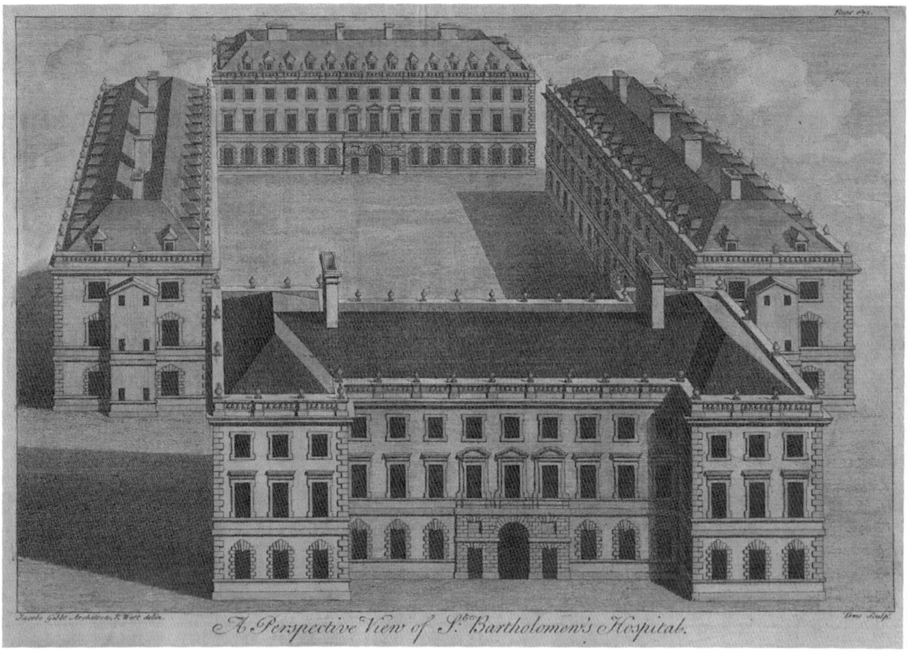

Figure 4. St. Bartholomew's Hospital. Copper line engraving on paper by Benjamin Cole, produced to accompany William Maitland's *History of London*, published 1754–6, hand coloured. Author's private collection.

was individual, face-to-face encounters that tipped the balance between distrust and confidence."[115] The balance was, however, tipped in favor of surgeons (versus physicians) for:

> The services provided by surgeons were far more tangible and appreciated (even where dangerous), thus constituting a better bond between the patient and professional. Partly because the quality of surgical training and skills improved during the century, surgery rose in esteem. At a pinch, the patient could make do without a physician; but when need arose, the surgeon was indispensable.[116]

According to Pott, a surgeon had to possess some intellectual knowledge, a willingness to let nature take its course in some situations, and the resolution and sensory abilities to carry out the job. Panicking was considered unmanly and resolution was needed. Surgeons needed to establish trust relatively quickly in situations involving emergencies, while treating chronic conditions required a different set of skills. Pott also addressed the issue of where a surgeon ended up practicing in the introductory lecture. If one practiced in the countryside, where there weren't physicians to consult (as in the city), it was no good being able to treat a compound fracture without knowledge of anatomy and diseases:

> Surg.n needs to do more than place the limb in an easy advantageous posture, or dressing and securing it, or the neatness and dexterity, these will not relieve the Patient of his Symptoms and principle complaint, he must have some medical assistance or he may sink from Diarrhaea, Dysentery, or Diabetes. It therefore behoves you to be acquaint'd with the means of removing these complaints, or you will find yourself greatly embarrass'd, and never will obtain the reputation of a good Surg.n.[117]

Pott spent considerable time in his lectures counseling his pupils on how to negotiate, persuade, and establish authority over patients in a polite but firm fashion. This had long been a difficult goal for surgeons to achieve as it depended not just on manifesting the physical prowess and dexterity to operate, but also on remaining calm and reflective when diagnosing and treating patients. Pott's pupils essentially needed to master a multi-part strategy.[118] Pott pointed out that evidence gained from an inspection of a patient's body or from listening to the story of their sickness had to be sieved and interpreted in much the same way as a lawyer would prepare for a court appearance.[119] Pott used his case histories to show that narratives of injury were frequently contradictory, as they were replete with economic concerns and emotional dilemmas. It was not so much that patients lied but that they told a version of events that put them in the best and most sympathetic light with their family, friends, employers, and medical men—and the versions often did not match. Patients also resisted certain diagnoses for their symptoms.

In *Treatise on the Hydrocele, or Watry Rupture, and other Diseases of the Testicle* (1767), Pott mentioned receiving a letter from Lincolnshire concerning a 35-year-old man who was enquiring about the castration of a presumably cancerous testicle. Was November the right time of the year to carry such an operation out? Pott replied that the "state and nature of the disease were of much more consequence toward determining the propriety or impropriety, of an operation, than the time of the year could be ..."[120] On receiving a second letter with details of the patient's ailment from a local medical man, Pott was advised about the length of the illness (a few weeks), the state of the testicle (enlarged, hard, and now painless), the fact that the man was married and subject to "scorbutic eruptions," his lack of appetite, and him being pale and wan. The man had taken cicuta (water hemlock) and an infusion of solanum (garden nightshade, not deadly nightshade), with the former not making any difference and latter making him very sick. As a result, "he was now determined for the operation; and that he would be in London in a few days."[121] When the man arrived in London in under a fortnight, Pott examined him and:

> I told him, that I had no doubt that his deafness, hoarseness, pain, spots, swellings &c. were all venereal; and that I was much inclined to believe, that the complaint in his testicle proceeded from the same cause.[122]

As might be expected the man did not take the diagnosis well:

> He did as venereal patients are frequently too apt to do; that is, he endeavoured to render my opinion improbable, by attending, that there had been an interval of some years since he had held any illicit commerce with any woman who he could suppose capable of injuring him; that he had been two or three years married; he only had a slight shanker, of which he was sure he had been well cured, &c.[123]

Pott told the man that he would take care of him only on the understanding that his enlarged testicle was venereal and advised him to see other "gentlemen of the profession" to confirm the diagnosis. The man returned to Pott and was successfully treated "and came out his mercurial course with a more healing aspect, and more flesh on his bones, than he went into it."[124] Pott thus avoided performing what proved to be unnecessary surgery.

Pott proffered further advice on how to behave once a surgeon told a patient that an operation was required. First, you must have "a clear Idea" of what you mean to do and the "Structure of the Parts affected & the Principles laid down by others." Second, "you must always carry in your minds" that you have "the power to increase" the patient's pain; given this, "a considerable part of your duty" is the "understanding (of) the doctrine of Irritability, & Insensibility of parts."[125] To aid pupils in these twin missions, Pott would describe more difficult operations in detail and focus on what could prevent them from being completed.

Pott repeatedly cautioned his students that practicing surgery on a corpse was not the same as cutting on the living. In couching for a cataract, for example, the geometry of the eye changed: "In performing this operation on a dead subject you'll find a very great Difference in regard to your facility or Difficulty in Depressing the Cataract, in proportion to the proper Distance you enter it from the Cornea."[126] Patients were naturally tense when they were being operated upon and this was also an issue for the surgeon. In the case of a Bubonocele (inguinal hernia) where the surgeon is struggling to reduce, or manually return the tissue to its original compartment, Pott recommended that you try to get the patient to relax by forcing them to pass out:

> If you find it impossible to reduce it, in all inflammations of Membranes & other Parts nothing equals plentiful bleeding; & here I cannot omit mentioning a Circumstance well worth attending to viz as a swooning produces a relaxation of the whole System, I would always do in such a Case bleed the Patient in such a Posture as may be most

> likely to produce that viz each & with great success in Children, who generally fainted on Bleeding.[127]

In his lectures, Pott offered guidance to surgery in general and to certain procedures in detail. In the case of the bubonocele mentioned above, he turned to the actual operation with the remark "I shall now give you the best method I can of performing the operation; & shall describe each Part which will occur to the Edge of the Knife as you go on." He stressed where to cut, how much to cut, and the purpose of the cut: to "see clearly what you're about."[128] Pott then recommended a technique to keep the site of the hernia in view:

> Use a round pointed incision knife and make one stroke/two assistants to be ready with soft Clothes to dip up the Blood, which is preferable to Sponges, for after taking the blood up two or three times, if you squeeze them ever so close, they will make the Part bloody instead of cleaning it, whereas in Clothes you'll always have a free clean Place to use for that purpose.[129]

Assistants were ever present in surgery, and Pott rarely mentions them or their roles. In this instance, his focus is on the use of cloths rather than sponges and not the surgical assistant.

Pott believed that once an operation began the surgeon must stay resolute and firm in order to ensure that the operator continued to act in the patient's best interest. To some extent these qualities are captured in a rare painting of an operation in progress from 1817.

Firmness was necessary to continue to probe, cut, and remove body parts as the surgeon's senses were assaulted with the cries of suffering, the feel of blood and other liquids splattering his clothing and face, the putrefying smell of opened intestines and abscesses, and the scrutiny of those who were watching the operation. Pott summarized the qualities required to operate as:

> When a Surg.n … is often call'd upon, [to operate] he must have other necessary qualifications Viz., a Eye, Hand, and temper, his Eye as God pleases to give him, his hand may if defective be owing to himself, & his intemperance, therefore it is commendable in Surg.ns to live a temperate life, his temper should be mild and engaging, humane and not rough to frighten the timorous Patient, but in the operative part be firm without appearance of brutality, which is always to be commend'd.[130]

To achieve firmness without the appearance of brutality meant maintaining authority throughout an operation. Pott became increasingly concerned that the chief threat to losing authority during surgery was the stress on celerity, or quickness, in operating, something he believed was a French import. In the Preface to *Observations on that Disorder of the Corner of the Eye, commonly called*

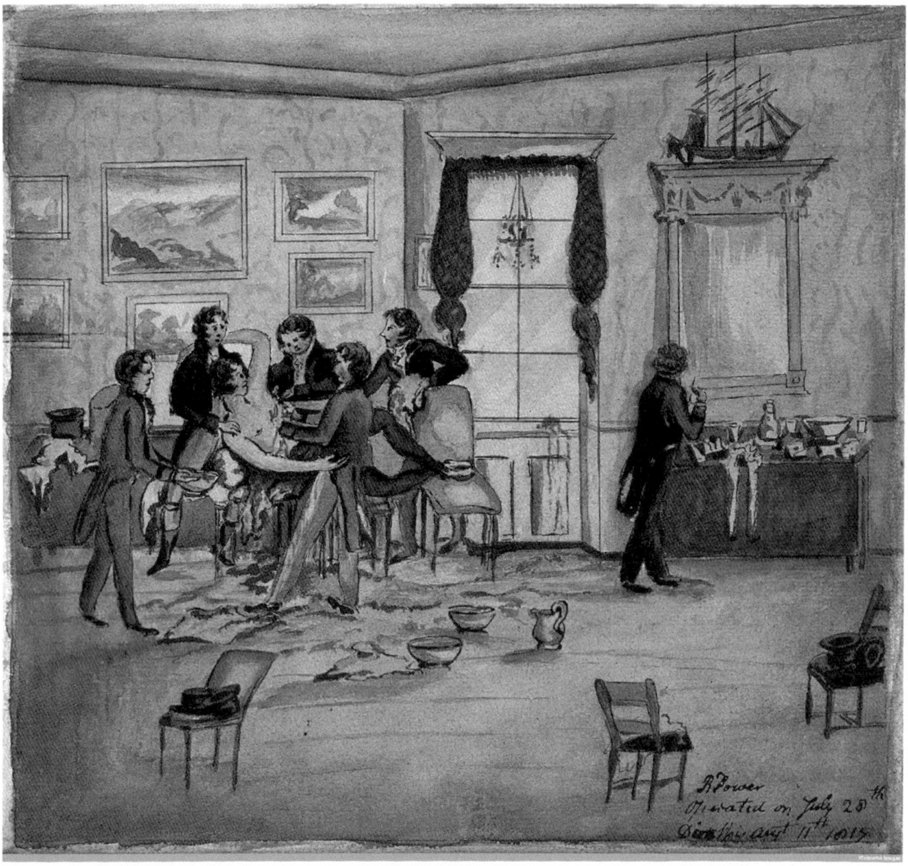

Figure 5. A surgical operation to remove a malignant tumour from a man's left breast and armpit in a Dublin drawing room, 1817. Watercolour, after Robert Power, V0016861. Courtesy of Wellcome Library, London.

Fistula Lachrymalis (1763), Pott drew attention to a new practice that particularly horrified him: bystanders at operations were using stopwatches to measure the motions of a surgeon's hand just like jockeys did with horse's feet. He remarked that this was:

> a practice which though it may perhaps have been encouraged by operators themselves, must have been productive of most mischievous consequences. Tute et celeriter [Safety and quickness] are both very proper characteristics of a good chirurgic operation; but tute stands as it should do, in the first place, as the patient who suffers the smallest injury, from the hurry of his operator, has no recompence [*sic*] from the reputation which the latter obtains from the by-standers.[131]

Pott condemned this absurd obsession with quickness in surgery as firstly based on a lie—quickness was no measure of dexterity in surgery—and secondly as a fashion imported from France where, as everybody knew, surgeons were renowned for their cruelty. In particular stopwatches were being used at capital operations such as lithotomies. While he was still apprenticed to Nourse, Pott had watched the great surgeon William Cheselden (1688–1752) operate at St. Thomas' hospital and no doubt had been impressed by the speed of his operating and the survival rates of his patients.[132] Pott realized the merits of speed but did not think this should be a primary factor in determining the quality of an operation.

The influence of French surgery on English surgeons, especially in terms of quickness in operating for the stone, is partly captured in the flamboyant life of Frère Jacques. In 1698 the English physician and vicar Martin Lister (1639–1712) went on a grand tour of the medical sights of Paris, where surgery was reckoned to be a high art form. At the huge hospital of La Charité and again at the Hôtel-Dieu, he witnessed Frère Jacques (Jacques Beaulieu) operate for the bladder stone.[133] Beaulieu was a French peasant and army empiric who wore a Franciscan's friar habit to ensure safety on his travels. No doubt it also served to cast himself in the role of Christ the Healer. Frère Jacques became famous for the speed in which he could remove a bladder stone through performing his new "lateral" operation. He cut through the perineum (the area from the scrotum to the anus) to get to the bladder, as opposed to going through the lower abdomen as lithotomy had been traditionally performed. In 1698 Frère Jacques was invited to operate on sixty charity patients in Paris using his new lateral technique. Louis XIV's surgeons were interested in finding out how fast Frère Jacques could remove a stone—and how many patients would survive the operation. Lister was among those in attendance and recorded his observations:

> I see him cut a second time in the *Hostel-Dieu*; and he perfom'd it upon nine Persons in three quarters of an Hour, very dexterously. He seemed to venture at all; and put me in some disorder with the Cruelty of the Operation, and a stouter *Englishman* than my self [might have fainted]. However I visited ... all [the patients] in their Beds [afterwards] and found them more amazed than in pain.[134]

Perhaps the patients' amazement could be put down to being in a state of shock. We do not know how fast he got the stone out of patients but we do know that just under half the people Frère Jacques operated on died from hemorrhage or infection due to bowel perforation and rectal lacerations. Seven died in one day at La Charité, and Frère Jacques accused the monks of poisoning them. Postmortems performed found no poison but instead evidence of cut bladders, rectums, and arteries. Another quarter of the patients were left with permanent incontinence and impotence. Louis XIV's doctors deemed the rest, just over a quarter, to be successfully cured. Despite these discouraging odds, surgeons continued to perfect the lateral operation and by the time Frére Jacques died a wealthy man in 1714, he had operated on at least 4,500 people across Europe.

Part of the push for speed in performing a lithotomy no doubt came from sufferers of disease. Bladder stones hurt a lot. They caused immense pain on urination and could block the urethra entirely, which would result in death. In 1727 the physician and poet Sir Richard Blackmore (1654–1729) described the miserable existence of a person suffering from "the Stone":

> Ere Night is half spent, he wishes for Day,when Day appears, he longs for Night; Distracted with his sufferings, he lyes wakeful counting the Hours, any one of which when protracted and multiplied by raging Misery, seems a numerous Train … He changes his Pillow, but not his Pain, new-makes his Bed, but keeps his old Inequitudes, and though he often turns from Side to Side, he never leaves his Agonies behind.[135]

Unfortunately bladder stones were common and often diagnosed early in life. Boys under the age of ten made up approximately half of the numbers operated on for bladder stones. Dietary issues such as lack of protein, high salt, sugar and fat intake, and dehydration led to stagnant urine and the formation of crystals in the urea. Samuel Pepys had a bladder stone removed in 1685 and gave a feast every year to celebrate his survival, while Isaac Newton died from bladder stone obstruction in 1727. Anxiety and public interest in lithotomy continued throughout the eighteenth century as evidenced by announcements in the newspapers of successful operations. The existence of stones could often only be surmised through extensive chronic pain in the region:

> *Public Advertiser*, London, Saturday May 21, 1774
> A few Days ago Mr. Thomas Bridgman, formerly Steward to the late Marquis of Tavistock, and since Steward to the Right Hon. Lord Clive, after having being grievously tormented for some Years with the most excruciating Pains occasioned by the Stone, had the Operation of Lithotomy performed upon him by Mr. Percival Pott, Surgeon to St. Bartholomew's Hospital, and is in a very fair Way of Recovery. What is remarkable, the Faculty were of different Opinions concerning his Complaint, not all agreeing that he had a Stone.[136]

In 1770 Pott told his pupils that surgery may have improved in the past fifty years, but "our successors will be as much astonished at our ignorance as we at our predecessors. Many useful improvements come from fools—(for example) Frère Jacques and the lateral operation."[137]

Pamphlets and books discussing new and faster operations, some translated from French, started to enter the medical market in England at the turn of the eighteenth century, and surgeons in London began to experiment with the possibility of a quicker procedure for removing a bladder stone.[138] The best known of these surgeons and the most adept was William Cheselden, the aforementioned chief surgeon at St. Thomas's Hospital. Cheselden was renowned for being fast in operating and designed his own instruments to help him develop even greater speed. He was as keen a dissector as Pott would be, and, like Martin Lister, he had observed surgeons working in Paris.

Cheselden took Frère Jacques' lateral perineal method of removing bladder stones and made it safer and faster. Dr. James Douglas noted, "He performs this operation with so much Dexterity and Quickness that he seldom exceeds half a minute …"[139] Chesleden's mortality rate in performing lithotomy was less than 10%, an obvious improvement from that of Frère Jacques. Four lusty assistants held the patient down, tied his ankles together, and removed the catheter that had filled his bladder with water. Chesleden quickly made a three-to-five-inch incision in the perineum, slit open the prostate gland, and inserted a sound to locate the stone after the catheter was removed. He then cut around the sound, scooped the stone out of the bladder with forceps or fingers and showed it to the admiring bystanders.

In 1763 Pott may have condemned the foolishness and ignorance of spectators who measured success in operating by how fast a surgeon cut by using the fashionable sport of thoroughbred racing as their guide, but spectators and their antics were there to stay. It was not enough to learn how to go through an operation unmoved by the cries of patients; now surgeons needed to learn how to ignore the distractions of having a rowdy audience. John Obadiah Justamond (d. 1768), surgeon to the Westminster Hospital, cautioned that operations were public events where "the effects of (the operation) evident to all present"[140] could lead to ridicule and prejudice. Pott's ever-lengthening remonstrations to his pupils to remember the patient is a living being and that neither showing off to the crowd nor winning the race to finish first would help the patient or the reputation of the operator, seems to have increasingly fell onto deaf ears:

> we ought [never] in any operation to be more expeditious than is consistent with the welfare of your Patient—for tho' it may attract the Notice of the Spectators, yet by being in a hurry, something of greater Consequences may be omitted than their opinion of your dexterity—as parts may be divided which ought not to be; so that the operation will not be attended we could wish; by which means the Surgeons Character is often more injured than if he had been longer about it.[141]

What we know of Pott's operative techniques suggest that he practiced what he preached—his pupils describe a self-possessed man who was capable of cutting, teaching, and belittling their answers to his questions all at the same time. As one pupil wrote in a poem composed in 1787 when Pott resigned his post of senior surgeon at St. Bartholomew's Hospital:

> Ye wretched creatures whom my walls contain (How much more wretched now shall be your lot), Cease to bemoan your agonizing pains, And join with me to moan the loss of Pott.
> Who with the keenest eye and steadiest hand, And the best judgment Nature could bestow, For fifty years has well supplied the land With wooden legs and such sad sights of woe.
> Heavens! when he lopp'd a limb to save a life, Or freed the bladder from the galling stone, Death fled affrighted when he seized the knife, And the weird sisters trembled at his frown.
> But he, serene, amidst the blood and cries Of the poor wretch with horrid tortures fired, Could calmly turn about and bless your eyes, Or damn them either, if the case required.
> Lives there a man who can supply his place With half die the dignity that he could boast?
> For who could operate with so much grace? Or with such blest assurance rule the roast?
> What now shall gain Bartholomew renown? For all my riches can avail me not;What brought each leaden-headed lad to town, What drew them hither but the name of Pott?
> Shall Pitts, Earle, Blicke parade my walls alone, And not a pupil follow at their heels?
> Shall Long and Harvey set a broken bone? Oh! no, kind Heaven, defend us from such ills
> Still Pott-shall grace the dictatorial chair, Still teach e'en blockheads in his art to shine;
> Still to my walls in flocks they shall repair, Still laugh at Hunter, and still pity Cline.[142]

Pott offered substantive remarks on several aspects of surgery and the comportment of surgeons—the patient-surgeon relationship, women's bodies, and dexterity and speed—that provide meaningful insights into how these topics were viewed in Georgian London. His case histories and lecture notes reveal attitudes and opinions that were prevalent among leading hospital surgeons and their pupils concerning their patients, peers, and reputations. The next chapter focuses on head injuries and sudden calamities that resulted from accidents and violence, situations which Pott and his pupils encountered in the metropolis. Here a speedy diagnosis was required, and often the patient was unconscious, meaning that it was impossible to get the patient's consent to operate.

CHAPTER THREE

"He Will Talk, Until He Dies"

Accidents and Violence

I shall by leave to illustrate what I have been speaking on with a Case.[1]

Case XXVII A boy about eight years old, the son of a Jew merchant in the city, received a blow on his head with a stick from his tutor. The stroke made him giddy for a few minutes; but as no blood was shed, and the pain soon ceased, he concealed it till it was discovered by his barber that his head was swollen in that part.[2]

Compound Fractures are easily cured in pure country Air, than in a Town. We labour under a great many disadvantages in the Hospital for want of it & many of the harmed will die in three or four days after the accident from Mortification—in this Case we never wait for Suppuration but amputate immediately—This is a doctrine I will abide by Gentlemen you will find success by embracing it.[3]

Case histories were key components in the education of pupils and fellow medical men in the art of surgery. Pott provided them in his lectures and especially in his published texts on head injuries, hydrocele and ruptures.[4] Case histories typically contained information on the context for the injury, the appearance of the injured body part, and the treatment and outcome of the intervention. They were far from being just brief accounts of diagnosis, treatment and prognosis, however. Pott constructed his narratives to also warn of common mistakes in surgery, criticize quackery, and teach the correct way to interact with other medical men and patients. Over decades of lectures he used his vast store of case histories to educate and occasionally amuse his pupils.[5] For example, in 1770 Pott told this vivid story during a lecture on chest wounds at St. Bartholomew's Hospital:

> … a case which I saw some few years ago will prove that all wounds of the lungs are not fatal. a [*sic*] Boy waiter at a Tavern running up stairs hastily with some knifes in his hand, which the boy fell upon, I was sent for and found a large wound on the right side, and from which when a candle was held to the part the air rushed out and immediately extinguish'd it; there was some haemorrage [*sic*] which ceas'd to flow of itself, it was stop'd lightly and speedily and the boy done well, it was never attend'd with any bad symptoms.[6]

The accuracy of Pott's accounts of his cases during his lectures is impossible to verify, as they were given orally and written down roughly by pupils who later copied them in fair hand. In the case of the waiter who fell upon a knife, however, we do have a published narrative of Pott's treatment of the boy. In *An Essay of the Cure of Abscesses by Caustic and on the treatment of wounds and ulcers; and a new method of curing the lues venera* (1779), Peter Clare states that he was apprenticed to Pott and accompanied him to treat this patient. Clare used his recollection of the case as a striking instance of how healing can occur by the first intention:

> During my apprenticeship, a youth about twelve or thirteen living at the Dog-Tavern, *Garlick-hill*, had the misfortune to fall upon the edge of a case knife, which penetrated the left lobe of the lungs, the air from which nearly extinguished the flame of a candle. The haemorrhage from the wound was considerable, till Mr. *Pott* placed the lad on his back, when the bleeding stopped. It was dressed lightly with dry lint; but fearing it might bleed internally, he made an unfavourable prognostic, and was most agreeably surprised to find his patient had no bad symptoms. He recovered in less than a fortnight; whence it was concluded the balsamic quality of his blood, uniting the wound by the first intention had affected the cure. He was bled at first, to guard against the symptomatic fever.[7]

The two accounts have some factual differences, most notably that Pott states it was the right lung that was stabbed while Clare claims the left. More interestingly, though, Clare includes Pott's initial prognosis, which was not good, while Pott simply states that the boy did well.

An analysis of Pott's case histories provides a historical prism of common complaints that affected the poor, the middling sort, and the rich. It also reveals glimpses of the social and economic conditions of life in Georgian London, especially the frequency of accidents, violence, and chronic conditions.[8] This chapter focuses on acute injuries.

Pott's peers considered the surgeon's book *Observations on the nature and consequences of those injuries to which the head is liable from external violence* to be extremely significant. First published in 1760 and considerably expanded eight years later, it went through three editions and was translated into French, Dutch and German. Jeremy Ganz notes that during the eighteenth century "at least 12 surgeons published on cranial injury, 6 of whom described significant clinical series [cases] on this topic."[9] Pott was certainly influenced by the work of the French surgeon Henri-François Le Dran (1685–1770), who claimed that the brain rather than broken bone was the source of the symptoms that followed trauma to the head. Pott remarked:

> What are the symptoms of a fractured cranium? is often asked; and there is hardly anyone who does not … answer, vomiting, giddiness, loss of sense, speech, and voluntary motion; bleeding at the ears, nose, and mouth, & c. … The symptoms just mentioned do indeed very frequently accompany a broken skull; but they are not produced by the breach made in the bone; nor do they indicate such breach to have been made. They proceed from an affection of the brain, or from injury done to some of the parts within the cranium, independant [*sic*] of any ill which the bones composing it may have sustained.[10]

In other areas of care of head wounds, Pott was not as convinced by Le Dran's theories on what to do. Pott argued that in any head wound, the preservation of the scalp should always be attempted through loosely suturing it back in place with a "slipknot."[11] Here he was going against the advice of other surgeons, especially French ones, who vehemently opposed suturing as they believed it led to "matter" developing underneath the stitches. Pott addressed this issue by recommending such matter be released through puncturing the scalp with a lancet to encourage the formation of abscesses. He believed abscesses were a collection of pus that had gathered, or could be encouraged to gather, in an inflamed part of the body. This view followed the work of Herman Boerhaave and his pupil Gerard van Swieten.[12] Abscesses could be good or bad, depending on the type of material that accumulated in them. Pott told his pupils how to differentiate between good and bad abscesses of the scalp. They were to notice how the scalp took the impression of a finger, its puffiness and color, and the amount of delirium and pain the patient had, including shivers and sweats.[13] If the signs were good, the abscess would, when opened, be full of good pus—yellowish white and of a thick ropey consistence—rather than bad pus—bloody, thin, of an offensive smell, curdled and cheesy.[14] The latter was the type of pus that flowed when Pott opened the head of a girl who died from being hit with a poker:

> A Girl about sixteen was knocked down by her mother with an iron poker of considerable weight; the latter immediately ran away and the former was brought senseless to the hospital. She had a large wound on top of her head, with a considerable fracture of the sagittal structure. The broken pieces were so large, and so loose, as to be easily removable without any perforation.[15]

After Pott removed the shattered pieces of bone, the girl was left with a two-inch hole in her skull and to quote her surgeon, was "perfectly senseless." Five days later Pott was becoming increasingly concerned that the girl was not waking up and decided to drain the blood collected around the wound. After this procedure, he ordered a nurse to hold a dressing in place while he visited his other patients. Pott returned two hours later to discover the girl coming around. By the next day she was asking for a drink. Despite these positive signs, the outcome was not good, for seventeen days after the girl was brought to the hospital she convulsed and died. Pott opened her skull and discovered a massive abscess of bad pus.[16] The girl was probably buried in a pauper's grave at Mount Hill Ground.[17]

Pott frequently saw patients whose head wounds, because they were becoming more and more inflamed, were causing high fevers and convulsions. In lectures he referred to this condition as commotion of the brain and told his pupils:

> In case of Commotion they do not sleep at all, or at a few minutes as a time … if the Patient is not kept in the dark, and out of sight of objects, he will talk, until he dies, and his Eyes appear like a person who has been kept awake by the most heartfelt Grief.[18]

He added that commotion of the brain is often mistaken for insanity, as the patient has a kind of "Maniacal Stare."

The aftereffects of a head injury were sometimes severe. He offered the case of a patient he knew who slipped and fell on his head: "I bled him till the Blood Almost lost its Redness, the man recovered after, but knew not the differance [*sic*] between an Onion and an Orange."[19]

Pott's text on head injuries graphically illustrates the dangerous nature of acute head wounds in the eighteenth century.[20] Out of the 42 patients Pott discusses, 25 died and 17 survived. Twenty-two of the patients were adult males, 8 were adult females, 12 were boys, and 2 were girls. Twenty-eight of the injuries were work related and 14 resulted from violence.[21] As Pott concluded in a lecture on head wounds, "We are very apt to be discouraged from the great degree of obscurity attending all Mischiefs of the Head."[22] Head injuries were always acute crises, even if patients and other medical practitioners did not always treat them as such.

Accidents and Surgery

Scholars have copiously examined work-related accidents within the context of the Industrial Revolution, knowing that they were common.[23] As Roy Porter has argued, however, the pre-industrial environment was equally as hazardous as the industrial one would become:

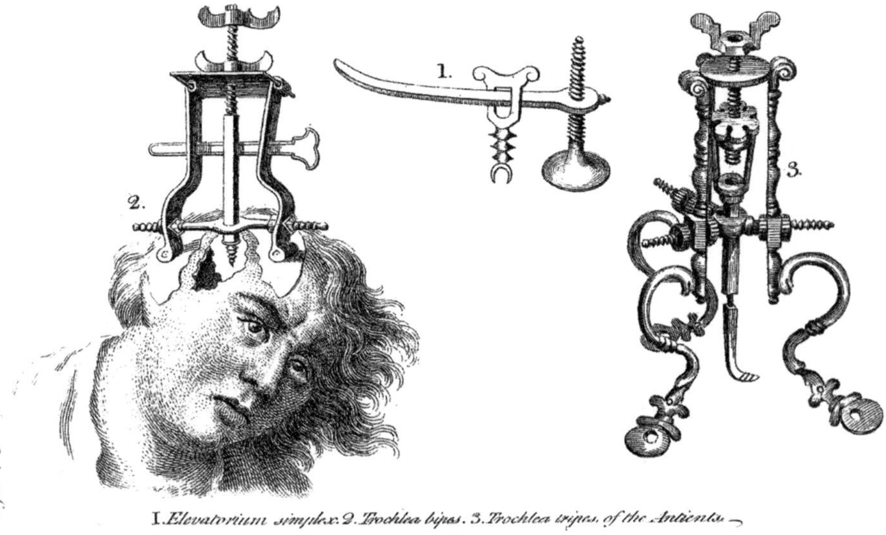

Figure 6. Trochlea, 1771 from *Illustrations on the nature and consequences of those injuries to which the head is liable from external violence*, London, by Percivall Pott. Facing page 205. L0007378. Courtesy of Wellcome Library, London.

> Roads were abominations, work was performed with unruly beasts of burden and under the heavens, there were the hazards of open fires, naked lights, or universal darkness, and everywhere hordes of infants ...[24]

Pott's case histories support such a conclusion. He recorded travel-related accidents involving pedestrians, horses, wagons, and coaches, such as the case of a boy of about 15 years "thrown over the head of a horse who went down with him ... He lived three days as if in a deep sleep and then died."[25] Children were crushed by carts and even gored by terrified animals awaiting slaughter at Smithfield Market, just outside the gates of St. Bartholomew's Hospital.[26]

Pott wrote about the case of a fifteen-year-old girl who was "tossed by an ox" and fell on her head: "As her dress was mean, and nobody knew any thing of her she was brought senseless into the hospital." Pott trepanned, or drilled a hole in the girl's skull, in order to investigate the extent of the wound and to drain any pooled blood. Despite the operation she died twenty days after the injury, "having been terribly shaken by spasms for several hours" at the end.[27]

London was the country's largest consumer market, the largest port, and had the largest pool of skilled and unskilled labour.[28] Not surprisingly the capital was an unhealthy place, and throughout Pott's lifetime the ratio of baptisms to burials has been estimated at below 70%.[29] In spite of this statistic the population of London grew from under 500,000 in 1700 to 960,000 by 1801.[30] The burgeoning opportunities in the metropolis attracted migrants, and historians such as John Landers have estimated that by the 1780s at least 23,000 Irish had settled in the eastern riverside parishes and were especially clustered in St. Giles-in-the-Fields near St. Bartholomew's Hospital, where Pott worked. In the East End, 15,000 to 20,000 Jews lived cheek by jowl.[31] The most common housing available was in rooms rented by the month, week, or night. The latter involved citizens simply providing a floor to sleep on for up to 20 people at a penny or two per night.[32] The majority of the poor labored in the clothing and textiles trades with building vocations coming in a close second, followed by leather and metalwork. By 1750 there were 500 master silk weavers in Spitalfields with 15,000 looms at work, while domestic service and the sale of drink employed thousands of girls and women. Hans-Joachim Voth has estimated that the average working day lasted 11 hours in the 1750s, and fatigue must have been ever present in the lives of most.[33]

Given the small cramped spaces in which Londoners lived, public houses and any open space or fields could attract unruly crowds. This is reflected in Pott's case histories, especially those concerning violence. As the population of the city grew, so did the need for buildings. Shoddy supplies and dangerous working conditions led to workmen and boys falling from hastily erected wooden scaffolding, poor quality ladders, and collapsing roofs:[34]

> I shall by leave to illustrate what I have been speaking on with a Case—I was sent for to a boy belonging to Christs Hosp.l when I came I found a fracture occasion'd by part of a scaffold falling on his head, I trepan'd him and from appearance judg'd it proper to divide the Dura Mater by which means a quantity of Coaglum was discharg'd and the boy instantly reliev'd, remains now in perfect health.[35]

When it came to head wounds, Pott based his arguments on the nature of blood and its relation to the development of pus on anatomical knowledge and experiential practice. He wrote that blood vessels connect the membrane of the dura mater to the inside of the skull:

> Proof of this is seeing the scalping of a living person of the separation of the skull from the dura mater of a dead one [especially if such person died apoplectic, or was hanged] prove beyond all doubt.[36]

After this anatomy-based proof, Pott turned to the issue of whether blood that leaked from the vessels really did become "the matter found on the surface of the dura mater ..." Pott believed this was untrue and that blood kept from air will not turn to pus:

> [It] is (I think) proved incontestably, by every day's experience, in many instances; in aneurisms by puncture; in retained menses, by imperforate vaginae; and in all ecchymoses. True pus cannot be made from blood merely; as may be known from the manner in which all abscesses are formed, and from every circumstance attending suppuration; and that the matter, found on the surface of the dura mater, after great contusions of the head, never was mere blood, I am as certain, as observation, and experience can make me."[37]

Pott acknowledged that a torn and flapping scalp "is sometimes very terrible to look at, and they who have not been accustomed to see it, may be inclined to think there is no remedy but excision ..."[38] But rather than removing the scalp, a surgeon should strive to reattach it as the sore that results from preserving the scalp is smaller, and the patient heals faster and has less deformity.

Clues to what Pott meant by "deformity" of the scalp come from a case history of a travel-related accident. A gentleman's coachman was thrown from his box on the road between London and Richmond. He remained sensible and was able to drive home. The next day, however, his master, a governor of St. Bartholomew's Hospital, "and a timorous man" according to Pott, sent the patient to the hospital for treatment.[39] After three weeks the coachman was "tired of the hospital" and permitted to go home. He returned two months later to have Pott look at his wound, which had not healed well and was discharging bad matter. It was described as the "size of a silver three-pence," and when probed, a loose piece of bone could be felt. Pott considered how best to proceed. He wrote that the removal of a circular piece of skin would leave a scar, which would not only be a great deformity, but a deformity which would be "liable to misconstructions ... and I made a longitudinal incision, sufficient for its (the piece of loose bone) extraction, and laying hold on it with a pair of forceps, brought it away."[40] The man survived. The probable explanation of the "misconstructions" to which Pott referred was that a circular scar on the head could be taken for what is now known as tinea capitis, or ringworm. In the eighteenth century it was called scald head and was stigmatized as a sign of dirt, poverty, and venereal infection. It was known to be contagious, and the coachman may well have lost his job if it looked like he was suffering from scald head rather than a broken head.[41]

Pott also addressed the issue of removing the scalp in women, pointing out to his pupils "as Hair will never grow on that Part again" they "ought to be guarded against" doing so and causing a scar and deformity.[42] In this case a bald and scarred spot could affect employment and marital prospects.

Head wounds were difficult to treat for many reasons, and prognosis was nigh on impossible. Patients who seemed to be doing well would suddenly turn worse and die, while others died quickly. Pott tells that "A porter at work at the water-side, was knocked down by a blow from an iron hook, at the end of a tackle belonging to a crane."[43] By the next morning he was blind and unable to walk. The porter was brought to the hospital, where Pott bled him heavily. He intended to trephine him the next day but the porter died in the night.[44] Pott also relates cases of a 24-year-old man who died five days after falling out of a two-storey warehouse after being hit by a crane and landing head down on a sugar hogshead[45] and a Hackney coachman who was thrown from his box in Holborn, fell on his head, and died three days later.[46] In lectures on the fractures of the cranium, Pott urged his pupils to operate sooner rather than later. He discussed survival rates of patients where their skulls had been perforated early versus those who were perforated later after suppuration had developed:

> and if you compare the number of those which, survive when the operation is Performed in the former state wth. those who perish in the Latter, you will find an amazing Difference, I do this to this to show you the Absolute Necessity there is in Perforating the Bone considering the Number on both Hands, to these Cases I shall, add another; In Case of Extravasation you have Indications and Symptoms and if You defer it until the latter, that is when Inflammation and Suppuration come on; I say when this happens you will find it frequently fails; and the patient do not stand that Chance he did, had you made use of the Preventive method …[47]

Operations on patients with head injuries were viewed as especially difficult because the person was often unconscious. It was far easier to operate on someone who was awake since their response to the actions of the surgeon provided valuable information.[48] Analgesics or hypnotics would destroy the control surgeons needed over the patient and the operation. It would also have put the patient to sleep—and in the eighteenth century sleep was regarded as a dangerous state, one that was closer to death than to life. In treating severe head injuries the surgeon was solely responsible for the outcome of the operation. No blame could be placed on an unconscious patient as they were unable to give consent for treatment.

In the case of a drunken drayman who had fallen asleep and trapped his head between the wheel and a post of his cart, Pott was forced to remove his bruised and severely mangled scalp. He lamented all the while that he could not save it. The man seemed to recover nicely, and Pott wondered how much his of loss of sense or "perfect stupidity" that he demonstrated when he was initially brought in to the hospital was due to the imbibing of liquor rather than the accident:

> On the 13th day he was so well, that having a large family to work for, he desired to be discharged from the hospital, and to be made an out-patient; but his sores were still so large, and I has so often been deceived by the salacious appearance of such cases, that I persuaded him to stay another week.[49]

Pott was right to be cautious, for eight days later the man developed a paralysis in his right arm and leg and died two days later. Pott opened the patient's head and described it as much diseased.

Signs indicating that a patient who had received "a smart blow on the head" was going downhill included, according to Pott, "acceleration, or hardness of pulse, restlessness, anxiety, and any degree of fever." The remedy was immediate, plentiful, and repeated evacuation by bleeding.[50] Patients often did not reach Pott in time for him to order this procedure, as was the case of a seventeen-year-old boy who fell from a scaffold while working with his father at the Mansion House.[51] His mother kept him home for two days, and then the boy returned to work only to fall ill five days later with a shooting pain in his head and convulsive fits:

> As it was not supposed that his fall had any share in that attack, no notice was taken of it: a few ounces of blood were drawn from his arm, and the apothecary who had the care of him gave him some of those medicines that are called nervous … at the end of three weeks he died, paralytic on one side, and convulsed on the other.[52]

The father called Pott only three days before his son died, asking him to look at a small swelling that had suddenly appeared on the boy's head. Pott probed it and discovered a large skull fracture with foul matter lodged beneath it. He told his pupils that he knew then that the boy would die.

Pott remarked, "all the best practitioners have agreed that the skull must be perforated in the case of a gun-shot wound due to the great contusion." Every other scenario where the skull was not obviously fractured or fissured was left to the judgment (and persuasion) of the surgeon except one: if the dura mater had become detached, trephine was necessary—it was the unicum remedium. Pott concluded:

> … some have been saved by [the trephine], none can escape without it; as there are no certain indications, no criteria, whereby we are enabled to judge, whether it will prove successful, or not, the event of each individual case can alone determine. When that is happy, the means are very justly commended; but when it is not so, they ought not therefore to be condemned; since they are built on rational principles, and are the only means in human power.[53]

Such judgment calls became more complicated because Pott, like other surgeons, frequently only saw patients long after their head wounds had occurred. Case XVI concerned a sailor who had received a severe blow on his head from a large splinter of wood during a battle against the French.[54] He continued to work for seven weeks and then began complaining of an unrelenting headache. The sailor was admitted to the naval hospital at Gosport, where he developed severe fits. He was transferred to St. Bartholomew's Hospital and placed under the care of Dr. William Pitcairn, who immediately had him bled and purged.[55] Sometime later the patient mentioned to Pitcairn that he had received a blow to his head ten weeks earlier. Pitcairn immediately called in Pott for a consult. On examining the sailor's scalp Pott noticed that the man convulsed when he pressed on a certain part of his head, although Pott could see no injury. He repeated the experiment the next day and again the following day. Pott recalled that the sailor was "so terribly convulsed, that I determined never to try it again."[56] He was at a loss and decided to trephine the patient as nothing had worked so far to relieve his fits: "During the time of the operation, the poor man suffered greatly from spasm; but that over he became easy and quiet." The discharge from his scalp was described as extremely offensive and three days later the sailor died, having developed a "peripneumony." Pott opened his head but found nothing of note to explain this "mischief."[57]

Pott included the case of the sailor in lectures to pupils at St. Bartholomew's Hospital. The surgeon's lively speech and engaging storytelling skills are well captured in the account scribbled down by an anonymous pupil:

> A Man who had received a violent Blow on the Head & it grew very uneasy upon the least touch it threw into rigours after a consultation I took a large piece of scalp off and was afraid I had killed the man by the pressure of the Knife the Scull appeared of a Blackish Colour and as it were worm eaten ... after sometime the man died.[58]

Pott emphasized the fact to his students that many patients, both rich and poor, went for weeks after an accident before calling him in or turning up at the hospital. He used this behavior to explain the poor outcome of most head injuries in his case histories. An elderly lady, for example, hit her head against an iron hook when her hackney landau hit a bump in the road[59] and ignored any pain for eight weeks before she had "to resort to laudanum for several nights in order to obtain a little broken rest." She was under the care of Mr. Daniel Brown of Little Britain,[60] and Pott went with him to the woman's home. Pott opened the swelling on her head, only to discover a hole in her skull through which to his surprise he could touch the dura mater with his finger. The elderly lady died three weeks later in a kind of fit.[61] Similarly the principal overseer of one of the great roads (the new turnpikes) was thrown down with great violence while he was giving directions to the laborers.[62] It was sixteen days until Pott was brought in at the request of the overseer's surgeon, the "late Mr. Bethune." Pott immediately operated, but it was too late and the man died five days later.[63]

Not all head injuries resulted in fatalities, even if they did not consult a surgeon soon after it happened. A woman who fell backwards down the stairs at home in September 1763 was not brought to the hospital until mid-December.

She had a swelling on her head the size of a "split Seville orange," which Pott opened and drained. The woman was discharged in March 1764. Pott had one of his live-in dressers care for her as she resided not far from his home and by late April she was well.[64]

In another case, the driver of a post chaise was thrown from his horse near Ware and hit his head on a stepping-stone in a brook. The passengers carried their driver to a public house where he recovered in half an hour and then drove them on to London. A week after the accident the driver vomited twice, fainted, and had a fever. His masters dismissed his illness as the consequences of poverty and drunkenness:

> From the hardship and the irregular manner of these people's living, his complaints were supposed to be owing to cold and intemperance, and he was treated accordingly: but on the ninth day, a tumor (swelling) appearing on that part of his head which had received the blow, a surgeon examined it ...[65]

The surgeon discovered a large fracture, and the coachman was finally taken to St. Bartholomew's Hospital a day later. There he complained to Pott that his head felt as "if it was squeezed between two trenchers."[66] Although he seemed stable for the week after the accident, this was not the case, and he died six days after seeing Pott.

Some patients with head injuries from work-related accidents did survive. They tended to be younger and included two laborers working with bricklayers, one of whom was knocked out by a large pantile and the other who fell from a high scaffold; a girl aged nine who fell from a high hayrick in Islington; a farrier's servant who had been kicked in the head by a horse; a lad, belonging to a horse dealer in Smithfield, who a horse threw against one of the sheep-pens; a boy aged about ten who fell twenty feet off a ladder; and a gentleman's servant who was riding carelessly and hastily through London and was thrown from his horse.[67]

Along with revealing the working conditions of his patients, Pott's case histories also allow glimpses into the leisure activities of Georgian children and youth. He recorded injuries from playing sports such as cricket, an especially brutal game, quoits, and cudgels.[68]

> CASE XLI A Child about nine years old received a blow from a cricket bat on the upper part of his forehead, which brought him to the ground, and deprived him of sense. I found him with a considerable tumor [a swelling] on his forehead, and considering the state he was in, would have removed immediately a part of the scalp; but a dabbler in surgery, who was a relation, undertook to cure him by an application [a medication]. On the third day I was sent for again, and found him nearly in the same state as I left him.[69]

Pott operated immediately—he scalped the boy, drained off the blood, and prescribed a laxative to ensure his body was open. In time the boy recovered. David Underdown, in *Start of Play: Cricket and Culture in Eighteenth-Century England*, describes cricket as a rough sport. It attracted large crowds and offered opportunities for gambling, and matches were played not only in local fields but also at the Artillery Ground and Kennington Common.[70] Another of Pott's cases also concerned cricket: "A lad about twelve years old, standing by a man who was playing at cricket, received a blow from the bat on his forehead."[71] The boy was knocked out, and as nobody came forward to claim they knew him, he was carried to the hospital. Pott bled him heavily, and as he was costive (constipated), Pott administered several purges, and the boy threw up a glyster.[72] The lad did well, so Pott discharged him after nine days. But five days later, the boy returned complaining of being dizzy and was readmitted. He became progressively ill with a high fever, shivers, and a throbbing pain in the forehead. Twenty days after the accident Pott opened the boy's skull in a last-ditch attempt to save his life. He found and removed a copious amount of putrid matter. The wound was then left open to keep it draining. A week later the boy was well enough to be discharged. Where he went afterwards and what finally happened to him, no one knew, as the boy appeared to have neither family nor friends.

Two other case histories involve games that resulted in head injuries. First, a young man playing quoits was struck by one of them on his head. (Quoits involved players pitching horseshoes at stakes in the ground and was no doubt popular with the farriers who serviced the 50,000 or so horses that trod the streets of the capital.) A farrier put a stitch in the large wound, and the man "vomited plentifully," which was looked upon as a good sign by both the players and spectators. The injured man was a farrier himself and returned to work the next morning. Five days later, though, he "was unable to stoop to shoe a horse on account of the pain in his head ..." The farrier had someone bleed him and bought some medicines to try, "but at the end of three days being worse and incapable of bearing the expense of remaining at home was brought to St Bartholomew's Hospital ..." Pott examined the head wound and removed the broken bone, which he found to be discoloured. "From the symptoms and signs I prognosticated no good ..."[73] He trephined him again the following day and discharged a great deal of matter. The farrier briefly became rational but expired that evening after over an hour of severe rigors.

Pott had more success with the second case:

> A Young man playing at cudgels[74] in Moorfields who received a stroke on his forehead; it did not seem to himself or the spectators to have been a severe one, but as

> it produced blood it was deemed by the laws of the game a broken head, and he was obliged to yield to his antagonist.[75]

The man appears to have returned to his game of cudgels. (A cudgel was a stick with a rounded end and was used as if sword fighting.) After the accident he went to work for the next twelve days until pain and fever brought him to the hospital. Pott saw him, opened and drained his head wound, and then bled fourteen ounces of blood from a jugular vein to drop his pulse rate and fever. Three days later Pott took another fourteen ounces from a temporal artery, stopping just as the patient fainted. The man rallied for a short while but then became as feverish and in pain as before. Pott searched for another wound, thinking from the poor state of his patient that he must have missed another injury to the skull, but didn't find anything. Deciding that he could again bear bleeding, Pott opened his temporal arteries "till his pulse failed so much and so suddenly that I was not a little alarmed."[76] The man eventually recovered, although he continued to be weak for a long time from the repeated phlebotomy.

The final case histories concerning accidents that Pott included in *Observations on the Nature and Consequences of those Injuries to Which the Head is liable from External Violence* involved children. We understand far less about accidents as a common cause of sickness, disability, and death in children than we do about other roots, Fevers of unknown etiology, the bloody flux (dysentery), scarlatina (scarlet fever), whooping cough, influenza, smallpox, and pneumonia killed perhaps 50% of London's children before the age of fifteen. Even surviving an illness could have permanent consequences; for example, scarlet fever left many children blind and deaf, and measles could cause severe scarring, bone loss, gangrene, and death, What little information we do have about accidents has been gleaned largely from coroners' inquests or trials.[77]

Pott's case histories suggest a chain of treatment options that better-off parents followed when caring for an injured child. First, they tried home remedies. A nine-year-old boy was playing under an empty cart and appears to have dislodged the stick that was holding up the shafts. One of the shafts hit him on the head and knocked him out. The boy went home where his mother "applied a bit of linen rag, wet with vinegar" to the bump on his head, kept him home for a day or so, and then allowed him to return to boarding school, as he appeared to be well. Five days later the boy complained that his head hurt and vomited up his breakfast, so the school sent him home, assuming that since "he had not had either smallpox, or measles" that "one of these diseases was to follow."[78] The family called in a doctor or "physical gentleman," as Pott refers to him:

> Three days more passed, and no eruption appeared: the fever continued much the same; he was frequently inclined to vomit, and what little sleep he got; was extremely

> disturbed. He was by order of the physician, let blood, had a blister applied to his back, and took some of the common febrifuge medicines.[79]

Leeches were also applied to the forehead, but the boy got worse with rigors and a high fever. At this point it appears that the parents finally told the physician about his blow to the head. (This follows the earlier cases about the length of time between the accident and mentioning the injury to a medical man.) Thirteen days after the accident Pott was finally called in to examine the boy's head. He found a flattish tumor containing a fluid and forcefully argued for immediately opening the skull:

> From the appearance of this swelling, from the date of the accident, the attack, (of rigours) violence and duration of the symptoms, I made no scruple to give my opinion, that the blow had been the sole cause of all the child's illness; that I suspected the skull under the tumour to be bare, if not injured; that I did also believe, that matter was forming, or formed, under the skull; and, that if the last conjecture, was true, the only chance the child could have of preservation, must be from the operation of the trephine.[80]

The parents refused to allow Pott to perforate the skull, as the bone was not broken. The physical gentleman "not having seen much business of this kind, and not rightly comprehending the true nature of the case, joined in opinion with the parents that such operation was not necessary." Three days later the boy died. "Having being contradicted, and (as I thought) somewhat improperly over-ruled, in the management of the patient while alive, I was the more importunate to get leave to examine him when dead."[81] Pott somehow received permission and confirmed that the blow to the head is what had killed the boy. He ended the case history with strong words about the delay in treating the boy with trephination. Pott admits that it probably would not have saved the boy by the time he was called in, "but still it was the only thing, that could with propriety have been done for him; and therefore it ought to have been done."[82]

The other case history Pott included in his work on head injuries follows the same pattern. A boy of about three- to four-years-old, the son of a merchant in Pott's neighborhood, was playing with his brother on a bed and fell on a soft bedside carpet. He complained of being sick and giddy but recovered after vomiting. Four days later the sickness and giddiness returned, and the parents called in Dr. Lee, "who not regarding the fall as having any share in his complaint, gave him an emetic, and ordered him some of those medicines which are called nervous."[83] Pott relates a sad list of worsening symptoms: the boy lost his sight, his right arm became useless, he could not stand, he became stupid (senseless), and eighteen days after the accident, the boy expired. Through autopsy, Pott confirmed the cause of death to be the fall from the bed.[84]

Violence and Surgery

Several legal records survive that tell of Pott being deposed or called as a witness to give evidence in cases where death may have resulted from violence to the head. The first time his name appears was in 1734 when a newly qualified Pott carried out a postmortem on the head of Mary Bernard, an old woman who had been beaten with a stick and left to die in a quarrel over sharing a cooked goose:

> Percival Potts, Surgeon. I view'd the Body externally, and found two Bruises, one above the Right-ear, and the other over the Right-eye. There was a large Fracture in the Skull, which began over the Right-ear, ran to the Orbit of the Eye, and thence to the upper Jaw-bone, and in two or three Places of it, small Pieces of the Skull were beat in. The Skull being remov'd, I found 8 Ounces of extravasated Blood, part between the first Skin and the Skull, another part between the first Skin and the Second, and the rest in the two lateral Ventricles of the Brain. The Skull being broke in, was the Occasion of her Death.[85]

John Bracket, a chandler, was found guilty of the manslaughter of Mary Bernard. Several witnesses testified to the good character of Bracket and the poor character of Bernard, stating she was often drunk and combative. The penalty for manslaughter was to be branded on the thumb with a "M," and Bracket in all likelihood received this punishment in the courtroom at the end of the sessions.[86]

The second case was twenty-five years later and involved a patient that Pott had actually cared for before his death:

> 24th October 1759
> *Percival Pott* one of the Surgeons of St. Barthomews [*sic*] Hospital and being Sworn upon his Oath says as follows:
>
> *William Walker* was brought into St Bartholomews Hospital on the Sixteenth of August 1759 and put under my Care.
>
> His skull was broke in two places, and he had all the Symptoms of a Concussion of his brain. He was trepaned [*sic*] by me and had all possible care taken of him, but died on the twenty second of October. His Death was most undoubtedly occasioned by the Injury done to the Skull and Brain
>
> Hold
> 24 Oct: 1759 [87]

It appears that Mr. William Tipton, the landlord at the Sign of the Fox & Birdcage on Great Arthur Street, had thrown Walker out a window. The two men knew each other well and had been playing bowls in a room above the alehouse, as three women who witnessed Walker's defenestration confirmed. Witnesses who had been on the hospital ward with Walker were also called to testify, including women who had cared for him and several other patients. One patient described Walker as "very much in Liquor when he was brought to the Hospital and very abusive with his Tongue." In all Walker spent nine weeks at St. Bartholomew's Hospital. The court asked Pott to explain his initial treatment of Walker:

> I had great reason to conclude his scull was broke, and on removing the scalp I found it so, in two places.
> Q: What part of the scull was it?
> Potts: They were both in the fore part of the head, and no doubt both produced by the same blow; the two places were little more than a finger's breadth distance. I trapan'd him immediately.
> Q: What is that? It is necessary the jury should know.
> Potts: That is making a hole in the scull, and taking a piece out.

Unsurprisingly, questions revolved around the mental status of the patient as much as his physical injuries. Was Walker ever capable of identifying Tipton as the man who had thrown him out of the window? And if he did, was Walker really in sound enough mind to do so? Pott stated that he never heard Walker "speak sensibly," even though he or his "young man" saw the patient once or twice every day. The "young man" was James Gordon, who described himself as "an apprentice to Mr. Potts." He would have been in the second year of his apprenticeship with Pott at the time.

Unlike case histories, court proceedings, with their concern about who did or saw what and when, make it possible to piece together the chronology of a patient's care from the time of their arrival to their death at the hospital. First, Gordon arrived within a half hour or so of being called in to the hospital to see Walker. He had walked from his lodgings (he does not state where this was) to St. Bartholomew's. Pott arrived a little later. Walker was then examined and admitted to one of the wards. The next day, about noon, Walker was trepanned, and Pott then ordered a "double watch" for the patient. This essentially meant that Walker would have one woman paid to watch him by day and another by night.[88] Mary Jones watched Walker the night he came in and for several nights following. She related that the patient "cursed and swore" during the first operation but was silent during a second trepanation. This suggests that she was either present or within earshot of both procedures. Little is known about the role of Georgian sisters, nurses, or watchers during operations, and they are rarely mentioned as being present in case histories.

Walker's mother and two of his friends were "put out" of the ward when the surgeons came to operate. This could have been because of the need to make space around the patient's bed for Pott to operate. It is not clear who ordered the visitors to leave, but it certainly points to the fact that in hospitals, as opposed to in homes, family and friends did not have an automatic right to be present during surgery. Walker's mother gut-wrenchingly described how her son:

> when he saw them put me out of the ward, he called Mother, Mother, several times, very loud, I heard him a pretty way off.[89]

Pott described Walker as being "so very ungovernable, and so irrational, that we were obliged to confine him with what we call a *strait waistcoat*." He reiterated that Walker "never gave me any thing like an intelligible answer in my hearing, but these people (the watchers and a patient) staid with him a great deal longer than I did; I do not speak this to invalidate what they have said." In the end the jury found Tipton not guilty and he was acquitted.[90]

In 1767, Pott performed two postmortems on Mary Gardiner or Gardener, a servant who was the victim of violence. The first is described in the coroner's inquest, and the second was published in the Old Bailey Proceedings.[91] The postmortem was to determine whether or not a head wound was the cause of death. Gardiner's mistress, Mrs. Harrison, who kept a winehouse, had criticized some roast beef that Mary had prepared. A quarrel ensued, and a frequent visitor to the home, Thomas Swinhoe or Swinner, slapped Mary in the face. She fell to the ground and hit the back of her head on the stone kitchen floor. Mary was laid senseless in her bed and died sometime during the night. Swinhoe sent for a surgeon, and Pott arrived with his twelve-year-old pupil, James Earle. Earle was deposed first and Pott second at the coroner's inquest. Both were asked to describe the external wound and its size. Pott peeled back the scalp, removed the skull, examined the membrane that covered the brain, and finally inspected the brain itself. He found no evidence of "any-Mischief done to the Brain or its Coverings, nor any apparent Cause of Death clearly deducible from the Accident."[92]

It seems that this examination was not enough to satisfy the coroner's jury for, as Pott related at the trial of Swinhoe:

> The next morning I received a letter from the Coroner, signifying the Jury were not satisfied with the examination of the head only, but desired I would examine the whole body, imagining she might receive some injury on some other part; I examined the body very carefully, both belly and breast, and indeed her whole frame; in the cavity of the thorax was a very large quantity of water; there was such an appearance, as implied a very irregular intemperate course of life.[93]

In the end, Swinhoe was acquitted.

In addition to his court testimony, Pott offers case histories that give glimpses of the violence which persons known and unknown could inflict on others in Georgian London. Case VII in his text on head injuries begins with a man having a quarrel with his wife that led to him striking her on the head with a mop-stick.[94] "The blow was a smart one, but as it neither fetched blood, nor brought her to the ground, it only finished with dispute, and no farther notice was taken of it." The woman went back to work "crying greens about the streets, and lived, (to use her own words) sometimes drunk, sometimes sober." In other words the woman sold vegetables from a basket she carried.[95] Jerry White notes that after domestic service and laundering and working with a loom, "street selling was the next great industry for women."[96] It tended to be done by women who were poor, frail, in desperate circumstances, and sometimes physically or mentally disabled. For green-sellers the income varied, depending on the quality of the vegetables they could afford to buy from farmers in Islington, the generosity of the clientele, and their own health (and sobriety).

A week after her husband struck her on the head, the woman felt more unwell than usual. She went to the hospital and was admitted as a physician's patient in one of the wards. Pott records that "the doctor wrote for her," or prescribed medications, probably febrifuges. Two days later:

> … the sister [nurse] of the ward, in cutting off the patient's hair, which was full of vermin, discovered a swelling, which she desired me to look at: it was flattish, about the breadth of the palm of a hand, and lay immediately across the sagittal suture.[97]

The woman became very ill and three days after admission was in intense pain, constantly thirsty, and "erysepilas [had] taken possession of part of her visage." Erysipelas was a fiery, painful, red rash and was also referred to as "Ignis sacer," "holy fire," and "St. Anthony's fire." Pott opened the swelling on the woman's head and trephined her skull. He found her dura mater discolored and covered with pus. The next day she was even worse: her whole face was fiery red and one eye was swollen shut. Pott trephined the other side of her skull, noting that the woman talked nonsense all the time and "called perpetually for drink."[98] He made a third hole in her skull and the large quantity of matter that flowed from it made him realize that the "event must turn fatal." The next day her right arm and leg became paralytic, and she "died on the 16th day since the accident."[99]

In another case of wife beating, a woman came to Pott's home. She told him that her husband had kicked her downstairs and broken her skull. Pott had her admitted to the hospital where she died thirteen days later, blind, paralyzed, and in pain. With no names and no dates it is impossible to determine what, if anything, happened to the husbands of these women.[100]

As with marital violence, many times we do not know if the violence Pott describes in a case history happened in a room, a tavern, or on the street:

> Two female inhabitants of St. Giles got drunk together, and quarreled; one of them threw a stool at the other, and knocked her down. The edge of the stool cut through the scalp, and broke the left parietal bone.[101]

Someone in the neighborhood reportedly dressed the wound, and the next morning the woman was brought to the hospital. She did well for a week but died twenty-three days after admission, even though Pott opened her skull twice to drain it. He discussed at length in this case history the pros and cons of perforating the sagittal suture covering the longitudinal sinus. Due to the density of blood vessels and the considerable hemorrhage that ensues, "the act of perforation, [may] considerably embarrass and perplex a young operator."[102] Pott meant that puncturing this area of the skull with the subsequent heavy bleeding could seem to be a foolhardy mistake to the operator as well as to anyone observing the operation. But he counsels that younger operators need to be aware, in spite of what older surgeons may have written, that such an operation is possible and indeed occasionally successful (if not in the case of this patient).

Pott used the case history of a lunatic's suicide attempt and another of a boy's attempt to escape after being beaten by his tutor to further teach his readers of the dangers and unpredictability of treating wounds to the skull caused by violent acts. The first case concerned a "Lunatic [who] threw himself from a window, two stories high, and in his fall, struck his head, against a sign-iron, and then against a slated pest-house."[103] Following this self-inflicted injury, the man was stupid for twelve hours but rallied when someone at the home where he was being kept let blood freely, although the man "shewed no signs of a right understanding."[104] The patient was confined in a strait waistcoat with people constantly holding him for two days and nights, until repeated phlebotomy and a heavy dose of opium led to sleep. Pott saw the man and reported that he awoke from this deep sleep, "perfectly tranquil, and perfectly rational."[105] In fact the man was so healthy that his "friends" would have permitted him to leave and go to the countryside if Pott had not overruled them. Who his friends were is unknown, but Pott may have been referring to the people who kept the lunatic in their house.[106] There is no mention of others residing there so he may have been the only patient. This was not unusual in private madhouses for the better off. Ten days after the man threw himself from a window, he became dull, languid, and complained that his head hurt and he could not sleep. Pott assumed he was returning to lunacy, as he seemed disordered. He asked the man's brother, who was an apothecary, to give him an opiate at bedtime. The next day the patient was even worse and told Pott that "he felt as if a cord was bound tight about his brain."[107] Pott opened one of the three wounds on the man's head, probed it, and found it to be in a bad state. He secured the consent of the apothecary-brother as well as the patient himself before removing a considerable portion of his scalp to reveal the cranium, which he found to be discolored:

> I bled him again, and desired that he might take freely of the salt of wormwood and lemon juice until the next day. That night he had a smart rigor, and the next morning finding him worse, and more disturbed, I made a perforation of the skull.[108]

Eventually Pott made a large hole in the man's skull and drained a considerable discharge of pus. The man then slept and with regular phlebotomy, recovered. Pott concluded by admitting he had misdiagnosed his patient, whose "want of sleep, his seeming anxiety, his taciturnity, and great unwillingness to answer any question"[109] were not caused by a returning lunacy but rather from a worsening head injury.

The other case concerning violent behavior and head injuries involved a child:

> A Boy about 8 years old, the son of a Jew[110] merchant in the city, received a blow on his head with a stick from his tutor. The stroke made him giddy for a few minutes; but as no blood was shed, and the pain soon ceased, he concealed it till it was discovered by his barber that his head was swollen in that part. In the middle of his head was a tumor, about the size of a common wall-nut: it was indolent, had a dull kind of pulsation, and palpably contained a fluid.[111]

Two surgeons, Mr. Serjeant Amyand and Mr. Shipton, appear to have directed Pott to open the boy's skull, and Pott carried out two operations under their supervision, the first to drain the wound and the second to remove a piece of bone from the sinus under the sagittal suture. The senior surgeons were likely Claudius Amyand (1680–1740), sergeant surgeon to George II and principal surgeon to the St. George's and the Westminster hospitals, and John Shipton of Brook Street in Holborn. Given that Amyand died in 1740, this case no doubt took place early in Pott's career. The boy survived the operations and in 1768 was still alive.

Turning now to cases of violence where the perpetrators were strangers to the victims rather than family members or servants, Pott provides the following history:

> A Poor-fellow crossing Tower-hill, got, before he was aware of it, into a mob, that was endeavouring to rescue a sailor from a press-gang. The man was knocked down. When the crowd dispersed, he was found senseless, and in that state was brought to St. Bartholomew's hospital, where he was immediately let blood and put to bed.[112]

Given that the surgeon whose week it was to be on duty at the hospital was Mr. Nourse, Pott's master, this case also probably occurred early in Pott's career.

The man was bled heavily for three days and then discharged, only to return nine days later to attend the weekly surgery where Pott screened people for admission to the hospital. Pott admitted him again, bled him, immediately ordered a glister to open his bowels, and demanded that he be kept in bed. The man died five days later.

Another case involved a watchman whose stand was in Whitechapel. The watchman got into a scuffle with some drunken sailors and received several blows and wounds to the head.[113] He was brought to the hospital the next day because he had lost a lot of blood and his head was swollen and bruised. The watchman had five wounds, but they all appeared to be superficial. Pott decided not to bleed him as he had lost a lot of blood already; however, he admitted him, as he "was more than sixty years old."[114] The watchman was recovering well but transgressed the rules of the hospital by staying out all night and was discharged. A few days later he was back with all the classic signs of a worsening head injury. Pott opened his skull, drained a small amount of matter, drew a little blood from one of his arms, and had "a glyster thrown up to procure a stool."[115] The watchman went steadily downhill. Pott opened his head twice more, each time draining a great deal of bad pus. He made a third hole in his skull deliberately large, as he suspected that the pus was so thick it could not drain from a smaller one. Pott expected his patient to die but the watchman survived. Much like a parable, Pott ends this case history with a lesson for his readers:

> Many, who see and are convinced of the justness, and propriety of it, (multiple perforations) want authority to vindicate them in proposing or executing it, and some part of the disgrace which has been cast on the operation of the trepan has arisen from this cause. Practitioners have in general been afraid to make more than one opening, and that generally a small one.[116]

Surgery was an art, and a decision to do or not to do something to a patient was often as subjective as it was objective. Pott reinforced this premise in his lectures on gunshot wounds. He began with disabusing his pupils of the common belief that only military surgeons had the skills to treat "wounds of this Nature" and give "relief to the part affect'd."[117] Pott told his students to first question the patient, if possible, to discover what kind of firearm caused the wound and the type of ammunition. Next they were to remove all the balls they could see, using forceps to enlarge the wound/s if necessary. Then they were to dress the area with a soft dressing that had been soaked in the "digestive balsam of Bartholomew's Hospital" and cover this with a "soft cooling cataplasm."[118] Pott surmised that the suppuration or the development of good pus in the wound would force any other balls out or that they would come away with the scab.[119] Surgeons recognized suppurative inflammation through several cardinal signs in their patients, such as hot flushed skin, pain, rigours and cold fits:

> Blood becomes putrid, with an offensive smell, putrid serum and crassamentum is discharged, and mixes with a thin serous secretion from the wounded surfaces and becomes whiter and thicker, by day 5 formed pus, and fever goes down.[120]

Pott was called in to the hospital during the Gordon Riots of early June 1780 and treated at least two patients who had been shot, both of whom were women.[121] Writings on the Gordon Riots describe the events of 6–7 June and give an inkling of what these patients may have witnessed and participated in. Initially most of the attacks in the city were directed at areas associated with Catholicism, such as Moorfields, but from 6 June they widened to include public buildings. The seventh of June is often called "Black Wednesday," since on that day a large distillery in Holborn owned by a Catholic named Thomas Langdale was burnt down, and the ignited gin ran through the streets, burning any who attempted to drink. That same night troops fired on those attacking the Bank of England and on those attempting to burn down the tollhouses on Blackfriars Bridge.[122]

The sightseeing gentry came the next day to see the conflagration and damage to property. Included among them on Thursday morning, 8 June, were Emily Pott and William Hickey, who rode out after breakfast as Pott made his rounds at the hospital. Emily was the mistress of Pott's troublesome son Bob, who was in India at the time. Hickey was Bob's closest friend and an acquaintance of the Scottish Protestant MP, Lord George Gordon, the man after whom the anti-Catholic riots were soon named.[123] Gordon was arrested on 9 June, taken to the Tower and charged with High Treason, but found not guilty at his subsequent trial.

Alice Kent, a 48-year-old married woman who "seems to have lived an irregular life," was admitted to the hospital during the first night of the riots. Pott saw her and confirmed that she had a compound fracture of the tibia and fibula resulting from being hit by a musket ball. The shot had left her ankle joint and heel (where the ball exited) shattered. "She was advised to suffer amputation which she positively refused." Her leg was put in splints and three days later had turned gangrenous. She was given Jesuit's Bark and opium every four hours, and the gangrene appeared to be slowing but shortly afterwards it killed her.[124]

The second woman that Pott treated was carried to the hospital on Black Wednesday:

> Hannah Stewart—21 Years of Age of a good habit of body a married Woman was brought into the Hospl on Wednesday nights the 7th Inst—with a compound Fracture of the Wrist Joint wherein both the Radius and Ulna were fractured, and the soft parts

> received considerable injury from a musket ball shot by one of the soldiers who was on duty quelling the disturbance, that the Ball appeared to have entered externally a little above the Head of the Ulna and Radius, lodging in an oblique direction through the Joint—which it easy much shattered, and produced a very troublesome Haemorrhage, which was soon stopp'd with a needle and ligature.[125]

Given that the bones were shattered, the usual treatment was to amputate:

> … but the woman not giving her consent—the arm was put in a Common Poultice—opiates were given to appease pain, her Body was strengthened by several purges—she also had been shot through both breasts—possible by the same Ball—her arm to-day looks less inflamed—but rather painful—her arm is swell'd and also painful. Mr. Pott saw it and order'd her to go on with the poultice—and some small fragments of loose bones were taken out on her admission.—her pulse is Quick, and she has a considerable degree of fever—Discharged Well[126]

Pott was all too aware of the argument it took for not only a surgeon to urge an amputation on a patient but for the patient to consent to such a traumatic procedure. To amputate meant making a choice that had both acute and chronic consequences. The operation and especially the aftermath was painful and sometimes fatal. If the patient survived, the loss of an arm or a leg changed their lives forever in socio-economic terms. Both of Pott's patients who were shot during the riots had refused amputation[127] with one dying and the other surviving.

Amputations

In mid-January 1756 Pott was thrown from his horse while riding along Kent Street (Old Kent Road) in Southwark and sustained a compound fracture of the lower leg, most likely breaking the tibia.[128] In his biography James Earle described the severity of the injury to his late father-in-law's leg. The bone was exposed and Pott:

> Conscious of the dangers attendant on fractures of this nature, and thoroughly aware how much they may be increased by rough treatment, or improper position, he would not suffer himself to be moved until he had made the necessary dispositions.[129]

Pott first sent a message to ask for two chairmen to bring their poles. As he lay on the pavement waiting for the chairmen to arrive from their stand in Westminster, Pott purchased a door from a bystander. He then instructed the chairmen to nail this door to their poles in order to make a stretcher. The chairmen carried Pott on this invention over London Bridge to his home on Watling Street, a distance of two miles. Making the long journey by foot while laying flat was far safer than trying to do so while reclining in a jolting carriage.

Once home, several surgeons quickly gathered to examine Pott's injury. The news was not good:

> the case was thought so desperate as to require immediate amputation. Mr. Pott, convinced that no one could be a proper judge in his own case, submitted to their opinion; and the instruments were actually got ready, when Mr. Nourse, who had been prevented from coming sooner, fortunately entered the room.[130]

Earle's account of Pott's dramatic rescue by Nourse from amputation is secondhand but we do have a firsthand account by one of Pott's dressers, a young man called Peter Clare:

> Several years ago Mr. *Pott* unfortunately met with a compound fracture of his leg by a fall from his horse, at the time of my living with him, and of course I was a witness to the proceedings in the cure. The accident was treated like a simple fracture, and the air excluded. His age was betwixt forty and fifty, and his constitution good; the wound healed without any sinus, and the callus was completely formed in eight or ten weeks. If relaxing means had been used, such as poultices, which are here improper for the reasons before mentioned, it is a question if this gentleman's many subsequent services would not have been lost to the community.[131]

Pott was well aware from personal and professional experience that agreeing to an amputation took considerable courage.[132] In a lecture given in 1769 on compound fractures, he listed six factors to be taken into consideration as to "whether the limb was saveable or not, Haemorrhage, Position, Setting, Dressings, & Bandage"[133] and whether the "bone/s are mashed or shiver'd etc."[134] Essentially the more trauma the limb had suffered, the less time should be taken in urging immediate amputation. But he knew it was difficult to persuade patients to lose a limb when:

> as every Man knows that … apparently desperate cases are sometimes cur'd & that People in every Circumstance I have mention'd have sometimes escap'd by Chance, so that Linbs are shatter'd & wounded as to render amputation the only probable means for the Preservation of Life, are now & then sav'd …[135]

Pott was among the lucky ones. He escaped amputation of the lower leg because Nourse, his old Master, thought it was possible to heal the wound. Nourse was right, and at the age of 43, Pott used his forced convalescence of several months to write his first book on the subject of ruptures.

Earle tells us that Pott sometimes used the success of his own case to strengthen the argument about the danger of letting air enter a wound, as it could cause inflammation, gangrene, and even death. In Pott's case, he was fortunate, for when the exposed bone "was returned into the proper place, a sort of valve was formed, which excluded air."[136] And air, as Pott forcefully reminded his pupils, was especially impure in London since it was shared by so many:

> Compound Fractures are easily cured in pure country Air, than in a Town. We labour under a great many disadvantages in the Hospital for want of it & many of the harmed will die in three or four days after the accident from Mortification—in this Case we never wait for Suppuration but amputate immediately—This is a doctrine I will abide by Gentlemen you will find success by embracing it.[137]

The foul air of St. Bartholomew's Hospital meant that limb removal was recommended immediately after injury. Other surgeons commented on this sad state of affairs, including provincial ones such as the Unitarian John Aitkin (1747–1822) of Warrington. In his *Thoughts on Hospitals* in 1771, Aitkin promoted the establishment of more rural infirmaries:

> Every Surgeon attending a large and crowded hospital, knows the very great difficulty of curing a compound fracture in them. This is so universally acknowledged, that the most humane and judicious of them have been obliged to comply with that dreadful rule of practice, immediate amputation in every compound fracture. Mr. Pott, than whom there is not in the whole professions a more unprejudiced patron of improvement, or a warmer advocate for humanity, has recommended this general rule upon the grounds of accurate and impartial observation. Yet, that it is not founded upon the nature of the case, but upon the added malignancy of hospital air, is evident from the different success in private practice and the country infirmaries.[138]

In a lecture on compound fractures given in 1777 Pott recalled "I had a compound fracture from a fall from my Horse."[139] The lesson he wished to impart to his pupils was that in a case like his, where the patient has "very good Habits, when the Wound is made even by the Bone, it will heal by the first Intention, which happened to myself …" Pott then warned them that the "great object of Consideration" concerns whether circulation can be maintained given the injury. If it cannot, "Gangrene & Mortification often come on within 24 hours."[140]

Essentially Pott had been very lucky in terms of the limited vascular damage he sustained from the fracture of the tibia and in that he escaped infection.[141] Despite his good fortune from going against the advice of every surgeon except one who inspected his wound and counseled that his leg should be immediately cut off below the knee, Pott remained convinced that amputation was generally necessary in compound fractures to save a patient's life. His response to stories of miraculous escape from the knife (including his own) was to point out that experience showed that attempting to keep a limb intact generally led to a lingering and painful death. In Pott's mind, the chance of death from amputation was by no means as great as that arising from foolishly trying to preserve a shattered arm or leg. In such cases "Amputation is vindicable upon every Principle of Humanity or chirurgic Knowledge."[142] This strong statement reflected Pott's role in a debate that arose in Europe during the eighteenth century, namely, was it best to amputate immediately after an injury occurred, or to wait for gangrene to develop and bones to separate from flesh? Parisian surgeons such as Pierre Dionis and Henri-François Le Dran argued for early amputation rather than waiting for a patient to recover from the shock of injury. Jean Louis Petit's invention of a better tourniquet also made fatal hemorrhage less likely while operating.

Largely as a result of Petit's tourniquet being so successful in stopping massive bleeding, amputations became more frequent and were seen as the treatment of choice following a compound fracture. As Pott noted, "you should know which is the best place to amputate, and be master of the circulation of the Limb." After describing how to mark the place to cut with a double strip of linen tape, Pott told his pupils that the "next circumstance is the tourniquet, Pettit's is certainly by much the best, as it will stand fixed, at any degree of lightness you please." Finally, only a small and light carpenter's saw should be used to cut the limb off "as it is the force of your arm that cuts through the bone and you need to feel how much force to apply."[143]

Many military surgeons, especially Johann Ulrich Bilguer (1720–96), the surgeon-general to Frederick the Great of Prussia, did not view amputation as the best option for compound fractures. From his experiences in the Seven Years War (1754–63) and as head of a large military hospital, Bilguer was convinced that amputations should be delayed in fractures caused by gunshot wounds until the blood supply to a main artery was compromised and/or gangrene had set in. He came to this conclusion because some soldiers who refused amputation actually survived and did well with a four to twenty-four month regimen of repeated cuts through gangrenous flesh until live flesh was found:[144]

> I make long incisions, not only on the mortified parts, but on those adjacent, which soon would be so. I make several of them … We ought always to cut to the quick; and if the bone be affected, the periosteum must be cut through, and the bone laid bare.[145]

Bilguer then recommended removing the mortified parts (to be recognized by their stench, color, and numbness to a bistoury) then packing the area with fomentations of herbs, oils, and vinegar, and finally applying a dressing. The theory was that such treatment would encourage copious drainage and healing by granulation. Bilguer first outlined this observation in 1761 when he received his doctor's degree from the University of Halle and published his thesis in Latin. It was translated into French and annotated by Samuel-Auguste André David Tissot in 1764, and later that same year was translated from French into English with the title *A dissertation on the inutility of the amputation of limbs*. Such a conservative and, as Bilguer himself admitted, tedious and painful approach to preserving a limb arose the ire of some surgeons, including Pott.

In 1770 an anonymous pupil recorded Pott's horrifying description of the symptoms that ensued from having a compound fracture:

> if the limb is not remov'd in a short space of time [they] are a violent symptomatic fever, thirst, a parch'd brown tongue, and very frequently a diarrhaea, the limb is at the same time in an inflammatory state, the Symptoms may continue 2 or 3 days, then instead of inflammation only the limb, will put in a Sphacelated appearance, the fever is increas'd attend'd with a Singulteus, Delirium, frequent faetid stools, colliquative sweats, and death is inevitably the consequence.[146]

Pott followed this description with the case of a foolish patient:

> An instance of this kind you have seen in this house lately, where Tibia & Fibula were much broken, the former protud'd considerably, so much as to make it an impossibility to reduce it, I advis'd the Man to submit to the operation, but he obstinately refus'd, at the end of four days he died, attend'd with the foremention'd symptoms ...[147]

John Heaviside's notes from Pott's course of surgery in 1781 captured the emotional nature of the debate on amputation and the emotional toll it was taking on Pott. Pott began by recommending "timely amputations" to save a patient's life if their scrophula was advanced—he believed it was a poison carried in the blood that would eventually poison the "whole system":[148]

> I should be sorry to be thought warmer on this Subject than I ought to be, because it tends to mutilate Mankind, but I am out of all Patience when I see People making general observations which will not apply to particular Cases by which honest judicious Practitioners are put into a very unfair light—[149]

In 1779 Pott published his *Remarks on that kind of palsy of the lower limbs, which is frequently found to accompany a curvature of the spine, and is supposed to be caused by it. Together with its method of cure* (discussed in chapter 4). Attached to this publication was a succinct essay titled *Observations on the necessity and propriety of amputation, in certain cases, and under certain circumstances.* This was a direct refutation of Bilguer's and Tissot's claims that amputation was rarely needed and was inhumane when it was carried out. Pott began the essay with a general dismissal:

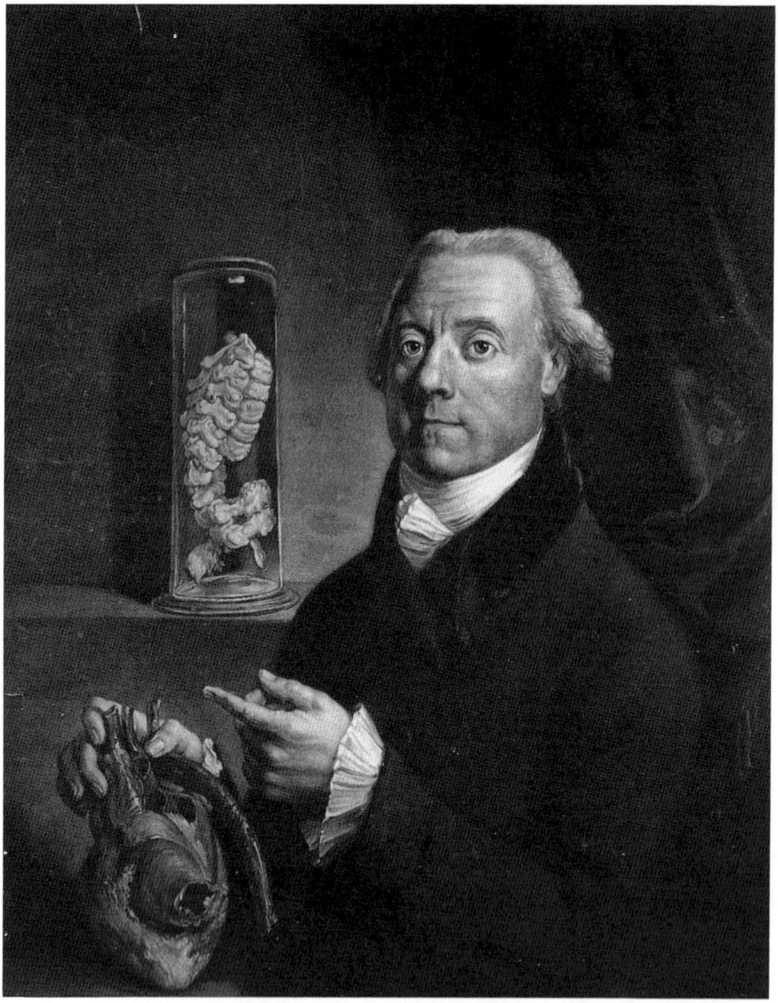

Figure 7. John Heaviside, Coloured mezzotint by R. Earlom, 1803, after J. Zoffany, L0017574. Courtesy of Wellcome Library, London.

> The boast of universal specifics, of remedies infallibly preventive of diseases, and of means whereby chirurgical operations may be rendered totally unnecessary, is the language of quackery, and not of science.[150]

For Pott, Bilguer's wholehearted condemnation of amputations accompanied as it was by a message about the cruelty of surgeons who performed such operations was enough to label him a quack. Throughout the essay Pott used terms that would have been recognized by his readers as those associated with mountebanks, including versions of the words bold, ignorant, weak, wicked, malevolent, and mischievous. Pott responded to the indictment of the operation with an acknowledgement of the permanent damage it caused a patient and the revulsion of those who had to watch such an operation. Yet it was sometimes necessary to save a life:

> The amputation of a limb is an operation terrible to bear, horrid to see, and must leave the person on whom it has been performed in a mutilated, imperfect state; but still it is one of those which becomes, in certain circumstances, absolutely and indispensably necessary.[151]

Amputation became mandatory once inflammation developed in a compound fracture from the "pernicious influence" of air entering the tela cellulosa.[152] But informing the patient of this need was a:

> very delicate part of the practice: for however pressing the case may seem to the surgeon to be, it will not in general appear in the same light to the patient, to the relations, or to the by-standers: they will be inclined to regard the proposition as arising from ignorance how to treat the case properly, or from an inclination to save trouble; or perhaps from a still worse motive, a desire to operate; and it will often require more firmness on the part of the practitioner, and more resignation and confidence on the part of the patient, than is generally met with, to submit to such a severe operation, in such a seeming hurry, and upon so little apparent deliberation; and yet it often happens, that the suffering this point of time to pass, decides the patient's fate.[153]

Such persuasion was complicated by the fact that amputation for scrophulous joints typically involved young children who could not give consent, "which inflicts a very distressing task on their nearest relations."[154] Besides tubercular joints, femoral and popliteal aneurisms often led to amputations. This was especially true among the laboring poor "who generally neglect" the aneurism "until it renders them lame and incapable of following their employment; and when it is got into this state it requires immediate attention."[155] Pott concluded his essay by attacking Bilguer for suggesting that advanced caries of the bones from "venereal, scorbutic or cancerous disease" can be cured by drying the bones out with the use of "bark, drying, burning, rasping and boring …"[156] The decision to amputate while the wound was fresh versus waiting to see how the affected limb did, continued on until the next century.

In 1787, the year before Pott died, the confusion and differing views concerning why and when to amputate is captured in a case that came before the Old Bailey law court.[157] In early June of that year, James Weston, a horse-hair weaver, assaulted William Cuit, the publican of the Falstaff, leaving him with a broken right leg. Just over two weeks later, Cuit died in St. Bartholomew's Hospital, and

Robert Pennington, one of Pott's former dressers, was called to give evidence. He told the court that he remembered the victim had been "brought (to the hospital) on a board about twenty minutes to one on the Sunday morning."[158] Pennington examined Cuit and found "a dislocation of the ancle [*sic*] with a fracture of the small bone. I told his friends that it would be mortal."[159] Pennington was then asked to explain why he gave this dismal prognosis and he provided two reasons: (1) the violence of the "accident," and (2) the fracture of the tibia had in turn broken the fibula (timpana in the transcript). In Pennington's view, this would undoubtedly lead to mortification in three to four days and death would quickly follow. The judge asked Pennington, "Would not amputation prevent that?" Pennington responded that he had consulted with another surgeon, Mr. Lock, who had confirmed that amputation was not a possible solution. The judge then asked, "Then there are not many instances where the bone and the flesh is shattered and mangled to pieces, which immediate amputation would cure?" to which Pennington answered: "Some, my Lord; but in compound dislocation, I never saw it; I have seen a good many, but I never saw it in compound dislocation." Still dissatisfied with this explanation, the judge pressed Pennington further and asked a logical question: if the dislocated ankle and fractured leg were amputated immediately, wouldn't that have eliminated any chance of mortification developing? Pennington replied, "No further than this, an inflammation generally takes hold of the whole system; if amputation is deferred, the stump will probably mortify."[160] Mr. Weston was found not guilty of manslaughter. Pott, as this chapter demonstrates, proffered a great deal of advice on wounds caused by accidents or violence and the question of amputation in such instances. The next chapter considers how eminent hospital surgeons such as Pott treated the tangled morass of chronic conditions that afflicted the poor and the rich of Georgian London.

CHAPTER FOUR

"A Poor Man Came to St. Bartholomew's"

Chronic Conditions

> Case V. A drunken, idle, fellow, who lived in the neighbourhood ... had a small omental hernia ... the hospital had, once or twice given him a truss; but being much oftener drunk than sober, he seldom wore it at all, and when he did it was seldom in the right place.[1]

> Mr. Pott's reputation in his profession is so universally established, that when he promises a radical cure of the watery rupture, and tells us he has been repeatedly successful in the use of a seton, we are satisfied the afflicted in this particular complaint, will pay a proper regard to so respectable an authority.[2]

In addition to discussing treatments for acute crises such as accidents and gunshot wounds, Pott described chronic ailments such as ruptures and hernias in his lectures and written texts.[3] These common conditions were often treated by others long before a patient came to the attention of Pott at the hospital or through a visit made to a patient's home.[4] Pott included numerous case histories of these chronic conditions in a *Treatise of the Hydrocele, or Watry Rupture and Other Diseases of the Testicle, It's Coats and Vessels* (1767). In one of these cases, he described a visit to a tavern to see a waiter "who was poxed with a true venereal sarcocele and a swollen testicle or hydrocele."[5]

J. Grigg attended Pott's lecture in the winter of 1781–2 and noted that according to Pott a hydrocele was an accumulation of fluid (not blood) in one of the coats

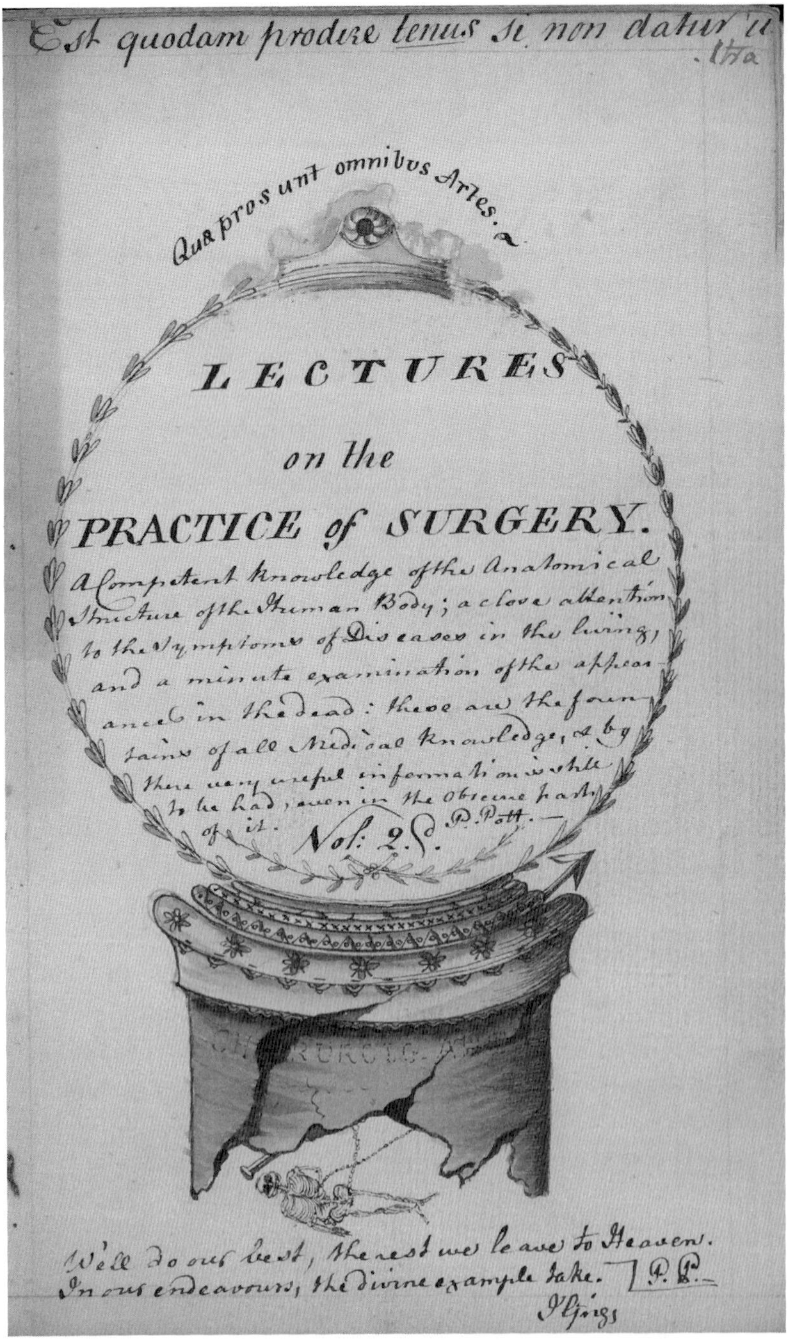

Figure 8. Pott, Percivall, Surgical Lectures, Vol. 2. Title Page. Taken down by J. Grigg. MS 3958, 1782, L0073681. Courtesy of Wellcome Library, London.

of the testis, while "a Venereal Sarcocele as I chuse to call it" was a late symptom of the pox, a smooth, hard and tense (painful) swelling "just at the lower part of the Spermatic Cord."[6] Pott cautioned his pupils that even though sarcocele was a late development of pox, they might have to search for other symptoms to validate the source of the problem (and to fully convince the patient that he in fact had syphilis). Pott recommended that they look for "Venereal mischief" by questioning the patient about pains "in the knees, shoulders, shins, sore throat, or appearances on ye Skin in consequence of dispersed bubo, (the characteristic copper-colored spots of syphilis) or ill treated Chancre."[7]

The waiter in Pott's case had agreed to give one of his acquaintances—a surgeon's mate on a man-of-war—a bottle of claret in return for draining the hydrocele.[8] The surgeon's mate repeatedly plunged a lancet into the waiter's scrotum and poked around with a probe. Instead of this leading to the release of the "water" that was assumed to be the cause of the swollen testicle, blood gushed out. Not surprisingly the waiter told Pott that he had been in wracking pain ever since. Pott treated him with phlebotomy, glisters, opiates, and febrifuge medicines. While these treatments cured him of his fever and pain, the waiter had "almost the whole testicle cast off in one large slough."[9] This loss of a testicle (a part Pott referred to as very essential to being a man)[10] resulted from an infection likely caused by the surgeon's mate puncturing and probing his scrotum.

Surgical Skills and Morality

Pott gave detailed instructions in lectures regarding the treatment of a hydrocele. He condemned the use of plunging a lancet into the scrotum (as the surgeon's mate had done), for not only did it show a lack of skill but often-resulted in generalized swelling or "anasarca":

> The taking hold of the Scrotum, holding it high in the fingers, or stabbing it with a lancet, with velocity, tho' the expulsion of the fluid is immediate & cannot lodge in the cells of the Dartos [muscle], yet the appearance is indelicate & unchirurgical, besides there is a strong proof of the impropriety of letting off the water with ye lancet, for if any quantity lodges, is produced anasarca.[11]

He remarked that some operators recommended introducing a probe (as the surgeon's mate had done) if the water "does not pass quickly enough ... but poking with this instrument is productive of great Inflammation, which tho' it had produced sometimes a radical Cure, is attended with great pain and confinement." The latter would result in a loss of income and social embarrassment. Perhaps Pott had in mind the waiter he had seen. Instead of lancet and probe, Pott thought surgeons should use a small trocar and then drain the water off with a cannula, thus demonstrating their delicate surgical skills. After all, one thing that differentiated surgeons from quacks was their intimate knowledge of anatomy. Pott informed his pupils:

> … the testicle does not hang like the clapper of a bell in the middle of the Tunica Vaginalis, but in the posterior part. Much mischief can develop from those who have thought it is a matter of no consequence where they plunged in the instrument.[12]

In 1780 Pott confessed to his pupils that he once removed a testicle believing it to be completely schirrous (cancerous), but when he got home and had a chance to exam the testicle at his leisure, he discovered if to be nothing more than a "common hydrocele."[13]

The majority of Pott's cases in *A Treatise of the Hydrocele, or Watry Rupture and Other Diseases of the Testicle, It's Coats and Vessels* concerned poor working men who came to St. Bartholomew's with swollen groins and hernias. They were worried about their livelihoods and frequently had tried other cures before they would become financially destitute. As Tim Hitchcock has vividly detailed in *Down and Out in Eighteenth-Century London*: "For the vast majority, livelihood depended upon their ability to do hard physical work … Poverty and disability went hand in hand."[14] Eventually the chronic edema of their groins coupled with the depletion of their funds by quacks would bring them to the hospital:

> A Poor man came to St. Bartholomew's hospital, and desired assistance for a swelling in his groin; for which he had, for a month before, been taking Jesuits drops and other quack medicines, till he had not a farthing left.[15]

In this instance Pott diagnosed a hernia humoralis of the testicle in his groin, drained it, and sent the now recovered man on his way.

Another poor man was brought from the vicinity of Rosemary Lane to the hospital with a painfully swollen scrotum that he had assumed for years was a water-rupture or a hydrocele.[16] Rosemary Lane, near Tower Hill, was the site of the Rag Fair, the market for used (and frequently stolen) clothes. It appears to have operated on a daily basis except Sundays from mid-afternoon until dusk. During the Rag Fair fencers and mountebanks were readily available to customers at public and lodging houses such as the Sun and the Wheathead or at stands on the street.[17] In desperation the poor man had paid a stage quack three guineas to cure him of a huge and painful swelling in the scrotum. The quack laid him on his back on a couch on the stage and thrust some kind of an instrument into the

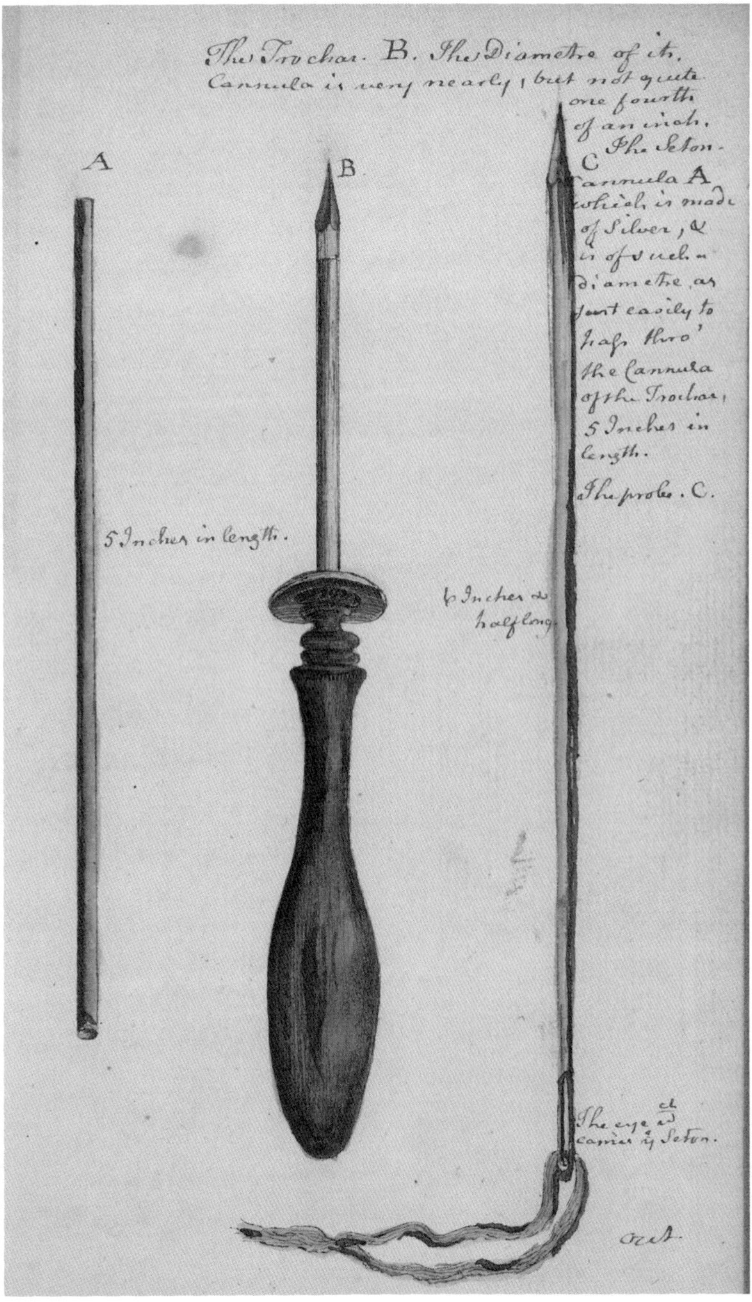

Figure 9. Illustration of surgical instruments, from Pott, Percivall, "Lectures on the Practice of Surgery," Surgical Lectures, Vol. 2. Trochars. Taken down by J. Grigg. MS 3958, 1782, L007368. Courtesy of Wellcome Library, London.

man's scrotum. Nothing came out but blood, and after the poor man had bled nearly a quarter of an hour, he fainted and was carried home by friends. The quack disappeared, and after two days of increasing pain and fever, the friends decided to bring the man to the hospital. Pott put him on an antiphlogistic regime, and he recovered.[18] He concluded this case history with "I suppose the reader will have as little doubt as I have, that all this mischief was produced by wounding the testicle, or epididymis."[19] Just like the waiter at the tavern, a raging infection had resulted from violent probing of the testicle.

Pott discussed ruptures (hernias) in *Observations and Cases Relative to Ruptures, etc.* and described the condition as common among the laboring poor.[20] Simon Dickie, in *Cruelty and Laughter: Forgotten Comic Literature and the Unsentimental Eighteenth Century*, has drawn attention to the throngs of disabled and deformed people visible in Georgian society:

> It is hard for us to imagine the almost phantasmagoric array of deformed bodies encountered every day on the streets of mid-eighteenth century London. Bodies twisted by hernias. Spines bent by rickets or tuberculosis. Noses eaten away by disease. Rotting gums and pockmarked faces. The inescapable sound of coughing, wheezing, and choking. Periodicals and polite correspondences persistently complain about the swarms of deformed beggars in every city street.[21]

Dickie highlights two areas where knowledge of the disabled is especially lacking—the "lived experience" and "just how many deformities were the predictable consequence of labour."[22] To a small extent analyzing Pott's case histories can provide useful insights here as they include references to the effects of physical deformities on patients' social and economic conditions.[23]

In the following account the possibility of marriage and the fear that a large abdominal rupture might negatively affect that prospect led a man to seek treatment from several healers, including Pott, who recalled, "A Young man, who worked as a journey-man with a silver-smith in Foster-lane, came to me three or four times on account of a rupture."[24] He attempted to reduce the rupture manually without success and subsequently recommended that the man use a suspensory bandage to keep the hernia in place. This was Pott's standard advice but:

> At the distance of about six months from his last visit, I was sent for to St. Bartholomew's hospital in a hurry, to a person supposed to labour under a hernia with a stricture. I found a man, who was only not dead [near death]; he had a dying countenance, a faultring pulse, a constant hiccough, and cold extremities.[25]

(A stricture was a narrowing of the gut from chronic inflammation and was a life-threatening event.)

After he examined the man, Pott considered his presence to be futile and made to leave, but the patient first wanted to reveal (or Pott encouraged him to say) how he had arrived in this miserable condition. The story, as Pott relates it, reads much like the confession of a dying man to a priest: "A few days before, having an intention to marry, and believing that his rupture would be prejudicial to him, he applied to someone recommended to him for relief."[26] After paying the person several guineas, the man received an ointment and a tight bandage to wear. Three days later the patient took the bandage off due to severe pain. He went to see his regular surgeon, who told him to "apply to his scrotum and groin a poultice made of boiled turnips and hog's-lard, and to come to him again the next day." As the patient was getting worse and was too ill to go see the surgeon the next day, his friends contacted the first healer who had treated the man. He demanded five more guineas to cure the journeyman. The patient could not pay this, and so his desperate friends contacted Pott. We do not know what Pott charged for a home visit but it was most likely shillings rather than guineas. When Pott examined the man, he felt what he termed "alarming crepitus," or crackling, "which infallibly denotes putrid air from gangrenous membranes."[27] Essentially the man had a strangulated hernia that had cut off the blood supply of the hernial sac, leading to gangrene of the sac and its contents. In *A Treatise on Ruptures*, Pott described the signs that a patient was sinking under this complaint and included these remarks on crepitus:

> … the eyes have now a languor and a glassiness, a lack-lustre not easy to be described … there is a crepitus to the touch, which will be easily be conceived by all who have attended to it, but is not, so easy to convey an idea of by words: this crepitus is the too sure indicator of gangrenous mischief within … the hiccough and the cold sweats continuing and increasing, with the addition of spasmodic rigors and subsultus tendinum, [twitching and convulsive movements] the tragedy soon finishes.[28]

The man died that evening. The following morning Pott dissected the scrotum and hernial sac and found them both foul smelling and gangrenous.

Pott's contempt for those he saw as predators on the pain of the sick is readily apparent in the following case:

> The late Mr. Hollingsworth[29] desired me to go with him to see a patient in the neighbourhood of Clerkenwell. It was a man, about fifty-five years old, who had a large ulcerated cancerous tumor in his right groin, with high callous edges; it always discharged a large quantity of a most offensive gleet [purulent discharge]; at times it bled profusely, and was always extremely painful.[30]

The patient recounted "he had showed it to two eminent rupture-curers; one of whom said, that it was a piece of caul [gut] and offered, for twenty guineas, to cure him by cutting it out. The other only sold him two bandages for it, neither of which he could ever wear.[31] Even worse, a cancer-curer had slipped out the patient's door just as Pott and William Hollingsworth drew up in a carriage. The cancer-curer had applied an escharotic (corrosive salve), "which by the patient's account, as well as by the appearance of the sore, had made terrible havock."[32] Pott added that the state of the sore meant nothing surgical could be done. Instead he recommended the patient take a tincture of Thebaic (or common Egyptian opium), "which advice he followed, during the short remainder of his life."[33] Pott remarked in *A Treatise on Ruptures* that the one good thing about being poor was that the destitute were less liable to being operated on by "rupture-doctors" because they lacked the money "to pay upfront for their murder."[34]

Pott was at times as critical of his fellow surgeons as he was of those healers he considered quacks. He referred to surgeons by name and poured as much contempt on their heads as he did on rupture-healers. Pott once told of a laboring man who had fallen down in the street with a load on his back. He was brought to the hospital with a suspected rupture from the fall, "having immediately perceived a swelling in his groin, and scrotum, which he had not before."[35] Mr. Freke was the surgeon on call that week, and believing the patient to have a rupture, he operated on him.[36] Freke was a senior surgeon who, according to Pott, "was a man not easily to be dissuaded from what he had a mind to do; and, having got the whim into his head, was determined to make the experiment on this, which he thought a fair case for the purpose."[37] Pott implies that Freke continued to operate even though it became clear to Pott and others attending that the patient did not have a rupture. The patient subsequently died.

Pott made other references to Freke as well. He tersely recounted another case where another one of Mr. Freke's patients died three days after undergoing a questionable castration,[38] and in yet another instance made a less-than-complimentary comment regarding Mr. Freke in a lecture:

> A man applied at the Hospital with a Cancerous Polypus, which had enlarged the nose to a considerable size, Mr. Freake thought proper to extract it, which he performed with considerable force and Brought out two Polypi, on introducing the finger up the mans the [*sic*] Septum … all the bones which from the nose were found dissolved and the nose itself fell down upon the face, having nothing left to support it; a dreadful Haemorrhage ensued which was with great difficulty suppressed, and the consequence of this rash operation, was a violent inflammation which seizing the cerebrum, suffered the patient to survive only thirty-six hours.[39]

Essentially, the growth had been acting as a scaffold for what remained of the man's nose. John Heaviside's notes from Pott's lecture course in 1769 offers further evidence of Mr. Freke's forceful manner:

> Boy with a polypus hanging from each of the nostrils, painful, hard, inflamed, & Mr. Freak undertook to cure him. Pulled off right polypus and nose collapsed, bled, high fever, died 3 days later of an inflammation of the brain. Polypus had been holding the nose up.[40]

Pott found that not just senior but also lowly assistant surgeons could cause problems with patients. Having persuaded a man who had come to the hospital to have his undescended left testicle removed, as it appeared to be diseased, Pott encouraged Mr. Charles Griffiths, "one of our then assistants," to look at the case. Griffiths did so and appears to have told Pott's patient that the swelling in his groin was not a testicle but a tumor of some kind and that it could be removed with internal medicine.[41] The patient left the hospital happy to avoid a castration. Pott, however, heard that several months later the man had presented himself at St. George's Hospital, and "the gentlemen there gave him the same opinion, and the same advice which I had given him; he submitted, and got a cure, by the removal of a testicle which had never been lower than his groin, and which was now become schirrhous."[42]

Other surgeons at the hospital regularly consulted Pott on hernias. Mr. William Sharp (1729–1810) asked Pott to examine a patient whose scrotum was so swollen from a large tumor that it hung halfway down to his knee.[43] The scrotum was ulcerated and lumpy, and the patient had pain in his back and felt tired and dispirited. Having examined the tumor, Pott and Sharp were uncertain about the chance of the man surviving its removal: "We communicated to him our opinions, our suspicions, fears, and uncertainty; and told him what hazard might possibly be incurred." The man asked them to go ahead with the operation.[44] They cut through the tumor and drained eleven Winchester pints of water, or twenty-five liters.[45] Pott would like to have made the opening even larger and drain off more, "but the patient was so lightened and so easy that he would not permit it."[46] A month later they were called back to see the patient as his swelling had returned. Pott noticed that his face was more pale and wan than before and that the man complained more of thirst and languor. Once again they drained the scrotum, but the wound never healed, and he died a fortnight later.

Pott dwelled on the question as to when to operate and when not to operate, mulling it over in many of his cases. In which situations should you succumb to the wishes of patients, family members, or friends over your own good judgment? In one instance, Pott was asked to meet Dr. Francis Joseph Pahud De Valangin (1719–1785), a Swiss physician, Mr. Thomas Godman (surgeon to the Charterhouse), and Mr. Bigue (possibly Jean Bigué) regarding the case of an incarcerated hernia:[47]

> Perhaps there is not in the practice of surgery a point which requires more judgment, firmness, or delicacy than to determine the precise time, beyond which this operation

> [for incarcerated hernia] should not be deferred, and for a surgeon to conduct himself so as to induce a patient to submit to it early enough for his preservation. The time in which a piece of gut will become gangrenous from stricture, or get into a state approaching to that of gangrene, is extremely uncertain, and depends on circumstances which no man can forsee.[48]

Pott advised against operating in this case, believing it was too late. He stated, "This was truly my opinion, and I gave it as such." The patient's wife demanded that Pott carry out the operation and "to avoid seeming to be either careless or brutal, I was prevailed on to divide the parts."[49] What he found was horrifying:

> The scrotum, integuments in the groin, and hernial sac were completely, and truly mortified; the portion of intestine, which certainly was not less than three inches, was in the same state, sunk, empty, [having burst] and as black as a coal; the offence (smell) was terrible; but the man suffered no pain as the parts were totally void of sensation.[50]

Pott left the rotten intestine intact, believing that the man would die soon. But the patient somehow survived, although he was left in a poor physical state.

Pott's reluctance to operate except when the condition required it or when the patient was insistent is confirmed in the letters of the influential writer Dr. Samuel Johnson (1709–1784).[51] In a brief note dated 20 September 1783, Johnson wrote to Reverend Taylor in Ashburne, Derbyshire, that he had a:

> dreadful disease that nothing but Mr. Pott's knife can remove, and the operation is not without danger, but I think it more prudent to venture, than to delay what must probably be done at last, and will be less safe, as it is procrastinated longer. I commit myself to eternal and infinite Mercy.[52]

Pott examined the enlarged testicle, which Johnson had presumed was a simple hydrocele, and told him that it was in fact a flesh swelling. Johnson was suffering from a sarcocele, or testicular tumor, that was presumed to be either cancerous or pre-cancerous. Pott informed Johnson that he would plan to remove the testicle after he returned from a visit to Lincolnshire. Johnson wrote to his close friend, the writer Mrs. Hester Thrale (1721–1821) that Pott had diagnosed the sarcocele after puncturing it with a trocar and warned Johnson that gangrene might set in if the sarcocele was not excised.[53] However, the swelling went down so much after being punctured that by early October Johnson was writing to Mrs. Thrale:

> Mr. Pot upon re-examination think it best, since Nature has done so much, to look quietly on, and see what it will do more. I proposed another orifice, which I think Mr. Cruikshank seems to approve, but Mr. Pot thinks not proper. The operation is therefore at least suspended, but the tumour is found not scirrous, [*sic*] and therefore

> not likely to corrupt any other part; and, say Pot, "one would not carry fire and sword further than is necessary."[54]

Johnson had been assured that the swelling was only local and wrote to John Mudge, a surgeon in Plymouth, that Pott told him it "indicates no depravity of the constitution" or cancer being present.[55] But Johnson was naturally worried, and while "it were madness to demand to solicite the excision" and he could "scarcely believe" that "the diseased part will cure itself," no matter what Pott told him. Mudge and the physician William Heberden seem to have vehemently pressed Johnson to have the sarcocele excised, while the surgeon and anatomist, Mr. William Cruikshank vacillated, and Pott stood firm.[56] Johnson reported in a letter to Mrs. Thrale on 27 October:

> I have this day a letter from Mr. Mudge; who, with all his earnestness for operation, thinks it is better to wait the effects of time, and, as he says, to let well alone. To this the patient naturally inclines, though I am afraid of having the knife yet to endure when I can bear it less. Cruikshank was even now in doubt on the event; but Pott, though never eager, had, or discovered, less fear.[57]

And on 1 November, "Mr. Pott bad(e) me this day take no more care about the tumour."[58]

Johnson's anxiety and desire to have the testicle removed while he felt strong enough to bear the operation versus his feeling some relief that his primary surgeon was advocating a wait and see approach is apparent in the letters he fired off to his friends and other medical men.[59] He was careful to write to Mudge that, "The operation is not delayed by any fears or objections of mine."[60]

One of the most frequently discussed medical encounters concerning Dr. Johnson and the Thrale family is that of Pott's diagnosis of Ralph Thrale (1773–1775). Hester Thrale kept a "Family Book" in which she recorded the health of her children and husband. Ralph was her ninth child, and his mother blamed her "vexations" or constant worries over the health of her family on his "heavy stupid & drowsy" state and the lack of "Wit sparkle in his Eyes like the Mother in Gay's Fables."[61] After Ralph's death in July 1775 Hester confided in the Family Book that she was scared to give Queeney, her eldest daughter, mercury for worms, remarking, "I think the Mercury Ralph took in the Small-Pox injured his Intellects. Tin and Wormseed are safer, if not so efficacious."[62] Ralph had been one-year-old when Daniel Sutton inoculated him, and Hester noted that he had a severe reaction and had barely the strength afterwards to cope with the discomfort of teething.[63] Here was a mother desperately seeking an explanation for her son's chronic condition.

In late spring 1775 Hester recorded a visit by Pott "the great Surgeon" to remove a polyp or growth from inside her husband's nose. After the operation was performed, Mr. Thrale insisted that Pott should see Ralph. Mrs. Thrale became distraught at the thought of Pott diagnosing her son and of the grave prognosis that might result:

> I was very unwilling, he was sick, he was asleep/I said/or any thing to keep him out of Sight; but come down he must, so I fetched him: ["] What d'ye talk of Sickness & Teething ["] cries out the Man immediately! "This Boy is in a State of Fatuity, either by Accident, or more probably from his birth, you may see he labours under some nervous Complaint that has affected his Intellects; for his Eyes gave not the Look of another Child sick or well.[64]

The diagnosis devastated Hester, who wrote in her Family Book:

> Oh how this dreadful Sentence did fill me with Horror! & how dismal are now the thoughts of all future Connection with this unhappy Child!" A Thing to hide & be ashamed of whilst we live: Johnson gives me what Comfort he can, and laments he can give no more.[65]

Scholars have famously described Pott as brutal for the way in which he told Mrs. Thrale that her son was irreparably damaged.[66] Certainly, as recorded in the Family Book, Pott appeared to be exasperated and out of patience with a mother who did everything she could to keep her son away from Pott. Mrs. Thrale's reaction to Pott's diagnosis was to remove Ralph from her presence. In contrast to his wife, Mr. Thrale appeared to suffer no qualms about Ralph's condition. Hester described him as "a happy man! he likes Ralph in his Sight as well as e'er a (any other) Child he has, and wonders/at/me for fretting that he is to be an Idiot."[67] Ralph was sent to Brighthelmstone with his nurse to try the sea air, but when his mother visited him there, she found him worse off. Ralph died in mid-July 1775, aged nineteen months. An autopsy found little Ralph's brain "almost dissolved in water & something amiss too in the original Conformation of the Head" and confirmed Pott's diagnosis and prognosis: Ralph was damaged from birth and had no hope of recovery. (He may have suffered from congenital hydranencephaly.[68]) Mrs. Thrale ended her description of the autopsy with "This poor Child is much better dead than alive.[69]

Pott treated another of Samuel Johnson's friends, James Boswell (1740–95), for symptoms of gonorrhea. The Scottish lawyer, author, diarist, and biographer of Johnson consulted Pott, along with other surgeons, on several occasions between May and October 1768.[70] In 1769 Boswell described Pott as "sensible, neat, and fine."[71] Pott treated him again for the same condition for the fee of one guinea in

July of 1785. After Pott's death, James Earle inherited Boswell as a patient and saw him on several occasions in 1790.[72] Earle treated Boswell's severe post-gonorrheal urethral stricture (caused by multiple bouts of the illness) with sounding, or the insertion of a probe to open the passage to allow urine to flow. This was a painful and potentially fatal condition.

Venereal problems were understandably stressful for patients. Mr. J. Spens of London wrote to William Cullen, an Edinburgh physician, on 6 June 1782 about his anxiety and anger at having a venereal affliction.[73] Spens explained that he believed that a recent bout of illness had "placed me in a very unpleasant Situation." Assuming he was experiencing a "fresh infection" Spens went to see John Hunter, who thought the symptoms were not venereal and prescribed Dr. James' Powders (a popular fever remedy), which only made him feel worse.[74] Hunter then had Spens take, "Mercury for 12 or 14 Days X. which did me no service. He then desired me to take nothing for a few Days."[75]

The unhappy patient, "in Vexation," went to see Pott, who had cured him of the Clap twice before (except for the Discharge) with four or five pills of "Balsamick medicine."[76] This time Pott gave him three pills, and Spens told Cullen that he had taken two of them but they had not helped. The pain and swelling in his testicle increased, and he found it impossible to urinate. Fearing a stricture the patient took forty drops of a strengthening balsam, which only made matters worse, and he was forced to insert a bougie to pass urine. Spens recovered briefly but now:

> in consequence of my having an Emission last night I have been once oblyged to use the Bougie and am not a little apprehensive I shall have to use it again—Mr. Potts has no Idea of going further than removing the Gonorrhœa. He thinks I must be satisfied with having a running—[that?] I am convinced wont do, because the slightest Cold, the smallest Deviation in my living Diet or the least excess in Drinking brinks on the Stricture by occasioning a Stoppage of the Discharge.[77]

Spens was desperate to get rid of the discharge, or gleet, and asked Cullen his opinion of the hot bath Pott had recommended if the stricture returned, noting that "it is a piece of great Luxury."

Spens continued with choice words about Hunter:

> Mr. Hunter in talking of my general Complaint is quite the Surgeon pulling but little faith in the Use of inward Medicines, He talk of knocking of excrescences in the Urethra as a Mason would in forming the Stone to the Building. and if you wont Allow Him the Use of the Chisel or [illegible], or in Other Words the Caustick or Bougie, He has but little Idea of curing the Disorder.[78]

Hunter thought that surgery was the only answer and that inward medicines such as those prescribed by Pott were only a temporary measure. Spens told Cullen that Hunter had told him about a Gentleman from Lisbon who was cured by "applying a Blister behind the Scrotum," and even though Hunter supposed this was for a temporary stricture, "however He is for my trying [it]." Spens asked Cullen if he thought this "might be tryed without Danger Because he [Hunter] acts with so bold a Hand." He added further remarks over the next few days, describing his pain, spasms, and the effect of the weather on his health, for a violent hailstorm had given Spens a "Slight return of the Influenza." He believed he was improving, though, thanks to Cullen's Balsamick Medicine. The pain had stopped Spens from riding, and he worried that he would gain weight as a result being prone to a fullness of habit. Spens must have been fraught because of the various offers for medical and surgical aid and promises of a temporary and perhaps even a permanent solution to his pain.

Dr. Cullen replied to Mr. Spens on 19 June 1782.[79] He sympathized with the patient's worries and poor condition before turning to the opinions of the surgeons Spens had consulted, "I am sorry to find it Mr Potts opinion that you cannot expect ever to be free of Some gleet and I am afraid he has some reason for thinking so but at the same time I am of your opinion that this would keep you always in a very ticklish State …"[80] Cullen recognized that the patient was as much concerned about the gleet as he was about the Clap or having gonorrhea. Pott had disappointingly told Spens that he didn't see any way to remove the discharge while Hunter had recommended an operation in such brutal terms that it had frightened Spens. Cullen's advice sidestepped the danger of criticizing Pott or Hunter and their treatments:

> You must first get quit of your gonorrhea and all the Symptoms which have any connexion with it Such as the pain of your testicles and as I suspect the daily Strictures. Your Surgeons one or other must judge of all this and when they Shall be of opinion that you are free of the gonorrhea I shall then advise what I think may be proper to obviate gleet & all its consequences.[81]

Cullen condemned Hunter's idea of a applying a blister or caustic to the scrotum and added that he saw no harm in Pott's recommendation of hot baths. The letter ended with advice about not rushing to take medicines whenever he feared he had a new infection or stricture, and for him to eat "a spare diet" to keep "down your fullness."[82]

In lectures on the diseases of the urethra, including "the gleet" or the discharge that accompanied gonorrhea, Pott told his pupils that:

> a great many people who have a desease, attend'd with a difficulty in making water, are subject to rigors … when you introduce a probe or a Bougie, they shiver violently and then get a fever—believes this occurs with disease of the neck of the bladder.[83]

Pott then gave a case about a gentleman on Carmon Street who had "a difficulty making water." He examined the man over his protests, as the patient fearfully told Pott that after treatment for the stricture he would experience shakes or rigors and a fever. Pott inserted a bougie but couldn't push it through the stricture. He then observed the patient, and as the man himself had predicted, "In about a Quarter of an hour he was seiz'd with such a severe Rigor, that I thought it would knock all his teeth out ..."[84] While he was on the subject of frightening sights that could occur when treating or examining the genitals, Pott followed this case history with a caution regarding phimosis—or when the foreskin of the penis cannot be retracted:

> Lect. 31. On the Phymosis
> When the prepuce can't be drawn back over ye Glans Penis from any inflammation or any other cause, it is call'd a Phymosis ... sometimes the Prepuce becomes gangrenous and this is very alarming to the young Surgeon.[85]

In 1780 Pott attempted to alleviate an acute episode of urine retention from having developed a stricture in Dr. John Fothergill (1712–80), a well-known Quaker physician. He managed with difficulty to pass a catheter but the condition returned and Fothergill died in great pain two weeks after Pott saw him.[86]

Operating on the bowels for hernias and strictures was likewise not to be taken lightly. Sometime between 1778 and 1781 Pott operated on a young woman for a suspected strangulated femoral hernia.[87] This was a medical emergency as the hernia was blocking blood supply and could lead to necrosis, dry gangrene, and death. The deliberate way in which Pott operated and the trouble he encountered while doing so is engagingly captured in the clinical notes for the case. The patient had first been treated with "costive applications," or medications for constipation, which proved unsuccessful. Her other symptoms most likely included nausea, vomiting, and crippling abdominal pain. The woman's perilous state is captured in a few sentences: "her pulse was small quick and fluttering ... and everything failing Mr. Pott determined upon the operation."[88]

The operation for strangulating hernia involved cutting down on the hernia, opening the hernia sac, and releasing the constricting ring. The case note states that Pott:

> began by making an incision towards the Labia pudendi thro' the skin and membrane adipose which was rather thick, he then came to some cellular substance which he carefully separated through and then introduced his probe in the puncture he had made to feel if he could in the cavity of the Labial Sac, but could not pass it up and down so freely as if he had been in one of the Herniated Sac, he then as cautiously replaced what was under it, when as soon as he had made a small opening into it out came a vast quantity of most offensive blackish matter with a faecal

> putrid smell, he then endeavord [*sic*] to raise his probe upwards but it wd. not pass through the ring.[89]

Pott attempted to force his finger and then his smallest probe through the ring but found that, "in every pass" the intestine was too tightly adhered to the ring. At this point Pott commented to the young house physician, who was observing and taking notes, that he could find no safe place to insert a knife in order to divide the ring without wounding the intestine and perhaps even piercing a nearby artery. Pott gave up trying:

> The intestine was black and in a gangrenous state it was left as it was found: Mr. Pott intending if she had lived 'till next day to divide the Intestine and give her the chance of an Artificial Anus.[90]

Pott was going to try to resection the bowel out of the abdominal wall and so create a stoma, or artificial anus (colostomy). Pott told the house physician that the intestine was in such an awful state because of the stricture. The house physician asked Pott, "if a probe could not be passed through the ring to divide it, how could an artificial anus be produced there?" This was an excellent question, and no clear answer is recorded in the book, perhaps because Pott was well aware that the young woman was dying. Even if Pott could have carried out a colostomy, chances were that the patient would not have lived long and the constant flow of fecal matter from the intestines would have been distressing and made her life miserable. Pott performed a postmortem examination on the young woman with Dr. William Pitcairn, one of the physicians at St. Bartholomew's Hospital, in attendance. The woman had been suffering from an inoperable femoral hernia.[91] Pott even tried to part the intestine from the ring during the autopsy but was unable to do so. He used the opportunity to satisfy his curiosity and to confirm the futility of having operated in this case.

A postmortem on another of Pott's patients with urinary blockage revealed the difficulty of ensuring a bougie did not fall out or be pulled out by a patient. The man, aged 39, was admitted to the hospital on 4 June in either 1785 or 1786. He had experienced pain on urination after receiving a blow to the perineum and scrotum and now was unable to pass urine at all. Pott inserted a bougie, which gave the patient some relief. But Pott related that the nurses neglected to check that the bougie remained in place, and when his dresser, a Mr. Robert, finally examined the patient, the bougie had been out for two days, and the man was in "terrible pain and distension of the bladder." Whatever had happened, the damage was done, and "Mr Robert the dresser, desired me to meet him [Pott] at 4 o'clock in the afternoon, when we found our patient very restless." They tried cathartics and bleeding to calm the man and had him placed in a warm bath, where he passed some bloody urine. The next day the patient was very ill, and he died on 22 June.[92] A paragraph "Appearances after Death" follows this account, which described the postmortem. Essentially the abdomen was opened, the kidneys laid bare, and the bladder opened. Inside it was found 2 quarts of bloody water, the bladder neck was inflamed and Pott could not get the probe in; a huge ulcer in the urethra had sloughed away, "which prevented the introduction of the catheter … this is sufficient I think to account for the death of the patient, and likewise satisfy me that nothing more could be done to save his Life."[93] Even if the bougie had remained in the ureter, there was no hope for the patient to recover.

Since hernias and hydroceles were chronic conditions, some patients, both poor and rich, naturally became regulars. They included "A drunken, idle, fellow" who had a small omental hernia. He had constantly been supplied with trusses, which he often wore wrongly, "but being much oftener drunk than sober, he seldom wore it at all, and when he did it was seldom in the right place."[94] Another gentleman had shown Pott his rupture many times over the years. It troubled him now and then to the point that he told Pott that he could not wear a truss to keep it in his abdomen and "the waistband on his breeches if buttoned tight was troublesome."[95] Suddenly the man became ill with all the symptoms of a stricture, or possibly an incarcerated hernia (he could not return the intestine to his abdomen when he was supine), and called Pott to his bedside in fear of his life. Fortunately Pott was able to reduce the hernia by hand.

In *A Treatise on Ruptures*, Pott wrote about ruptures that could not be reduced—that is, pushed back into the abdomen:

> Irreducible ruptures generally occur from long-term neglect of them, patients have contented themselves with wearing a suspensory or bag-truss … People in this situation should be particularly careful not to make any attempts beyond their strength, nor aim at feats of agility; they should take care to suspend the loaded scrotum, and to keep it out of the way of all harm from pressure, bruise, etc. When the tumor is very large, a soft quilted bolster should be worn at the bottom of the suspensory to prevent excoriation, and the scrotum should be frequently washed for the same reason …[96]

Pott added that just because these chronic hernias appear stable, the patient should not be misled into thinking that they would always remain so. The treatment Pott generally used to return a hernia that could not be pushed back by hand into the abdominal cavity was a tobacco smoak-glyster, or clysma fumiosum.[97] He used this technique in the belief that tobacco fumes reduced ruptures by quieting peristaltic motion.[98] Pott described one successful treatment:

> When about half an hour had been spent in the continual impulsion of the smoak, the man cried out, My rupture is going up: and, in the space of two or three minutes, it did so, with a noise which was heard by every one in the room.[99]

In 1780 Pott's former apprentice, Peter Clare, described the machines used to push tobacco smoke into the rectum:

> The particular machines for conveying the tobacco are either a pair of bellows with a worm tube, or large syringe, by which means great quantities of the smoke of this powerfully stimulating plant are thrown into the inflamed but torpid intestines, frequently procuring a copious evacuation of their indurated contents, and a return of the *hernia*, when all other means had been tried with out success.
>
> Some surgeons prefer the infusion of the tobacco to the fumes, which are injected glysterwise, and with equal success.—The infusion is made by pouring one pint of boiling water on one drachm of tobacco.[100]

As Pott blithely told his pupils, "We can throw into the Rectum such Substances that we cannot throw into the Stomach …"[101] But Pott cautioned that tobacco can be abused and made too strong; friends of the patient should look out for "a Sickness and Stupour so common to young Smokers."[102]

If tobacco did not work to encourage the gut to calm and return to the abdomen, "a composition of salt, honey and aloes, boiled to the proper consistence of a suppository" could be tried. "By these I have seen very alarming ruptures returned, when they have been thought capable of being relieved by nothing but the chirurgical operation."[103]

Pott included cases of hydrocele and hernia at the end of several case histories because they amused and fascinated him and he assumed the same would be the true of his readers. One concerns a poor fellow who worked with a farmer at Islington and came to the hospital with a hugely swollen scrotum:

> The man said, "Sir, I can get rid of it all by pissing, but it fills again in a few hours, especially if I drink." Upon my seeming to disbelieve what he said, he took up his scrotum, and squeezing it together with some violence, discharged the whole by the urethra.[104]

Pott's final case history in *Observations of Ruptures* describes a rare ovarian hernia.[105] The patient was a 23-year-old woman who had been admitted to the hospital because of two small swellings in the groin. She had not been able to work as a servant for two months because of pain from the tumors. Pott described the woman as in full health, large breasted, stout, and with regular menses. She was originally Nourse's patient, and Nourse had tried in vain to push the swellings back into two openings he found in her groin "that they had clearly passed out." Pott was called to the ward to try to push them back, and then Mr. Peter Sainthill, another surgeon, did the same. Both were unsuccessful. The woman was desperate and "being incapacitated from getting her bread, and desirous to submit to anything for relief, it was agreed to remove them." The operation was successful with a "body so exactly resembling a human ovarium" being extracted from each swelling.[106] Pott ended this case history with evidence that he had continued to follow the patient for quite a long time:

> She has enjoyed good heath ever since, but is become thinner and more apparently muscular; her breasts, which were large are gone; nor has she ever menstruated since the operation, which is now some years.[107]

Pott rarely included what might be considered even mildly salacious material in his lectures or works. However, an anonymous student recorded the following account in a lecture on diseases of the uterus. Pott described an imperfect vagina that had been mistaken for a prolapsed uterus. When he cut into it:

> half a common pail of blood of a thin serous nature was discharged, the belly shrunk amazingly and you might have put a child of six months old into the Vagina, but before the woman left the hospital, it contracted to the size of a woman who has had 3 or 4 Children, the patient was twenty-two years of age, and I suppose had, had menses since sixteen or seventeen—I remember another case, where the patient had the face, breasts and every other distinction of a female except a Vagina and Uterus, neither of these existed, nor any thing to supply their place, and this person, never had any signs of Menstruation.[108]

In the *London Magazine* of May 1771, a review appeared of Pott's *An Account of the Method of obtaining a perfect or radical Cure of the Hydrocele or Watery Rupture, by Means of a Seton*. Pott had been experimenting with first piercing the tunica vaginalis or serous covering of an enlarged testicle, draining off the fluid with a cannula, and then inserting a seton consisting of "ten or twelve strings of candle-wick cotton."[109] Pott's goal was to irritate and inflame the walls of the tunica vaginalis and of the inner tunica albuginea, and encourage them to join together over the course of ten to fourteen days. This would close the space that the build up of the fluid had created and, hopefully, prevent a recurrence of the "watry rupture." It also would preserve the testicle. Pott argued his case in typical fashion: first, by describing the anatomy of the parts; second, by pointing out the confusion that reigned over what treatment to try to cure testicular swellings from the time of the ancients to the present; third, by explaining which surgeons' ideas he had been impressed by (Monro secundus) and which he had found lacking (Cheselden); and finally, by detailing his new simple method of permanently curing the problem with examples of cases from the hospital. The *London Magazine* summed up Pott's account of his method with:

> Mr. Pott's reputation in his profession is so universally established, that when he promises a radical cure of the watery rupture, and tells us he has been repeatedly successful in the use of a seton, we are satisfied the afflicted in this particular complaint, will pay a proper regard to so respectable an authority.[110]

As seen in this section, ruptures and hernias were generally not life-threatening conditions unless a strangulation or permanent stricture occurred. Pott preferred to operate when the need to do so had been established for certain, because the patient's condition made it difficult for them to earn their living or to appear in public. Uncertainty, Pott wrote was far worse for a surgeon to deal with than hazard or the danger that carrying out an operation might cause more pain and suffering for the patient.[111] Whether hazards existed in operating could be answered with experiments on patients using new methods, but uncertainty could not be removed and would (and should) always trouble the conscience of any surgeon.

Deformity and Paralysis

In 1779 Pott published his *Observations on the Necessity and the Propriety of Amputation in certain cases, and under certain circumstances* (discussed in the previous chapter). It was sold with another essay, *Remarks on that kind of Palsy of the Lower Limbs which is frequently found to accompany Curvature of the Spine, and is supposed to be caused by it. Together with its method of cure.* For the price of one shilling and sixpence, Pott offered his advice on amputations and also told of his experiments in making artificial abscesses on children and adults with crooked spines or paralyzed legs. On the title page of the two works, Pott includes a quotation from the Praefatio of *Medicinae Historia Sanorum Regimen*, Liber 1, by the Roman medical writer, Aulus Cornelius Celsus: "Verumque est ad ipsam curandi rationem nihil plus conferre quam experientiam" (And it is true that nothing conduces more to the rational method itself of curing than experience). This aptly summed up the underpinnings of Pott's statements concerning how to treat what would become known within a few decades as "Pott's palsy."[112] Pott remarked:

> The disease of which I mean to speak, is generally called a palsy, as it consists in a total or partial abolition of the power of using, and sometimes of even moving the lower limbs, in consequence, as is generally supposed, of a curvature of some part of the spine. To this distemper both sexes, and all ages, are equally liable. If the patient be an

> infant, it becomes as object of constant, though unavailing distress to its parents; if an adult, he is rendered perfectly helpless to himself, and useless to all others, which, of all possible states, is surely the very worst.[113]

Pott first explained how palsy (meaning some to all loss of voluntary motion) manifested itself in infants (under the age of two), children, and adults. He discussed how parents, nurses, and patients themselves gave reasons for the symptoms of weak legs and a bent spine. In infants the explanation concerned delayed development, for "the child is uncommonly backward in the use of his legs, or is thought to have received some hurt at birth."[114] Where a child was already able to walk, the disease slowly affects their gait and they complain:

> of being very soon tired, is languid, listless, and unwilling to move much, or at all briskly; in no great length of time after this he may be observed frequently to trip, and stumble, although there be no impediment in his way; and whenever he attempts to move briskly, he finds that his legs involuntarily cross each other, by which he is frequently thrown down ...[115]

Eventually the knees would give way, and the feet droop down. In adults the disease progressed more quickly with stiffened ankle joints and a loss of sensation in the legs. It is not until the curvature of the spine was noted, however, that the patient and their family or friends realize that this is not simply a nervous palsy from a back injury but something far more serious.

Mechanical devices such as "steel stays, the swing, the screw chair, and other pieces of machinery" were tried "in order to restore the spine to its true and natural figure."[116] James Lind of Fleet Street was one proprietor who provided such devices, and in 1734 his trade card advertised the manufacture and sale of:

> all Sorts of Instruments for Lame and Crooked. Likewise Steel or Belt Trusses for Ruptures in Men, Women, or Children proceeding from any Cause Whatsoever. Also Streight Stockings, Steel Stays, Collars, Ham-Screws & Swings to prevent Children being crooked.[117]

Lind, like others in the business, provided physicians, surgeons, and families with devices to correct or prevent deformity.

If pressed, Pott most likely would have referred his patients to Holmes & Laurie, who were conveniently located on Bartholomew Close, adjacent to the hospital, although he had little faith in the utility of their products for some diseases. Their trade card advertised them as "workmen" to the major hospitals in London who could provide steel springs, trusses, collars, neck-swings, strait stockings, and steel bodices. Mrs. Holmes was available to attend the "Female Sex."[118]

Yet Pott commented that none of these devices could help a patient with this type of palsy and that the person will live in pain, unable to breathe or eat properly, with "involuntary flux of urine and faeces," until they:

> die in an exhausted emaciated state; or, which is still worse, drags on a miserable existence, confined to a great chair, or bed, totally deprived of the power of loco-motion, and useless both to himself and others.
>
> This in an infant is most melancholy to see, in an adult most miserable to endure.[119]

Having captured the pitiful existence of those suffering from this condition, Pott then revealed how he had come to muse on the cause of these symptoms and a possible remedy. He had been touched by:

> An affecting instance of this distemper in the person of a very promising youth of fourteen years old, with whose family I was nearly connected, induced me to think more of it than perhaps I otherwise would have done; and the restoration of the use of his limbs, immediately after a seemingly accidental abscess near the part, engaged my attention still more, and became a matter of frequent, though not very satisfactory contemplation; I say unsatisfactory, because it served only to increase my doubts, without leading me toward a solution of them.[120]

Pott came to the conclusion that the palsy or paralysis of the legs was not due to some problem with the spine but rather to a predisposing factor that had yet to be discovered. In essence "we had most probably mistaken an effect for a cause."[121] In the following pages, Pott outlined his rational system of observation and experience that led to this realization. First, he had never seen nor knew of a malformation of the spine or a crooked back that led to the legs being paralyzed. Second, Pott returned to a topic that he wove throughout his lectures—the foolishness of fashion and women:

> That none of those strange twists and deviations, which the majority of European women get in their shapes, from the very absurd custom of dressing them in stays during their infancy, and which put them into all directions but the right, ever caused any thing of this kind, however great the deformity might be.[122]

Yet as Sorge-English has shown, British females in the eighteenth century used stays throughout their lives, and boys wore them until they were breeched between the ages of three to four.[123] Pott's use of the term "European" may have been a response to the writings of the French physician Nicholas Andry de Bois-Regard (1658–1742). In 1741 Andry published *L'orthopédie ou l'art de prévenir et corriger dans les enfants les difformités du corp*, which counseled parents on how to prevent and correct spinal deformities in children, among other topics. It was translated into English as *Orthopaedia or the art of correcting and preventing deformities in children* in 1743.[124] In his work, Andry recommended exercise and the attachment of weights to the pull the body into shape.

Some London physicians opposed swaddling and stays, including William Cadogan (1711–1797), who in 1750 addressed his pamphlet *An Essay on the Nursing and Management of Children from their birth to three years of age* to a Governor of the Foundling Hospital. Four years later he was appointed one of the physicians to the hospital, and his ideas were put into practice. Cadogan advocated loose, light clothing for infants, rather than swaddling:

> besides the Mischief arising from the Weight and Heat of these Swaddling-cloaths, they are put on so tight, and the Child is so cramp'd by them, that its Bowels have not room, nor the Limbs any Liberty, to act and exert themselves in the free easy Manner they ought. This is a very hurtful Circumstance, for Limbs that are not used, will never be strong, and such tender Bodies cannot bear much Pressure ...[125]

As a surgeon Pott did not address swaddling leaving it instead to his physician brethren.

Based on observations of living and dead patients, Pott was adamant in his *Remarks on that kind of Palsy of the Lower Limbs* that this palsy was not caused by a blow or a fall, or by the dislocation of vertebrae. On dissection Pott had found "thickened ligaments, carious bones and a quantity of sanies [blood-tinged fluid] lodged between the rotten bones, and the membrane investing the spinal marrow."[126]

Having made his case, Pott turned to a discussion of how he had developed a cure for palsy. The idea had come from a conversation with Dr. Thomas Cameron,[127] a physician to the Worcester Infirmary. Cameron mentioned that he had read a passage in Hippocrates about four years earlier and "noted a passage where he speaks of a paralysis of the lower limbs being cured by an abscess in the back or loins." Cameron had tried this treatment with some success and referred Pott to Mr. Henry Vaughan Jeffrys,[128] a surgeon "of eminence "at the Worcester Infirmary, who had also successfully treated a case.

Pott returned to London and carried out his experiment of making a counter irritation of an artificial abscess close to the curvature of the spine. The first patient was an infant who had lost use of "its legs for about two or three months." Pott made a cut in the flesh on one side of what he termed the projection, and inserted a dried pea. Essentially Pott was making an issue, or artificial draining wound. He:

> gave strict charge to the mother to take care that the pea was kept in; the woman, who had no faith in the remedy, did not take the proper care, and consequently the discharge was not equal to what it should, and mighty have been; but notwithstanding

> this neglect, at the end of about three weeks or a month the child was manifestly better, and began to make use of its legs; it was then seized with the small-pox and died.[129]

In another instance, a tall, thin man on crutches, aged about 35, came to Pott. He told the surgeon that he thought his injury came from lifting a heavy weight, and remarked that his legs and thighs were cold and "nummy [*sic*]."[130] Pott carefully made a seton and inserted a silk thread into cuts he made on each side of the curve in the man's back. The wife was instructed in how to change the dressing, and Pott then visited the patient every three to four days. He was delighted when after six weeks of drainage from the setons that the man reported more sensation in his legs and was using his crutches less. The man and his wife, though, distressed Pott by their lack of faith in his treatment:

> The setons had now, from not having been properly managed, worn their way out, and I would have converted them into an issue, but as neither the patient nor his wife had ever believed that the discharge had had any share in his amendment, but on the contrary that he would have been better without it, he would not submit to what I proposed, and I left him.[131]

To Pott's annoyance, when three weeks later he bumped into the patient walking in the street with just a "common cane" and asked him what he had been doing to look so well, "he told me that the sores had continued to discharge till within a few days, but that he had drank a great deal of comfrey-root[132] tea, with isinglass[133] and supposed that had cured him."[134] Pott scoffed at this remedy of herbs and dried fish air bladders, adding that he had successfully treated several patients in the last year including a twelve-year-old boy, "whose case was so truly deplorable, that I made the experiment merely to avoid the appearance of inhumanity, by discharging him as incurable, without trying something."[135] The spine of the boy was so curved that when he was held up by the arms, "the extremities of his groin touched the floor."[136] After three months of using caustics to keep wounds open and draining near his spine, he could now walk without assistance and was some inches taller.

Pott concluded his thirty-nine pages of remarks with a summary of the methods he used to make and keep a wound open. He had a preference for issues made by caustics over those made by incision or a seton, describing the latter as "painful and nasty." Pott may have learned from the two cases where the mother and wife did not cooperate and follow his instructions that setons did not last long and incisions took a long time to come to suppuration. Pott used caustics to create an eschar, or dry scab, that would fall off after a few days. He would then cut out the middle of the exposed wound and place a pea or more often a large dried kidney bean in it. To further encourage the wound to stay open and continue to drain significantly, Pott sprinkled finely powdered cantharides (a blistering agent from Spanish fly) every few days. The goal was to keep at least one wound open until the patient was totally recovered. This would take several months in most cases.[137]

Information on Pott's experiments with tubercular patients from ca. 1777 to 1779 can be gleaned through analyzing cases in his lectures and accounts by surgeons who were with him at the hospital during this time. Among these surgeons was John Jebb (1736–1786), a clergyman and a physician who was a former pupil of Dr. William Pitcairn at the hospital and had attended the lectures of William and John Hunter. In early 1779 Pott signed Jebb's Royal Society nomination certificate. Three years later Jebb published *Select Cases of the Disorder commonly termed the Paralysis of the Lower Extremities.*[138] The work was dedicated to Pott as "At an early period of my medical studies, you pointed out the path to substantial science …" Jebb explained that "the cases are transcribed from "notebooks where he took down the symptoms and appearances" and "some of the cases were under the immediate management of Mr. Pott."[139] Jebb's offered glimpses into how he was influenced by Pott in the practice of surgery. He announced that he intended to confine himself:

> to the evident symptoms; and the patient's narrative, being fully satisfied, that to describe disorders according to the forms in which they really evidence themselves to the senses, with a careful attention to the patient's feelings, is the most likely method of acquiring both a knowledge of their causes and of their cure.[140]

This stress on symptoms, stories, senses, and feelings resonates in Jebb's description of the patients that he took care of most likely under direction from Pott. One case in November 1777 concerned T.C., a 32-year-old man who, by the time he came to the hospital, told Jebb that he had "tried the cold-bath, mercurial frictions, tincture sacra, volatile liniment, a strengthening plaister to the loins, and the screw-chair." Jebb added that the "cold-bath and screw-chair were evidently hurtful."[141] He probably was responsible for applying the caustics to T.C.'s back on both sides of the "protuberance," as he describes the increased "twitching" in the man's thighs and legs that quickly followed. Over the course of six months in the hospital, T.C. gained some sensation in his feet and some control over his walking. This gradual progress continued with the recovery of the "power of expelling flatus per anum."[142] Eventually the man was discharged as being well.

Another case, that of a 21-year-old man called R.B., did not end so well. The man had fallen from a hayloft, and Jebb saw him in June 1778. He recorded his pulse as "generally 140 but once 180 strokes in a minute."[143] (Pott did not record the beats of the pulse in any of his accounts of patients, a practice more often seen among physicians than surgeons in the eighteenth-century.) R.B. died, and Jebb was disappointed that the man's friends were unwilling to "allow examination into his parts."[144]

Jebb also told of another of Pott's patients, a boy of about ten, R.S., who a year earlier had received a blow to "the pit of the stomach" that knocked him to the ground. He recovered but a week later started to complain of a loss of sensation in his legs, followed in another week by the "second dorsal vertebrae becoming protuberant." A few days later, his feet became "rigid and pointed down."[145] Dr. Pitcairn, to whom Jebb was a pupil, managed the boy's care for nine months, and when the boy was still in a terrible state, "at length he recommended him to the treatment of Mr. Pott." Jebb tells that the disease had ravaged five or six vertebrae and that the boy's back was so curved that his chin permanently rested on his breast: "The appearance was so unpromising, that Mr. Pott declared, he was induced to make trial of the caustics, merely because he would leave nothing undone in a case so truly deplorable, but that he could scarcely expect any advantage from their use." This remark suggests that R.S. may have been the pitiful case of the twelve-year-old boy that Pott described as his third experiment in *Remarks on that kind of Palsy of the Lower Limbs*. R.S. was in all likelihood Richard Simpson.

In Wellcome MS 4337, the book of clinical notes taken by one of the house physicians at the hospital from 1778 to 1781, a case is described in King Ward under the care of Pit., or Dr. Pitcairn. It is given in full below:

> King Pit.
> 1778 19, may Rich.d Simpson—8 years of age a fine & fair complexioned boy—has a palsy in the lower Extremity from a particular curviture in the spine inwards—nearly from the Ileum to the lower vertebrae of the neck. Feels no kind of pain—and has not the least sensation either in his Legs or Thighs. Is unable to move his legs, and in short they are wholly useless. His Belly and Stomach project very much outwards, partly from the pressure of the spine, and they seem themselves to be swelled. He has had this complaint 10 months, and was very healthy until then. Says his Brother kicked, and that this leaning in the spine followed.
> Has stools reg. and makes urine free.
> RxCalom. f .ij.o:n
> Lin. Vol. (Take 2 fluid ounces of Calamine, apply as a liniment)
> 19 Dr (Pitcairn) saw him, and has left him to Mr. Pott.
> 1 June Mr. Pott has done nothing for him yet.
> 11—Two Spaces were made are on each side the spine—and he seems to have been relieved by them.[146]

The patient was referred to Pott on 19 May and wasn't treated until 23 days later. Pott may have been deciding that R.S.'s case was hopeless but thinking that everything should be tried to treat the boy anyway. We can pick up the story of what happened to Richard after the caustics were applied to his back by returning to Jebb's account. The boy could move the great toe of one foot after a month and was "exhorted to attempt to move the other. ... The ancle joint got better, curve diminished and was discharged after 10 months."[147] Richard Simpson, variously described as an 8-, 10-, or 12-year-old boy, spent a total of 19 pain-filled months in the hospital and was treated first medically with a mercurial rub and then surgically with Pott's experimental issues.

A few brief references to how patient's dealt with their fate, allow glimpses of what it took to lay forlornly in a hospital bed for several months. In May of 1779, J.R. "spent 18 weeks laying in bed with wonderful patience, without perceiving the minutest alteration in the symptoms of his complaint. ..." Jebb remarks that Mr. Pott "paid remarkable attention to his case, repeatedly encouraging him to persevere."[148] After eight months he was discharged as being well. M.B., one of the few women mentioned in either Pott's or Jebb's accounts of cases of the curvature of the spine, died aged 47 in February of 1779, and a J.D. passed away the same month just a few days after the caustics were applied. Case 8, T.R. was dissected in October of 1778.

Jebb included a few more examples of patients with curvature of the spine in *Select Cases of the Disorder commonly termed the Paralysis of the Lower Extremities* (1782). In one instance a laboring man left the hospital to return to his employment before the caustics took effect. He returned and petitioned for assistance but was treated "by a person not under the immediate inspection of Mr. Pott." This person burnt the skin "three inches below the protuberance" rather than at the sides, and despite the drainage continuing over several weeks, the patient's condition did not improve. It was only when the caustics were "reapplied properly" that he recovered.[149] A girl with protuberant vertebrae and St. Vitus's dance was cured with caustics, but a man who had "been much devoted to venereal indulgences and had a defect of vital power" was less fortunate and died.[150]

Jebb also wrote of a boy about seven-years-old who was in the hospital in early 1779. Jebb tried to get the hospital to apply caustics "according to Mr. Pott's directions, but my remonstrances were in vain."[151] He implies that the death of the boy eighteen months later "when he was bent almost double" was due to an improper diagnosis of a condition called *conglobate glands*. This was a term used in Georgian surgery for the lymphatic glands of the thoracic region. Jebb wrote that:

> Not only an erroneous description of a disorder, but even the assigning of an improper name to a complaint, as Mr. Pott has repeatedly observed, leads to an improper treatment of that disorder; and thus the art of medicine often perpetuated the evils, which it is its object to remove.[152]

Two foreign-born doctors observed and commented on Pott's treatment of patients at St. Bartholomew's Hospital, Dr. Arnold Barthélemy Beerenbroeck (1751–1824), an Antwerp-born physician who studied in Louvain, Paris, and Leyden, and Dr. Johann Hunczovsky (1752–1798), a Czech-born surgeon to the Emperor of Austria and director of the Josephinum, a military surgical teaching institute in Vienna. Beerenbroeck quickly translated Pott's *Remarks on that Kind of Palsy* into French and had it published in Brussels in 1780. Two letters from Hunczovsky in London to Alexander von Brambilla in Vienna have survived that describe in words and drawings Pott's treatment of curvature of the spine. Brambilla (1728–1800) was Body Surgeon to the Emperor Joseph II and in 1778 had been appointed Sole Superintendent of the Army Health Service.[153] He was also responsible for sending Hunczovsky to London in 1779 to gain further medical training. In 1783 Hunczovsky published *Medicinisch-Chirurgische Beobachtungen auf seinen Reisen durch England und Frankreich, besonders ueber die Spitaler* (Medical-Surgical Observations in travels through England and France, particularly in hospitals), which included a few pages on Pott's palsy. Brambilla, however, had already published *Instrumentarium Chirurgicum Viennese* in Vienna in 1780, which included a description of Pott's methods.

Hunczovsky wrote his first letter (in Italian) to Brambilla in June 1779 to report that Pott was using cauterization to treat curvatures of the spine that caused paralysis of the legs. He told Brambilla that Hippocrates had observed that paralysis was cured when an abscess was formed near the site of the curvature and that a surgeon named Jones had read this and experimented with some patients in England. Hunczovsky may have confused Jones and Jeffrys here. He continued:

> Mr. Pott introduced this method of treatment for similar ailments in St. Bartholomew's Hospital; not all, but some are cured. Two of these patients are being treated at the moment, one aged 37, the other 14; the former fell on his spine three years ago and became paralysed in the lower limbs; the tumour which is now formed by the vertebrae developed imperceptibly. The latter suffered the same accident in infancy.[154]

To help Brambilla envisage where Pott had applied the caustics, Hunczovsky drew sketches of two patients, one a man and the other a boy, sitting up in bed with their bare backs revealed and two eschars visible on either side of their spines. He added that several weeks of suppuration had benefitted both patients and that the boy was starting to walk unaided. His second letter in August 1779 confirmed that the patients were nearly cured and had been sent to convalesce in the countryside.

Pott's treatments were gaining prominence throughout Europe. The surgeon's *Remarks on that kind of Palsy of the Lower Limbs* (1789) was quickly translated into French, and in 1782 Pott issued another essay on the disorder titled *Farther*

Remarks on the useless State of the Lower Limbs, in consequence of a Curvature of the Spine. Notably he had dropped the word palsy from the title. Pott commented on the success of his publication and that he had "received such manifold and repeated testimony of the success of the proposed method" from "eminent practitioners, not only in this town and kingdom, but in many other parts of Europe." For Pott this was empirical proof that the treatment he had suggested could now be considered as a "universal" cure.[155] The focus of the publication was to give a fuller picture of the morbid anatomy of the vertebrae. It included six engravings of the changes he had observed in the bones as the disease progressed. Pott also outlined how difficult it was to diagnose the disorder based on the multitude of symptoms that could be manifested, remarking that "In an adult it passes for rheumatism, or gravel, or a sprain."[156] The true cause of the disease lay not in the helpless state of the legs; therefore machinery, "particularly the swing and the screw … always have been and ever must be unsuccessful."[157] Pott now recommended that the sores be made large enough to hold several peas, and the discharge should be maintained by "means of orange peas, cantharides in fine powder, aerugo aeris (verdigris—a corrosive), or any such application as may best serve the intended purpose, which should be that of a large and long continued drain."[158] Finally Pott named what he believed to be the underlying cause of all the problems, namely scrophula or tuberculosis:

> That is, that same kind of indisposition as occasions the thick upper lip, the tedious obstinate opthalmy, [*sic*] the indurated glands under the chin, and in the neck, the obstructed mesentery, the hard dry cough, the glairy [slimy] swellings of the wrist and ancles [*sic*], the thickened ligaments of the joints, the enlargement and caries of the bones, &c., &c., &c.[159]

The French physician Claude-François Duchanoy (1742–1827)[160] translated *Farther Remarks* into French in 1785, and it was published in Paris as *Du mal vertebral ou de l'impotence des extrémités inférieures, qui reconnoît pour cause un vice de Colonne Epinière; avec le moyen de la guérir*. French medical men praised both of Pott's essays, and by the early nineteenth century Pott's palsy was referred to as "La Maladie du Pott" and a little later as "Paraplegie Pottique."[161]

Pott continued to be interested in cases of spinal curvature and paralysis of the legs until the end of his life, as a volume of transcribed lecture notes by an anonymous pupil show. At the back of the book several cases from the 1780s are listed, including two concerning curvature of the spine. One details the last few months in the life of Thomas Baker, a sixteen-year-old.[162] He was admitted to the hospital on 4 October with a history of spasms in his legs and a "small projection of the ninth dorsal vertebrae from the neck"[163] that had gotten much bigger in the preceding six months. The boy developed a hacking cough that brought up blood-streaked pus along with night sweats. On admission the curvature of Thomas's spine was so large that "he could not bear the present incumbent weight of his trunk, he could not walk without supporting the upper part of his body with his hands upon his knees …[164] and he was to all appearance in a dying condition."[165] Pott diagnosed him as having scrophulous, and caustics were applied. Thomas appeared to get much better but when the issues stopped draining, he fell victim "to his last enemy."[166]

The case that preceded Thomas Baker's concerned a fourteen-year-old boy and was listed under one word—"Paralysis."[167] He was admitted in January 1786 when his friends were advised to send him to the hospital because for the past five weeks he had been unable to use his legs. He was admitted under the care of James Earle. One week later Pott:

> advises a caustic to be applied to each side of the spinous processes of the os sacrum … 'he issue was made so large as to admit 12 pease, after it had discharged for 3 weeks the boy began to find a numbness with a gentle perspiration attack. …[168]

The boy recovered and within seven weeks could walk well with sticks but a note at the end added that he should perhaps have issues made to help the paralysis in his arm.

A War of Words: William Hunter and Percivall Pott

From 1756 to 1764 William Hunter and Percivall Pott engaged in a war of words over who had first identified and, therefore, had the right to discuss in print, a condition known as congenital or congenial hernia. While this dispute has been examined from the viewpoint of who was in the right, an analysis of the ways in which the argument progressed reveals in a microcosm the competing claims of hospital surgeons and anatomy schools to new knowledge in Georgian London.[169] As Roy Porter declared, William Hunter viewed his Windmill School "rather like the lyceums of classical philosophers, as a self-defining community of the *cognoscenti*, [where] Hunter regarded unfolding his discoveries within the walls of his 'private college' a bona fide form of 'publication.'"[170] Essentially for Hunter, knowledge gained from viewing specimens in his school was private property and needed to be defended if stolen.

The dispute over who first discovered how an inguinal hernia, generally seen in infant boys, was formed began in February 1757 when Pott had published a short treatise titled *An account of a particular kind of rupture, frequently attendant upon new-born children; and sometimes met with in adults; Viz. that in which the intestine, or omentum, is found in the same cavity, and in contact with the testicle.* It was dedicated not to another medical man but to Nicholas Linwood, Esq. (d. 1773), a London wine merchant and former director of the East India Company. Pott at this time was still recovering from his horse accident and was likely dependent on the generosity of others to sustain him and the family through this period. The treatise was anatomical rather than surgical in tone, although Pott did include a handful of cases towards the end. This became important in the dispute that followed, for Hunter accused Pott of stealing his idea about how the congenital hernia developed in the fetus and was manifested in the adult body from specimens that his brother, John, had shown Pott at the Windmill Street anatomy school in 1756.

Before tracing the chronology of the countering claims of ownership to this anatomical discovery, it is necessary to explain what a congenital, or congenial, hernia was. Pott described it thus:

> The Congenial Hernia as it is now called, is that particular kind of hernia, in which the portion of intestine or omentum, which occasions the tumor, instead of being found alone in the hernia sac [as in a common rupture] is found in contact with the naked testicle; the bag containing them being formed by the *tunica vaginalis testis*.[171]

By 1763, when Pott wrote this definition, several charges had been leveled against him by the Hunters and their friends. Pott acknowledged this in the paragraph following his description of the hernia:

> On this species of rupture, a few years ago I published a small tract; [An Account of a particular kind of rupture, & c.] on which some reflections were made in the Critical Review, insinuating that I had borrowed the subject or matter of them from Professor Haller, or Dr. Hunter. [March, 1757][172]

Pott stated he ignored the insinuations of plagiarism, as he believed the criticism had not come from William Hunter himself but instead from one of his pupils. It was not until Hunter had published his *Medical Commentaries No. 1* with further accusations of Pott's behavior that Pott responded, concerned that silence might imply that he was guilty of such malevolent acts. In his defense Pott laid out a series of ideas and actions that led him to the discovery of the congenital hernia and which point to an uneasy relationship between hospital surgeons and anatomy school owners.

First, Pott acknowledged that other prominent surgeons had speculated on the formation of the congenital hernia, including Samuel Sharp (ca. 1709–1778). Pott had not been convinced by Sharp's explanation of the issue and added in a jibe at Hunter's ungentlemanly behavior that "Mr. Sharp has too much good sense to be offended when I say that this account did by no means satisfy me."[173] Sharp was senior surgeon to Guy's Hospital and a renowned writer of works on operative techniques. In 1746, due to ill health, he relinquished a course on anatomy, surgery, and bandages that he offered to a society of naval surgeons in Covent Garden to his sometime pupil William Hunter. Sharp's course became the foundation of Hunter's anatomy school.

Pott continued his account that sometime in late 1753 or early 1754 he had gone to hear Hunter give a "publick lecture at Surgeons Hall on male parts of generation."[174] He went because "Hunter was an ingenious enquirer into the animal economy and had the opportunity to inspect many dead bodies."[175] Pott asserted that Hunter didn't give any new information in the lecture, and he returned home to continue his examination of fetuses at different stages of development to try to understand how a congenital hernia formed in some infants. Pott had been looking at what he called "a treatise in French and Latin from 1726 by Reneaulme Lagaranne[176] on herniae." Lagaranne supposed that ducts in the abdomen connected to the testicles, and Pott, inspired by this remark, "immediately opened the bellies of some foetuses of different ages, which I had by me in spirit, and found the ducts exactly as described by Lagaranne."[177] At this point Pott shared his thoughts with "two or three friends and a very inquisitive young gentleman, who was at that time my dresser at St. Bartholomew's hospital."

> He said that he had a day or two before thrown some injection into a boy, born dead, at the full time, that he would bring him to my house, and that we should examine it together. We did so and found the ducts open on each side.[178]

The young gentleman who carried a corpse to Watling Street may have been Peter Clare as he was Pott's dresser in 1754.

Pott strongly believed that William Hunter was unable to accept criticism of his theories and would not participate in a collegial network of fact-finding, like Pott and his friends were willing to do. So, Pott turned to the scholarly process itself and gained "pleasure" from the probability of his investigation "discovering a truth." He sought opportunities to view more bodies, note their appearances on paper, draw them, prepare specimens, and finally, show the papers and presentations "to many of my friends, and among the rest to Mr. Serjeant Hawkins, Mr. Sainthill, the late Mr. Nourse, and the late Mr. Webb …"[179] This group encouraged Pott to continue his research, after which Pott organized his notes, showed them to his friends again, and then went to see Dr. Hunter at his home. This may have been sometime in late 1756, and again Pott stated that he learnt nothing new from his conversation with Hunter:

> Having always entertained a high opinion of Dr. Hunter's *anatomical* abilities, I called at his house designing to have told him on the subject: the doctor was not at home, but his brother Mr. Hunter was, and with him I had some talk. The same gentleman also shewed me one single preparation, tied down, in a glass, in spirit, exhibiting the situation of the testicles of a foetus pretty near the time of their passing from the abdomen into the scrotum, of which kind, I had then several at home, and which many of my friends had seen.[180]

The visit was short, the words "congenial hernia" were never uttered, and moreover John Hunter revealed little as he spoke with "the most cautious, apprehensive reservedness."[181] Pott went home and sent his treatise to press with not a syllable changed. Shortly after it appeared William Hunter accused Pott of two acts of intellectual and anatomical theft. The first was that he had not acknowledged in the treatise that he had conversed with John Hunter in 1756, and the second was that Pott had not cited in his work on ruptures *Opuscula Pathologica,* a 1755 text by Baron Albrecht von Haller (1708–1777), the Swiss physician, anatomist and physiologist. Pott criticized the first charge for being rude and hasty and was particularly concerned that William Hunter had told "his *tale* to the young people at his lecture-room," which he found to be disingenuous and unmanly, meaning that Hunter had chosen not to approach Pott directly, even though he was someone "who called Pott a friend."[182] He quickly dismissed Hunter's second charge by stating that he had not read Haller's book in Latin or French prior to publishing on ruptures, and what business was this of Hunter's anyway as he "has really nothing to do with [it]."[183]

Additional accusations of theft and plagiarism in Pott's *An account of a particular kind of rupture frequently attendant upon new-born children, and sometimes met with in adults* came in a review published in the March 1757 issue of *Critical Review.* Although anonymous, it is likely that Tobias George Smollett (1721–1771), the periodical's editor and a surgeon by training, penned the piece.[184] Smollett, importantly, was also a friend of the Hunters.

The lukewarm review questioned Pott's finding, since it was based on only a few cases and dissections. The review noted that:

> it was possible for part of the intestine to be pushed into the sacculus with the testicle as it enters an opening in the abdominal muscles in the foetus or new-born child. The sacculus became the tunica vaginalis—meant to only hold the testicle.[185]

This was nothing new in the writer's opinion and "even in this part" Pott "seems to be grasping at what does not belong to him; and we can see in the performance itself, the marks of restraint, and of a burdened conscience."[186]

When it came to accusations of plagiarism, the reviewer noted that Pott did not acknowledge Haller's account of the congenial rupture, but more importantly, claimed that Pott "learned all that he has published at second-hand, and imperfectly from Dr. *Hunter's* lectures." This information came to the attention of the reviewer in a letter "from one that calls himself a pupil of Dr. *Hunter*." The charge was that Dr. Hunter had shown preparations and drawings made by John Hunter of the congenital hernia in his last three courses, meaning that their discovery dated back to 1755. The letter added that Dr. Hunter had told Pott and others of his discovery and made no secret of it. The *Monthly Review* of May 1757 also questioned in a brief description of the treatise as to whether Mr. Pott had really made any new discovery.[187]

The *Critical Review* of December 1763 took Pott to task again in a discussion of the second edition of *A Treatise on Ruptures* (1763). The writer noted that Pott had added a new section on the dispute with Dr. Hunter over the congenial rupture where "he alledges that he is unjustly accused of plagiarism from Haller" and he complains of the treatment he has received from Dr. Hunter.[188] Neither side is chosen as the winner.

In July 1764 the same periodical published a review of William Hunter's reply to Pott's second edition of *A Treatise of Ruptures*. The piece begins badly for Pott:

> In the first section, the doctor proves Mr. Pott's assertion of not having learned the opinions he has published concerning congenial ruptures from baron Haller's book, to be extremely unlikely if not absolutely false ...[189]

The evidence for this remark is that Pott could not prove that he had discussed his idea with any "apprentice, pupil, or friend" before Haller's book came out. The periodical noted approvingly that Hunter had compared passages quoted "from the baron and from Mr. Pott ... in his Medical Commentaries, part i. p. 73 & 74."[190]

> The next section is employed in what passed at a visit Mr. Pott paid to Mr. J. Hunter; in which every allegation against Mr. P. are as clearly proved as ever they were against any culprit at the Old Bailey, and that upon the evidence of credible witnesses.[191]

The review concludes with the opinion that Hunter's *Medical Commentaries* "is written with such perspicuity, accuracy, and spirit, that it cannot fail of amusing a reader who is not concerned in the dispute."[192]

The *Monthly Review* of February 1765 included a two-page piece on Pott's second edition of *A Treatise on Ruptures*, admitting that they were only doing this because the altercation between Pott and Hunter was ongoing.[193] The essay detailed Pott's defense of his discovery and William Hunter's response to it.[194]

While Hunter's "considerable severity, keenness, and even stinging ralliery" was criticized, his counterarguments to Pott's points were praised and:

> if it be recollected with what difficulty and peril the fame of anatomists is achieved; by their living, like hyenas, from the graves, and their being surrounded by putrefaction, it must dispose every considerate man to leave such adventurers in the unenvied possession of their utmost acquirements, of every kind.[195] Hunter is declared the winner "but his essential triumph would not have been diminished by a temperate exertion of it ..."[196]

Hunter had fired the last shot in this salvo and had subsequently been damned with faint praise.

The exchange highlighted the unsavory nature of anatomy and the potential vindictiveness of those who practiced it for money and fame.[197] Pott stayed silent on the matter after defending himself against the charges of theft in the second edition of *A Treatise on Ruptures* (1763).[198] Similarly no mention was made of the Hunters in the third and fourth editions of the treatise that appeared in 1769 and 1775. So how did this public debate affect Pott and his reputation? The Epilogue considers what Pott's legacy became through the eyes of the generation of surgeons who came after him and what it meant to be declared "The Best Surgeon in England."

Epilogue

Pott's Legacy: Then and Now

… none contributed more powerfully than Mr. Percival Pott, to the improvement of the practice of surgery in England. His life, indeed, forms a sort of epoch in the history of the profession … he was in his time the best practical surgeon, the best lecturer, the best writer in surgery, the best operator, of which this large metropolis could boast.[1]

By the lot of human nature, few men can now record his talents as lecturer: and vain would be the attempt, upon this occasion, to describe the elegance of his language; the animation of his manner; the perceptive force, and effect, of his truths, and doctrines.

Well may he be holden in memory as one of the brightest ornaments of St. Bartholomew's Hospital.[2]

The history of carcinogens is usually traced back to the identification by Percivall Pott (1714–88) of scrotal cancer among chimney-sweeps in 1775.[3]

A few weeks after Pott's death in February 1789, the surgeon Jessé Foot (1744–1826) composed a eulogium for the *European Magazine*.[4] Foot began with a quote from Shakespeare's *Hamlet*, "He was a man, that take him for all in all, we ne'er shall look on his like again" and praised Mr. Pott's "most active mind" joined to "the most unremitting attention."[5] Foot was no friend to the Hunters, and this has to be taken into account when considering the words he crafted. After noting that Pott "arrived at the summit of his profession alone" … "without any particular patronage," Foot added:

> His wheels have now and then been attempted to be clogged by jealous opponents, which in the end served to path him forward in his career, instead of checking him; for every explanation in surgical opinions that he was engaged in, tended to confirm the new truths which he had adopted and to make them seen in a stronger point of view.[6]

Foot explained away Pott's supposed faults—while Pott could be seen as "abrupt," this was due to being "quick and decisive in his opinions." This remark came after a sentence praising Pott for having "the strictest professional integrity," defined as an unwillingness to linger and attempt to treat impossible cases or to use flattery in order to convince a patient to succumb to surgery. Foot implied that Pott had not received the approbation he deserved for his "system of Surgery,"[7] noting that some medical men were hypocritically praising it after Pott's death, something they should have been doing when he was alive:

> He retained a most vigorous mind to the last, although he was advanced in years; for he was a subject (as it was his usual expression) of Queen Anne. The writer of this attended his last course of lectures, which he gave to a crowded Theatre during the latter winter. And he may truly say, that he did not know which to prefer, as he was as much absorbed in admiration of his close reasoning, select dialect, judicious technical expression, as by his thorough surgical information.[8]

The eulogium included details not found elsewhere of Pott's funeral procession on 29 December 1788. The hearse was accompanied by "five mourning coaches, with many of the Faculty in their private carriage, and more would have joined the solemn farewell, had they known when it would have been."[9]

Pott's legacy had to be created and his reputation secured, and as argued in chapter one, this goal characterized James Earle's biography of his father-in-law. In August 1791 the pro-Hunter *Critical Review* published a review of Earle's *The Chirurgical Works of Percival Pott, F.R.S. a new Edition, with his Last Corrections. To which are added A Short Account of the Life of the Author, a Method of curing the Hydrocele by Injection, and occasional Notes and Observations.*[10] The anonymous reviewer questioned Earle's opinion of the greatness of Pott in reforming surgery. While acknowledging that, "To Mr. Pott modern surgery is greatly indebted," this was only because he essentially did what was expected of an elite hospital surgeon—he wrote books, tried to cause little pain, and came up with "simple and efficacious plans."

> Yet perhaps the great reformation in surgery, the civic crowns with which Mr. Earle endeavours to decorate his tomb, are not exclusively his due. The improved plan was

already began; for Heister, LeDran, and Cheselden, were much more mild, gentle, and humane than their predecessors. They began to see, that pain was not always the means of curing pain, and that to relieve was rather the surgeons office than to torture.

If we compare them with their predecessors they were lenient and humane; if we look at them in Mr. Pott's work, they were severe and unrelenting. This is the light, in which Mr. Earle considers, the medium through which he has surveyed them. But it ought to be remarked, that Mr. Pott cited those parts in which reformation had yet made little progress, and if he had been giving a general character, might not greatly have differed from us. In a polished nation, though in consequence of luxury, diseases may be more frequent, the remedies are more mild and gentle.[11]

Having demolished Earle's claim that Pott was the first to reform surgery, the reviewer concluded with a lukewarm summary of Pott's achievements:

Though Mr. Pott was not the first to reform, he greatly contributed to disseminate milder and more humane methods of cure. Many of the more abstruse parts of surgery, which from their intricacy and uncertainty had been left to quacks and old women, he explained familiarly, and scarcely in any instance has he written, without essentially instructing mankind.[12]

The reviewer posited that Pott was essentially not one of the greats and was also somewhat boring:

The life of this eminent surgeon contains few singularities. He labored diligently to attain a knowledge of his profession, and he was rewarded by a great degree of public confidence.[13]

Earle's life of Pott was also mocked for its laudatory style in *The Lounger's Common-Place Book* of 1796. The anonymous compiler of this alphabetical compendium of anecdotes was Jeremiah Whitaker Newman (1759–1839).[14] A surgeon and satirist, Newman revealed that he relied on one of Pott's "enthusiastic admirers" for much of the article and the man (Earle) had stated that Pott's legacy was considerable, "his life was a national blessing, his death a national loss; he enlarged the bounds of art, human malady shrunk before him; he was eyes to the blind, and a feet to the lame."[15] Newman then punctured the balloon with a story that he acknowledged was probably untrue but was too good not to include in his book. Newman had gotten it from a surgeon who had known Pott and claimed that Pott dismissed people of "*unpromising* appearance"[16] when they came to his home asking for aid:

If a patient ever presents himself to Pott," said the wit, after a second bottle; "if a patient calls, whom he suspects of not having a five guinea fee in his pocket, he always

> has his hand in the direction of his watch string, and the following, or some such speech ready cut and dried at his tongues end." "I must beg of you *my friend* to be as concise as possible, for I am to be at Lady Harrington's[17] [the old Countess was at that time an excellent patient] exactly at two, and am a very material evidence, in an important cause in the court of King's bench, where I must be precisely at three, so that you see I have not a moment to lose.[18]

It turned out that in this case the scruffy servant who Pott turned away with his well-worn excuse was in fact related to a Lord who had suffered an accident while hunting and urgently needed a surgeon to attend him. The snobbish Pott, therefore, lost a lucrative fee.

Earle was a proud man who was not shy about promoting himself, as his extant letters reveal. In September 1801 he wrote to Lady Mary Holdernesse (1721–1801) to inquire if she would help him procure a Baronet.[19] She unfortunately died a few weeks after Earle sent his letter, and he had to wait until 1807 to be knighted. In his writings on surgery Earle viewed himself as Pott's heir, though not necessarily an uncritical one. In *Observations on the cure of the curved spine and the means of lessening the effects of fire on the human body* (1799), Earle stated the purpose of his book was to improve on Pott and to specifically question his father-in-law's disapproval of mechanical ingenuity in managing palsy. In *Observations*, Earle advertised his own designs for spinal restraints. Then, in the 1808 edition of Pott's *Chirurgical operations*, Earle commented on and referenced his own cases to prove Pott either right or mistaken in his treatments. In the third volume Earle went into great detail on how ideas had changed on palsy of the lower limbs since Pott's work on the condition. As in 1799 he opposed Pott's condemnation of the use of mechanical devices to straighten spines and drew attention to a machine he had invented "that elevates the head, support, the thorax, pass down the spine and strengthen it as a splint does a broken limb." Earle also boasted of his own skills in treating head injuries and especially drew attention to the positive reaction to his work. A man who fell down in a fit from a loaded wagon and was run over by a wheel had a scalp and facial wound which, with its mixture of mud and blood, resembled "a dirty quagmire, in which the wounded portions were loose and floating." After Earle treated him the man was left with "little scar or deformity that astonished all who saw the wound. I may add that the man, before the accident, had been reckoned handsome, and the front view of his face afterward still retained its comely appearance."[20]

Surgeons such as William Hey (1736–1819) and John Abernethy (1764–1831) who had attended Pott's lectures, read his works, and walked the wards with him, also referenced the great man in their publications and lectures. Hey, a senior surgeon to the General Infirmary in Leeds, referred to Pott as "that excellent surgeon" on the first page of his massive *Practical Observations in Surgery, Illustrated with Cases* (1803). He was discussing fractures of the skull and was intent on examining Pott's strenuous recommendation to excise a "circular portion of the scalp in all cases where the application of the trephine became necessary."[21] Hey thought this was not so but as "the opinion of such an author must have great weight in settling the practice in these cases," he must examine "the grounds of this opinion …"[22] Throughout *Practical Observations*, Hey cited Pott's opinions, advice, and apprehensions. On the subject of strangulated hernia he mused that "if Mr. Pott is right that the operation only kills 1 in 50 if done immediately perhaps ought to operate sooner versus trying bleeding, cold baths, opium, tobacco clysters."[23] He stated candidly that he had experimented on patients following the example of successful cases from Pott's books. The results were somewhat mixed, as seen in this case of a strangulated hernia:

> I have always been afraid of large wounds of the omentum; but as the excision of a gangrened portion, by cutting through the adjacent sound part, stood so strongly recommended by Mr. Pott, of whose judgment I had a very high opinion, I determined to follow his example in this instance. I cut off, therefore, all that had a morbid appearance, and the remainder, as soon as I ceased to hold it, retired spontaneously into the abdomen.[24]

The patient violently hemorrhaged venous and arterial blood for several hours and remained in "an uncertain state for two weeks after the operation."[25] Hey summed up the experiment with: "This case clearly shews, that large wounds of the omentum are attended with danger."[26]

Norman Moore tells us that Abernethy sat in "Mr. Pott's old chair" at the meeting of the Medical and Philosophical Society of St. Bartholomew's Hospital on 1 October 1799, and "talked as he often did of Percivall Pott for whom he had a warm admiration, and related cases."[27] Similarly Abernethy's lectures at St. Bartholomew's hospital included anecdotes that captured Pott's style of communicating information and set up Abernethy's improvements on treating certain conditions:

> The old Surgeons were terribly afraid of opening large abscesses—Hence Mr. Pott used to say—The Man who escaped with a lumbar abscess was as fortunate as the Man who drew a 20,000 prize—And truly in the way which they formerly opened them there were dangerous indeed.[28]

In published works Abernethy would refer to patients he had seen Pott treat. Under the heading of the "Consequences of Venaesection," Abernethy first commented on the dangers of people using "bleeding-shops in the city." Having a vein in your body opened in such a setting could lead to phlebitis and damaged nerves if they were punctured by mistake. Abernethy then included the case of a patient with an injured nerve that he had seen Pott treat successfully. This was quickly followed, however, with criticisms of the content of Pott's lectures on the subject of venesection:[29] "In the lectures of that eminent surgeon, I had heard dangerous and fatal consequences attributed to the injury of a nerve in venaesection, but I learned no other distinctions of cases."[30] Abernethy continued that he intended to distinguish (by giving many examples) rather than generalize like Pott had done—in other words, he was critical of Pott for not including enough case histories in his lectures to allow a surgeon to distinguish between different types of problems that he could encounter in patients who had been improperly bled.[31]

Samuel Cooper (1781–1848) spent decades compiling and publishing multiple editions of his massive *A Dictionary of Practical Surgery: containing a complete exhibition of the present state of the principles and practice of surgery, collected from the best and most original sources of information and illustrated by critical remarks.* The *Dictionary* first appeared in 1809, nine years after Cooper had spent time at St. Bartholomew's Hospital in order to qualify as a surgeon's mate. Cooper refers to Pott's works on nearly every page, and many parts are transcribed word for word. Cooper's surgical *Dictionary* instantly became the textbook of choice for students in Britain, Europe, and America, and continued to be revised and issued until 1838.

Pott is praised throughout the work as the man responsible for having improved the practice of surgery in England. Cooper took Earle's biography at face value for what it said about the barbarity of surgery before Pott humanized it; Pott's books, however, received the most praise, though this was not blind praise:

> Where shall we find more sensible, or more truly practical observations on the treatment of abscesses, than in his excellent treatise on fistula in ano? Where shall we meet with better remarks on the local treatment of gangrenous parts, than in his valuable tract on the mortification of toes and feet? What author abounds with so many just observations on injuries of the head, blended it is true with rather too great a partiality to the trepan, the so frequent necessity for which is now less generally acknowledged? His description of the inflammation and suppurations of the dura mater, and of the treatment, is matchless. The account, which he has left us of the disease of the vertebrae, attended with paralysis of the limbs, is perhaps his most original production. His celebrated essay on fractures was also very original, and has had in this country considerable influence over the treatment of these injuries; but, as there can be no doubt, that the effects of position were exaggerated in this part of his writings, and that surgeons ought still to make every possible exertion to render their apparatus for broken bones more effectual. (See *Fractures*)[32]

Cooper ends with the judgment that Pott, in his time, was "the best practical surgeon, the best lecturer, the best writer in surgery, the best operator, of which this large metropolis could boast." Pott is then compared to:

> Another character of still greater genius and originality, though of inferior education, was the ever memorable John Hunter, surgeon to St. George's Hospital, who was at once eminent as a surgeon, ananatomist, a physiologist, a naturalist, and a philosopher. If Pott materially improved many parts of the practice of surgery in England, and evinced himself to be the most skillful operator of this time, John Hunter was also not less importantly employed in extending the boundaries of physiological knowledge, and in the investigation of human, and particularly comparative anatomy.[33]

For Cooper, Pott and Hunter contributed to surgery in different ways, with Pott being the better surgeon because of his skills in operating and knowledge of illnesses and Hunter being a researcher of rare brilliance in anatomy and physiology. The latter of course had much less to offer a compiler of a dictionary of practical surgery.

On 14 February 1815 Sir William Blizard (1743–1835), a former pupil of Pott and John Hunter, delivered the Hunterian Oration to the Royal College of Surgeons in London, which was published in 1816. Blizard was surgeon to the London Hospital, founder of its medical school in 1785, and president of the College of Surgeons in 1814 and again in 1822. He chose as his topic for the oration the lives of eminent surgeons and devoted a large section to Pott. Blizard praised Pott first for his knowledge of classical authors and then for the beauty of his language and his strong and elementary ideas:[34]

> His descriptions of the various species of hernia, and his suggested processes of relief, will remain standards of practice, unshaken by the noble displays of anatomical ingenuity, of accurate observation, and of solid reflection, of living ornaments of this College.[35]

Blizard also praised Pott for the gentlemanly way in which he conducted operations and "for general information and benefit, in the dignified style of hospital practice."[36] He concluded:

> By the lot of human nature, few men can now record his talents as lecturer: and vain would be the attempt, upon this occasion, to describe the elegance of his language; the animation of his manner; the perceptive force, and effect, of his truths, and doctrines.
>
> Well may he be holden in memory as one of the brightest ornaments of St. Bartholomew's Hospital.[37]

This judgment of Percivall Pott as the best practical surgeon of his era, a gentleman, and a writer of clarity and elegance continued throughout the nineteenth and early twentieth centuries.[38] He was, however, invariably compared to John Hunter as Hunter's reputation grew and Pott's declined.[39] For example in a biography of Abernethy from 1853 George Macilwain remarked:

> When Abernethy entered into life, the best representative of the regular surgery *of that day* was Mr. Pott, who was contemporary with the period of Mr. Hunter's labors. Mr. Pott was a good surgeon, an eloquent lecturer, a scholar, and a gentleman, and he gave some surgical lectures at St. Bartholomew's Hospital. We have perused two manuscript copies of these lectures … There are ripples of a more humane and scientific surgery, and many parts that are suggestive of onward study … but we do not perceive anything in Pott's lectures in the shape of a science … there are no steps, no axioms by which we can reach the platform of more general propositions.[40]

Macilwain continued that it was John Hunter who created the science of surgery through positing hypotheses and carrying out repeated experiments.

Sir James Paget (1814–1899) in *The Hunterian Oration* of 1877 exclaimed that: "I have little doubt that Percivall Pott was the best practical surgeon of the time. I think it certain that he was the best in this country; I believe he was the best in Europe."[41] But his works, unlike Hunter's, show no evidence of "the science and exposition of principles" of surgery.[42] This characterization of Pott as a doer of surgery and Hunter as a thinker of surgery became even more sharply defined in the later nineteenth and twentieth centuries. It was concurrent with Pott's relationship to John Hunter moving from what it had actually been—that of a pupil who attended some of Pott's lectures in 1751—to being one of the surgeon's primary students. In a medical essay from 1907, "Remarks on Hernia—Particularly in Children," Pott was referred to "as John Hunter's teacher and professional rival. A man who, as a practical surgeon, was as illustrious as Hunter was as a scientific one."[43] James Robinson in an article on the history of St. Bartholomew's Hospital in 1993 notes that an important and significant contribution of Pott's may have been overlooked:

> John Hunter, probably the greatest scientific surgeon of any era, learned his trade at the feet of Sir Percivall; it is also possible that he gleaned from the master the importance of the scientific and research approach and may have inherited Pott's dislike of operating. Pott described amputations as "terrible to bear and horrible to see," an accurate description before the days of anaesthesia and antisepsis.[44]

In fact there is no evidence that Pott disliked operating, unlike William Cheselden or William Hunter.

Today Pott's legacy consists principally of two things: (1) the world would have been deprived of his many elegant books if he had not fallen from his horse in 1756, and (2) he is the father of occupational medicine due to his essay on chimney sweeper's cancer in 1775. No mentions of cancer scroti appear in either Foot's eulogium or the *Critical Review*; the *Critical Review*, however, did include a snide remark about the story of Pott's cool and calculated response to his accident:

> The venial error of too eagerly accumulating extraordinary qualities has lessened a little the merit of Mr. Earle's work. The accident, and his behaviour in consequence of the compound fracture, required only a little firmness, and the classical elegance of Mr. Pott's writings is to found chiefly in the eager partiality of his biographer's mind.[45]

Pott's accidental fall from his horse and the story of the events that followed it, namely the construction of a stretcher from a door and chair poles and the near escape from amputation, are not found in his works. What evidence we have points to them as being embellishments of James Earle's account. While the accident certainly happened, the fortuity of it leading to Pott becoming a prolific author was made only after Pott's death.

Pott has been most celebrated since the mid twentieth-century for a short chapter in his *Chirurgical observations relative to the cataract, the polypus of the nose, the cancer of the scrotum, the different kinds of rupture etc.* (1775). Scholars have described Pott's essay on scrotal cancer as a milestone in various scientific fields from occupational and environmental health to epidemiology and the prevention of cancer.[46] In the essay Pott established a causal link between the development of cancer later in life to exposure to a substance in the environment, namely soot that collected in the rugae, or wrinkles, of climbing-boys' scrotums. Legislation over the next 100 years to restrict some of the crueler practices of employing child sweeps aged four to seven years to climb narrow twisted flues is claimed to have flowed from Pott's discovery.[47]

To understand how and why this connection has been made, it is best to begin with an analysis of what Pott was actually arguing in his short piece on chimney-sweepers' cancer. Pott began the essay with an acknowledgment of the work of Bernadino Ramazzini (1633–1714), an Italian physician who had published a treatise, *De Morbis Artificum Diatriba,* in 1700 in which he described disorders associated with 54 different occupations. Pott wished to drawn attention to an occupational disease "not publickly noticed" before. He added that "The trade call it the soot wart."[48] He described how it first appeared in the lower scrotum and became a painful hard sore. Pott commented that he had never seen it develop before puberty, and that is why both patients and surgeons had generally assumed it be a venereal disease. Mercury rub treatments had grim results. Pott saw how the testicle enlarges and became hard as the disease traveled up the spermatic process to the abdomen, where it settled in the inguinal glands and affected some of the viscera before painfully starting to destroy the surrounding parts. Pott's language mirrored that of Ramazzini and especially of the reformer's Jonas Hanway in its compassion for those stricken with occupational diseases:[49]

> The fate of these people seems singularly hard; in their early infancy, they are most frequently treated with great brutality and almost starved with cold and hunger; they

> are thrust up narrow and sometimes hot chimnies, where they are bruised, burned, and almost suffocated; and when they get to puberty, become peculiarly liable to a most noisome, painful, and fatal disease.[50]

Pott then turned to a treatment for the disease and stated that castration is insufficient to stop the spread of the cancer: the scrotum must be removed where the sore is. Otherwise the disease will come back in a few months and spread, as Pott had seen in several patients who came back to the hospital very ill. What caused the disease, according to Pott, was "a lodgment of soot in the rugae of the scrotum." This was good news since it meant that it was not "a disease of habit"[51] and the patients were generally young and in good health, which made it easier for them to bear surgery. They were "Not old men with acrimonious fluids, or women who have ceased to menstruate with cancer."[52] And Pott had even more good news:

> as the scrotum is no vital organ, nor can the loss of a part of it ever be attended with any, the smallest amount of inconvenience; and if a life can be preserved by a removal of all that portion that is distempered, it will be a very good and easy composition; for when the disease has got head, it is rapid in its progress, painful in all its attacks, and most certainly destructive in its event.[53]

Pott's essay was not widely noticed in his lifetime. The only significant contemporary mention of it I have found is in The *London Review* of April 1775. In comments on Pott's newly published *Chirurgical Observations relative to the Cataract, the polypus of the nose, the cancer of the scrotum, and the mortification of the toes* the anonymous reviewer remarked:

> The subject of the *third* tract, called in our hospitals the *chimney-sweeper's* cancer, though a real and as peculiar distemper as any of the *morbi artificum*, has hitherto been neglected by chirurgical writers. Mr. Pott points an easy, and effectual mode of cure, if timely taken; which he advises, because when the disease has got head, it is rapid in its progress, painful in its attacks, and most certainly destructive in its event.[54]

When I first began researching Mr. Percivall Pott and read that nowadays he is most famous for having discovered the first causal link between an occupational hazard and a disease, I assumed, wrongly, that this observation was the pinnacle of his work. Far from it, since no evidence suggests that Pott campaigned for better conditions for climbing-boys or for any kind of legislative protection. His essay on cancer of the scrotum is about a local disease that could be cured if caught early. Compared to his treatise on palsy of the lower limbs, which details cases, different treatments, and was reissued with new content, cancer of the scrotum was of only limited interest to Pott. His interest and skills lay in the whole field of what he, and his colleagues, called practical surgery.

For nearly fifty years in Georgian London, Pott lectured and wrote with rare clarity and precision about what a surgeon saw, did, and thought about. He situated himself both as a skilled surgeon from treating thousands at Saint Bartholomew's Hospital, and as a gentleman who could treat the elite. Analyzing Pott's character, values, and actions challenges the prevailing view in historiographical works on surgery before the era of general anesthesia as a realm of screaming patients and larger than life, eccentric operators whose primary aims were to operate as fast as possible. What emerges from an academic biography of the man rated the best surgeon in England is a more complex picture of the varieties of approaches to taking care of patients.

Pott's life tells us much about the day-to-day business of being a surgeon in a highly competitive market over several decades. He knew and commented on the difficulties of establishing a practice, the cutthroat nature of being elected to hospital posts and the patrons who had to be cultivated to maintain success. Pott was highly unusual, if not unique, in the number and length of the case histories he provided. He had a leading role in crafting the image of a professional surgeon as one who treats the multitudes at a leading hospital, teaches the next generation of surgeons and establishes a successful private practice devoted to the important families of the day. Pott's writings and actions are key to our understanding of how healthcare developed in eighteenth-century England.

Notes

Introduction: "What Brought Each Leaden-Headed Lad to Town, What Drew Them Hither but the Name of Pott?"

1. *St. Bartholomew's Hospital Journal*, April 1928, p. 107. These are lines from an anonymous poem written in 1787 when Pott retired from practice at Saint Bartholomew's hospital. The whereabouts of the original manuscript is unknown.
2. Bynum, William F.: "Physicians, Hospitals, and Career Structures in Eighteenth-century London," pp. 105–28. In: Bynum, William and Porter, Roy (eds.), *William Hunter and the Eighteenth-Century Medical World*. Cambridge University Press: Cambridge, 1985, see p. 107.
3. In 1986 Harold Cook memorably described seventeenth-century English medicine as a "medical marketplace" where patients/consumers demanded and bought medicines and services from practitioners within an unregulated system. Cook, Harold: *The Decline of the Old Medical Regime in Stuart London*. Ithaca, NY: Cornell University Press, 1986. The debate about the usefulness of this concept has led to several new works including Jenner, Mark S. R. and Wallis, Patrick (eds.): *Medicine and the Market in England and Its Colonies, c.1450–c.1850*. Palgrave Macmillan: Basingstoke, 2007, and Brown, Michael: *Performing Medicine: Medical Culture and Identity in Provincial England, c. 1760–1850*. Manchester University Press: Manchester, 2011.
4. See Lawrence, Christopher: "'Democratic, divine and heroic': The History and Historiography of Surgery," pp. 1–47. In: *Medical Theory, Surgical Practice: Studies in the History of Surgery*. Lawrence, Christopher (ed.), Routledge: London, 1992. For a progressive view of the history of surgery see Wangensteen, Owen H. and Wangensteen, Sarah D.: *The Rise of Surgery: From Empiric Craft to Scientific Discipline*. Dawson, Folkestone, 1978.

5. Lawrence, Susan C.: "Educating the Senses: Students, Teachers and Medical Rhetoric in Eighteenth-Century London," pp. 154–178. In: *Medicine and the Five Senses*. Bynum, W. F. and Porter, Roy (eds.), Cambridge University Press: Cambridge, 1993, see p. 160.
6. Osteomyelitis of the frontal bone associated with a purulent collection under the periosteum, causing swelling and edema over the forehead.
7. Sternbach, G.: "Percivall Pott: Tuberculous Spondylitis." *The Journal of Emergency Medicine* Vol. 14, No. 1, 1996, pp. 79–83. Pott's disease is a reactivation of latent disease, frequently years after the initial infection and produces a characteristic kyphotic deformity. Also see Hakulinen, E.: "Mannen Bakom Syndrome: Percivall Pott." *Läkartidningen* Vol. 82, No. 34, 1985, pp. 2784–5 and Callahan, Charles W.: "Construction Crew Discovers Grave of "Tiny Tim," *The Journal of Infectious Diseases* Vol. 176, No. 6, 1997, pp. 1653–1654. Children aged 3–10 years were often infected by adults with TB pneumonia. The bacteria lodges in the spine and causes pain, stiffness, general wasting, fatigue, and intermittent fevers. As the spine crumbles the height of the trunk is reduced. Paraplegia can result from compression of the spinal cord.
8. For an imaginative use of Pott's essay on scrotal cancer, see Labianca, Dominick A. and Reeves, William J.: "Science Literacy at Brooklyn College." *College Teaching* Vol. 37, No. 4, 1989, pp. 135–137.
9. *Dictionary of National Biography* Vol. 46, 1885–1900. Percivall Pott by D'Arcy Power, 1896.
10. Lawrence, Christopher: "'Democratic, divine and heroic': The History and Historiography of Surgery" in *Medical Theory, Surgical Practice: Studies in the History of Surgery*, Lawrence, Christopher (ed.), Routledge: London, 1992, p. 10. Also see Schlich, T.: "The Emergence of Modern Surgery," pp. 61–91. In: Brunton, D.: *Medicine Transformed: Health, Disease and Society in Europe, 1800–1930*. Manchester University Press: Manchester, 2004.
11. Wear, Andrew: *Knowledge and Practice in English Medicine, 1550–1680*. Cambridge University Press: Cambridge, 2000. Porter, Dorothy and Porter, Roy: *Patient's Progress: Doctors and Doctoring in Eighteenth-Century England*, Polity Press; Cambridge, UK, 1989; Porter, Roy: "'Expressing yourself ill': The Language of Sickness in Georgian England," pp. 276–299. In: *Language, Self and Society: A Social History of Language*. Burke, P. and Porter, Roy, Polity Press: Cambridge, UK, 1991; and Payne, Lynda: *With Words and Knives: Learning Medical Dispassion in Early Modern England*. Ashgate Press: Aldershot, 2007.
12. Snow, Stephanie: *Blessed Days of Anesthesia: How Anaesthetics Changed the World*. Oxford University Press: Oxford, 2008.
13. Schlich continues that it "has been almost totally disregarded, so much so that, in the end, it is of secondary importance whether surgeons or some other occupational group are being dealt with." Schlich, Thomas: *The Origins of Organ Transplantation: Surgery and Laboratory Science, 1880–1930*. University of Rochester Press: Rochester, 2012, p. 9.

Chapter One: "Climbing the Ladder": Business and Surgery

1. X54/1, "Diary Containing Memorandums relating to avocation, Accounts, Correspondances [*sic*], Anecdotes, &tc. Which may serve as a reference on my private concerns." *Barts and The London Hospital NHS Archives*, f. 42. Harvey (1759–1829) came from

County Donegal. The diary includes an autobiography covering the years 1759–1821 in which this description of Pott appears. Harvey also pasted a portrait of Pott into the diary.

2. Harvey's diary contains the only extant pupil records for St. Bartholomew's Hospital for this era. Harvey was senior surgeon from 1807–24 and appears to have kept notes primarily for financial reasons, since he had to share pupils' fees with other surgeons. On some of the contents of the diary, see Ruston, Sharon: "One of the 'modern sceptics': Reappraising Shelley's Medical Education." *Romanticism* Vol. 9, No. 1, 2003, pp. 1–20.
3. Hanover Square is in the heart of Mayfair. It was one of the first Georgian Squares to be built in the 1720s in the West End. The houses had plain fronts with elaborate interiors, gardens, stables and servant quarters in the back. As a successful hospital surgeon with a large private practice, Pott was not unusual in steadily moving west as his fortune grew. George Frideric Handel, the composer, lived just off the square, and from their opening in 1774 the Hanover Square Rooms became the leading venue for musical performances in London. See Longstaffe-Gowan, Todd: *The London Square*. Yale University Press: New Haven, CT 2012, and Curl, James Stevens: *Spas, Wells, & Pleasure Gardens of London*. Historical Publications Ltd.: London, 2010.
4. Harvey, Diary, f. 52.
5. James Earle (1745–1817) had also been a live-in apprentice of Pott's from 1762–9.
6. Chaplin, Arnold: *Medicine in England during the Reign of George III*. Henry Klimpton: London, 1919, states that there were 274 surgeons, 149 physicians and 351 apothecaries resident in London in 1783 (p. 133). Earle would follow in Pott's footsteps and become a surgeon at St. Bartholomew's hospital. His writings also mirrored Pott's in terms of subjects: *A Treatise on the Hydrocele*, 1791; *Practical Observations on the Operation for Stone*, 1793; *Observations on the Cure of Curved Spine*, 1799; *On Burns*, 1799; *A New Method of Operation for Cataract*, 1801; *Letter on Fractures of the Lower Limbs*, 1807; and *On Haemorrhoidal Excrescences*, 1807.
7. For an older example see Lloyd, G. Marner: "The Life and Works of Percivall Pott, 1714–1789, Wix Prize Essay 1933." *Saint Bartholomew's Hospital Reports* Vol. 46, 1933, pp. 291–336. The entry on Pott in the *Dictionary of National Biography* relies primarily on Earle as does Shand, William: "Percivall Pott, FRS (1716–1788)." *Trauma* Vol. 2, 2000, pp. 291–295 and Ross, John A., "Percivall Pott, 1714–1788." *Paraplegia* Vol. 24, 1986, pp. 287–292. Lloyd, however, does criticize Earle's biography: "Though giving a record of Pott's life and works, a poor picture of the man is painted. It lacks the colours of the eighteenth century; it lacks the tone of contemporary Medicine; it lacks the background of Georgian London," 292. The best contemporary short biography of Pott is Fu, Louis Kuo-Tai: "Notable Names in the History of Surgery: Percivall Pott (1714–1788)." *Annals of the College of Surgeons of Hong Kong* Vol. 4, 2000, pp. 110–122.
8. Modern references to Percivall Pott give the date of his birth as January 6, 1714 rather than Earle's date of December 26, 1713. However, when Pott was born the Julian calendar was in effect and the legal year started on March 25 (Lady's Day). Pott was baptised on January 11, 1713 at St. Christopher le Stocks on Threadneedle Street. Baptism Record, P69/CRI/A/001/MS04421, Item 002, St. Christopher Le Stocks, Composite register, *London Metropolitan Archives*. The church was demolished in 1781 due to the expansion of the Bank of England. In 1752 England and Wales adopted the Gregorian calendar that set the New Year as beginning on January 1.

9. This probably was John Pott (b.?1642). His second wife was Susan Stracey, "the daughter of a fine pot-maker at the sign of the Wheatsheaf in Gracechurch Street." See CLA/002/02/01/2733, John Pott, Citizen and Grocer, The Inventory, 4th Sept. 1705, Cornhill, *London Metropolitan Archives*. The inventory is thirteen pages long and shows that John Pott's total estate at death was valued at £2253.13.5. It included dried goods such as currants and wet goods such as olive oil. Pott was a Warden of the Grocers' Company as was Sir John Houblon who witnessed the inventory. Freemen like Pott who died leaving orphans had an inventory taken which would be exhibited in the Court of Orphans.
10. A Scrivener and Notary was a lawyer who had passed the examinations of the Worshipful Company of Scriveners of London. Scriveners and Notaries specialized in international trade, and this may have been another connection to the Houblon family in particular, and to the Huguenot community in general.
11. The marriage certificate records that the wedding took place on the 23rd of November 1712 at All Saints, Edmonton, Middlesex. See DRO/040/A/01, Item 004, All Saints, Edmonton, Composite register, *London Metropolitan Archives*.
12. Registers of baptisms, marriages and burials for the British Factory at Lisbon are held by the *London Metropolitan Archives*. Unfortunately they only begin in 1721 (and end in 1806). Lt. Benjamin Houblon died in Lisbon in December 1708, according to probate. His estate was divided with one third going to his wife and two thirds to his daughter. See prob. 11/505, 263, *The National Archives*. His father, Sir John Houblon (1632–1712), was a merchant and specialized in trade to Portugal and Spain. In 1710 a Percivall Pott was listed in the land tax records as a lodger of Sir John Houblon. Perhaps this is where Sir John's recently widowed daughter-in-law, Elizabeth Houblon, caught the eye of Pott's father. MS 11316/33, John Houblon Esquire, London Land Tax Records, *London Metropolitan Archives*.
13. The history of the Bank of England is well told through manuscripts and artifacts located in the bank's museum. During my visit there in March 2012, a helpful guide pointed out where the long and narrow Tudor houses would have stood before the bank was built in 1734. Formerly it was housed in the grocer's Hall. On the Houblons see Houblon, Lady Alice Archer: *The Houblon Family: Its Story and Times*. Archibald, Constable and Company Ltd.: London, 1907.
14. Wilcox was chaplain to the English Embassy and married Jane (d.1725), the daughter of John Milner, British consul at Lisbon.
15. I would like to thank Councillor Ian Armitt, JP, for putting me in touch with Dr. Mike Still, Assistant Museum Manager of the Dartford Borough Museum. Dr. Still performed an exhaustive search in an attempt to locate the school. Also I am deeply grateful to Mr. Malcolm Scott of the Horton Kirby and South Darenth Local History Society for a similarly exhaustive search of records. He provided the following valuable information: "Not only is Darenth parish in the diocese of Rochester but the manor of Darenth had for several centuries been held by the Dean and Chapter of Rochester Cathedral … In view of the close connection (to the Bishop of Rochester) I wonder whether Percivall might have been sent there to be educated by one of the clergy (who would have been appointed by the diocese) in a private capacity rather than to a school as such." Email message to author, July 12, 2013.

16. Nourse's one publication was *Syllabus of Anatomy and Chirurgery in twenty-three Praelections* in 1729. He probably delivered the lectures at the Barber-Surgeons' Hall though Nourse did not formally become Demonstrator of Anatomy there till March of 1731.
17. Branches of the Pott family continued to work in trade. A cousin of Percivall Pott's was the biggest vinegar salesman on the excise list in 1781. He probably owned a manufactory on Mansel Street, Whitechapel. See Walfpord, Edward: *Old and New London*, Vol. 6, Cassell, Petter & Galpin: London, 1878. Also see SC/GL/PEN/001/095, a drawing of the large and impressive manufactory of "Messrs Potts, vinegar merchants, near the Southwark Bridge by J. B[uckler] del., 1827," *London Metropolitan Archives*. Robert and Arthur Pott of Monkwell Street, vinegar makers, were left twenty guineas for funeral expenses in Pott's will. On apprenticeship, see Leunig, Tim, Minns, Chris and Wallis, Patrick: "Networks in the Premodern Economy: The Market for London Apprenticeships, 1600–1749." *Journal of Economic History* Vol. 71, No. 2, 2011, pp. 413–443. Apprentices resided with their master while training, but received little or no wage, and their board and clothing had often to be subsidized by parents or sponsors.
18. Lawrence, Christopher: *Medicine in the Making of Modern Britain 1700–1920*. Routledge: London, 1994, p. 63. Nourse was apprenticed to John Dobyns, a surgeon at St. Bartholomew's Hospital.
19. "Entry from the Freedom Admission register for Edward Nourse, September 1730, Indenture signed by Edward Nourse, surgeon and Percivall Pott, apprentice," COL/CHD/FR/02/579, *London Metropolitan Archives*.
20. Gray, Drew D.: *Crime, Prosecution and Social Relations: The Summary Courts of the City of London in the Late Eighteenth Century*. Palgrave Macmillan: Basingstoke, 2009, p. 160. Also see Minns, Chris and Wallis, Patrick: "Rules and Reality: Quantifying the Practice of Apprenticeship in Early Modern England." *Economic History Review* Vol. 65, No. 2, 2012, pp. 556–579.

    Minns, Chris and Wallis, Patrick: "The Price of Human Capital in a Pre-industrial Economy: Premiums and Apprenticeship Contracts in 18th Century England." *Explorations in Economic History* Vol. 50, 2013, pp. 333–350. The latter discusses the up-front payment known as a "premium" that English apprentices in the eighteenth century paid. Finally, Wallis provides an excellent overview of apprenticeship in "Apprenticeship and Training in Premodern England." *Journal of Economic History* Vol. 68, No. 3, 2008, pp. 832–861.
21. Wall, Cecil: *The History of the Surgeons' Company, 1745–1800*. Hutchinson: London, 1937, p. 37. Pott apparently had a decent command of Latin: "He had a fine copy of Albucasis … from which he more than once quotes. He had read Falloppius, and had looked into Hippocrates, Paulus Aegineta, and Rhazes." Moore, Norman: *The History of St. Bartholomew's Hospital*. C. Arthur Pearson Limited: London, 1918, Vol. 2, p. 642.
22. Earle, James: *The Chirurgical Works of Percivall Pott*. London, 1790 (in 3 volumes), Vol. 1, p. viii.
23. Earle, *The Chirurgical Works*, Vol. 1, p. xii.
24. Earle, *The Chirurgical Works*, Vol. 1, p. xii.
25. Earle, *The Chirurgical Works*, Vol. 1, p. xii.
26. "On April 7, 1739, [Pott] was a candidate for the post of assistant surgeon and got 41 votes, His opponent, John Townsend got 202, while five others did not go to the ballot.

Pott was elected assistant surgeon to St. Bartholomew's on March 13, 1745. He received 109 votes, while Stafford Crane got 48, Francis William Manaton 26, Philip Stephens 8, and Robert Young declined the ballot. See Moore, *The History*, Vol. 2, p. 641. The other surgeons elected while Pott worked at the hospital were: Stafford Crane, 1748–84; Robert Young, 1749–83; Anthony Bigg, 1749–50; Thomas Griffiths, 1750; William Sharp, 1755–1778; Edmund Pitts 1760–1791; James Earle, 1770–1817; Charles Blicke, 1779–1815; William Long, 1784–1807; and Ludford Harvey, 1784–1824.

27. Ward, Candace: *Desire and Disorder: Fevers, Fictions, and Feelings in English Georgian Culture*. Bucknell University Press: Lewisburg, 2007, quotation from p. 50.
28. Pott "used sometimes pleasantly to say to his pupils that they might remember they had been dressers to a barber-surgeon." Moore, *The History*, Vol. 2, 640. This is purely anecdotal evidence of course.
29. Moore, *The History*, Vol. 2, p. 640. This is of course anecdotal evidence.
30. Dobson, Jesse: "Percivall Pott." *Annuals of the Royal College of Surgeons of England* Vol. 50, 1972, pp. 54–65. Quotation from p. 55.
31. Wall, *The History*, p. 36.
32. The same year Pott had been granted the livery of the Barber-Surgeons Company after paying the customary fine of 10 shillings. This made him eligible to run for the post of assistant surgeon.
33. Harvey, Diary, f. 55. The following year Harvey was successful and became an assistant surgeon, but he then began to fret about the long wait that might ensue until one of the senior surgeons hopefully retired or died. Harvey was correct to worry: "1807 in August made Principal Surgeon at Barts on the resignation of Mr Long after waiting for it a period of 23 ½ years, and it was an event to me of the greatest importance as it brought to me an additional Income of 700£ a year" (f. 69). Mr. Heavyside, or John Heaviside, had also been a pupil of Pott's for four years probably 1766–1770. Susan C. Lawrence mentions Harvey's stressful career in *Charitable Knowledge: Hospital Pupils and Practitioners in Eighteenth-century London*. Cambridge University Press, Cambridge, 1996, pp. 64–5.
34. Porter, Roy: "Medical Lecturing in Georgian London." *The British Journal for the History of Science* Vol. 28, No. 1, 1995, pp. 91–99.
35. Wall, *The History*, p. 83, states that dressers like apprentices were attached to particular surgeons. They saw accidents "if the surgeon for that week at the hospital trusted them." John Collins Walker wrote to his family in America while he was studying at Guys Hospital in 1799–1800: "There are two kinds of students in the hospitals … the one called 'dressers,' and the other 'walkers.' The first have the advantage of practicing on all the simple surgical cases, and dressing all wounds themselves: the others merely see what is done. Of course, the former have vastly the greatest opportunities: but the expense is likewise double; as the walker pays £25, the dresser £50. Though I do not like to pay so much money for one object, I believe I shall enter as a dresser; for, as I intend to become a surgeon, I think the acquiring [of] a facility and steadiness in manual operation of the utmost importance." Cooper, David K. C.: "John Collins Warren (1778–1856): An American Surgeon in London." *British Medical Journal* Vol. 345, No. 7888, 2012, pp. 42–43. Quotation from 42.
36. Peachey, George C.: *John Heaviside*. St. Martin's Press: London, 1931. He was a pupil of Pott's for 4 years, from about 1766–1770. Heaviside bought No. 14 George St, Hanover

Square in 1787 and opened a museum. Also see Chaplin, Simon David John: "John Hunter and the 'museum economy', 1750–1800." Unpublished dissertation, University of London, May 2009. I am grateful to Dr. Chaplin for sharing this with me.

37. Pennington came from Alford in Lincolnshire. He practiced as a surgeon in London and developed a special interest in man midwifery.

38. John Abernethy (1764–1831) was a Londoner and an apprentice of Charles Blicke (1745–1815) at the hospital. He was elected assistant surgeon in 1778 when Blicke was elected to replace Pott, and in 1815 on Blicke's death, Abernethy became a senior surgeon. James Hutchinson was a Quaker from Pennsylvania who had received his education from apothecaries and chemists. His uncle sent him to London where he was put in the care of the Quaker physician, Dr. John Fothergill, who advised Hutchinson to study surgery as so few of his countrymen had focused on this science versus that of medicine. A signed receipt for 50 guineas from Pott shows Hutchinson paid to become his dresser a month after he enrolled at the hospital in September 1775. Hutchinson also paid to attend lectures on anatomy and surgery by William and John Hunter, on physic, chemistry and material medica by George Fordyce, a doctor at St. Thomas's Hospital, and on midwifery by Dr. Thomas Denman, physician and accoucheur at the Middlesex Hospital. See Bell, Whitfield, J.: "James Hutchinson (1752–1793): Letters from an American Student in London." *Transactions & Studies of the College of Physicians of Philadelphia* Vol. 34, No. 1, 1966, pp. 20–25.

39. Bell, *Letters*, p. 22.

40. Bob Acres, a dedicated coward, was a character in Richard Sheridan's play *The Rivals*. It was first performed in January 1755 at Covent Garden Theatre.

41. This story appears to have been originally published in the *Medical Times and Gazette* Vol. 1, 1869, p. 361 as "Something About One Of The Old School." J. F. Clarke (who was probably the person who sent it to the *Medical Times and Gazette*) included it in *Autobiographical recollections of the medical profession*. J. & A. Churchill: London, 1874, pp. 353–4. Also see Thornton, John L.: *John Abernethy: A Biography*. Simpkin Marshall Ltd: London, 1953 pp. 23–4. Pennington ends the anecdote with "We were closely associated for nearly fifty years afterwards, but we never had an angry word. Dining with him some forty years after in Bedford Row, the old quarrel between us accidentally cropped up. 'Well,' said Abernethy, 'the truth of the case was this—the moment I saw you uncover your biceps, I was certain I should be thrashed, and so, my boy, I surrendered at discretion.'" *Medical Times and Gazette*, p. 361.

42. Susan C. Lawrence's quantitative research is invaluable here in providing some context. She notes that 11,059 pupils signed up to walk the wards in London hospitals between 1725 and 1815. See *Charitable Knowledge*, p. 108.

43. See Wall, *The History*, pp. 84–5. Pupils were not attached to any particular surgeon and that makes them difficult to trace. They had to provide evidence of having served a 5 years' apprenticeship (this was waived after 1745) and to pay a fee for 6 months to a year. These fees were pooled and divided among the surgeons and apothecaries at the hospital. Pupils were entitled to attend all operations and could visit the wards with surgeons but could only watch what they did and ask questions.

44. John Jones refers to Pott several times in *Plain concise practical remarks on the treatment of wounds and fractures*, John Holt: New York, 1776. Jones was one of the founders of the

New York Hospital, became the first chair of surgery at King's College (now Columbia University) in 1767, and attended George Washington and Benjamin Franklin after he opened a practice in Philadelphia. See Peltier, Leonard F.: "Percivall Pott and Pott's Fracture." *Surgery* Vol. 51, No. 2, 1962, pp. 280–286. William Pryce practiced surgery at Redruth from 1760–1790 and opened the first hospital in Cornwall. See Stone J. L & Hockley A. D.: "Percivall Pott and the Miners of Cornwall." *British Journal of Neurosurgery* Vol. 16, No. 5, 2002, pp. 501–6. Henry Park wrote *Method of Treating Diseases of the Joints of the Knee and Elbow, in a Letter to Mr. Percival Pott*, London, 1783. Park spent three years at St. Bartholomew's Hospital studying with Pott from c. 1761–4. At age 23 he was appointed surgeon to the Liverpool Royal and came to recommend full excision of a joint in cases of chronic infection rather than amputation of the limb. See Cohen, Lord: "Liverpool's Contributions to Medicine." *The British Medical Journal* Vol. 1, No. 5440, 1965, pp. 945–948.

45. See Digby, Anne: *Making a Medical Living: Doctors and Patients in the English Market for Medicine, 1720–1911.* Cambridge University Press: Cambridge, 1994, p. 52.
46. See Lane, Joan: "Eighteenth-Century Medical Practice: A Case Study of Bradford Wilmer, Surgeon of Coventry, 1737–1813." *Social History of Medicine* Vol. 3, No. 3, 1990, pp. 369–86. Wilmer wrote *Cases and Remarks in Surgery*, London, 1779 and *Practical Observations on Herniae*, London, 1788. He studied with Pott in about 1758 and later vehemently criticized Pott's treatment of compound fractures in *Cases.*
47. Wadd, William: *Nugae Chirurgicae or A Biographical Miscellany, illustrative of a Collection of Professional Portraits*, London, 1824. William Wadd was the eldest son of Solomon Wadd (1745–1821), who had been a pupil of Pott's in c.1766. See *The Gentleman's Magazine and Historical Chronicle* Vol. 91, February 1882, p. 184. William Wadd was apprenticed to James Earle in 1797.
48. Bloom, H. T. G., Richardson, W. W., Harries, E. J.: "Natural History of Untreated Breast Cancer (1803–1933) Comparison of Untreated and Treated Cases According to Histological Grade of Malignancy." *The British Medical Journal* Vol. 2, No. 5299, 1962, pp. 213–221, see p. 214. The ward was funded by a friend of Howard's, the brewer Samuel Whitbread (1720–1796).
49. Wilson, William James Erasmus: *The History of Middlesex Hospital During the first Century of its Existence.* John Churchill: London, 1865, p. 123.
50. On the diversity of surgical education in the eighteenth century see, Lane, Joan: "The Role of Apprenticeship in Eighteenth-century Medical Education in England," pp. 57–104 and Gelfand, Toby: "'Invite the philosopher, as well as the charitable': Hospital Teaching as Private Enterprise in Hunterian London," pp. 29–152. In:. Bynum, W. F. and Porter, Roy (eds.), *William Hunter and the Eighteenth-Century Medical World.* Cambridge University Press: Cambridge, 1985.
51. Board of Stamps: Apprenticeship Books, Series IR 1; *The National Archives.* From 1710 to 1804, apprenticeship premiums were taxed at 2.5% on fees up to £50, and at 5% over £50. The Commissioners of Stamps recorded the payments and the names of the master, apprentice and trade.
52. Board of Stamps. For general comments on apprenticeship see Levene, Alysa: "'Honesty, sobriety and diligence': Master-apprentice Relations in Eighteenth- and Nineteenth-century

England." *Social History* Vol. 33, No. 2, 2008, pp. 183–200. Levene argues that contrary to their reputation poor apprentices were generally well behaved.

53. The Court of Examiners met every two weeks to examine candidates. See Harland, Kathleen: "Royal Naval Surgeons Afloat and Ashore 1700–1750. "*Transactions of the Naval Dockyards Society Publications*, Vol. 6, 2010, pp. 9–30. Also in the same volume, Crimmin, Pat: "The Shortage of Surgeons and Surgeons' Mates c.1740–1806: 'An Evil of a Serious Nature to the Service.'" *Transactions of the Naval Dockyards Society Publications*, Vol. 6, 2010, pp. 49–55.
54. See Wall, Cecil, Cameron H. Charles, Underwood, E. Ashford: *A History of the Worshipful Society of Apothecaries of London*. Vol. I, 1617–1815, Oxford University Press: London, 1963, Vol. 1, pp. 190–1. Exam book Reference COS/2/1, 1745–83, *Royal College of Surgeons*, lists the date, sometimes the examiners present, names of those examined, and the qualification granted such as diploma, India service, naval surgeon, regimental surgeon, mates etc.
55. See Wallis, P. J. and Wallis, R. V.: *Eighteenth Century Medics*. P. J. Phibb: P. J., 1988 and Board of Stamps. The lower cost for Rayley suggests that he had already served at sea as a surgeon's mate or formerly been apprenticed to another master. He would then need to complete only half an apprenticeship with Pott. See Minns, "Rules and reality" on the fluidity and prices of apprenticeships.
56. The barbers kept the original hall, and it was several years before the surgeons had one of their own built. Moore, *The History*, Vol. 2, p. 638 states that the full name of the new company was "The Masters, Governors, and Commonalty of the Art and Science of Surgery." For further details on the separation see Cope, Zachary: *The History of the Royal College of Surgeons of England*. Anthony Blond: London, 1959.
57. See Hamilton, Bernice: "The Medical Professions in the Eighteenth Century." *The Economic History Review* Vol. 4, No. 2, 1951, pp. 147–162 and Pelling, Margaret: "Corporatism or Individualism: Parliament, the Navy, and the Splitting of the London Barber-Surgeons' Company in 1745," pp. 57–82. In: *Guilds and Associations in Europe, 900–1900*. Gadd, Ian and Wallis, Patrick (eds.), Centre for Metropolitan History, London, 2006. Moore, *The History*, Vol. 2, p. 639 also describes the Company as never having much prestige and being old-fashioned.
58. Pelling, "Corporatism," p. 62.
59. Hamilton, "The Medical Professions," p. 150.
60. Hamilton, The Medical Professions, p. 150. Cope makes this argument too in "The History," p. 9.
61. Pelling, "Corporatism,"p. 63. The surgeon William Cheselden and his son-in-law, the physician and MP, Charles Cotes, were prime movers in the split. Cheselden became Master of the Company of Surgeons in 1746.
62. Pelling, "Corporatism," p. 65.
63. Pelling, "Corporatism," pp. 73–4.
64. Power, D'Arcy: *Memorials of the Craft of Surgery in England compiled by John Flint South*. Cassell & Company: London, 1886. p. 381.
65. He was under warden again in 1767 and 1769.
66. Winslow, Forbes: *Physic and Physicians: A Medical Sketch Book, exhibiting, The Public and Private Life of the Most Celebrated Medical Men of Former Days; with Memoirs of Eminent*

Living London Physicians and Surgeons. Londman, Orme, Brown, and Co.: London, 1839, Vol. 1, p. 312. I have not found this passage in lecture notes from Abernethy's courses. In 1767 Pott referred to the examination of surgeons at the Barber-Surgeons' Company. He told his students that "In the old method of examining Surgeons was to ask how many Tumours there were, answer was four." MS0071, Box 1. Anonymous, "Mr. Pott's Surgical Lectures, October 2nd 1767," f. 2. *Royal College of Surgeons of London, Royal College of Surgeons.*

67. On the turbulent life of John Wilkes, see Cash, Arthur: *John Wilkes: The Scandalous Father of Civil Liberty.* Yale University Press: New Haven, CT, 2006.
68. The White Hart off Cavendish Square was near to where Foot lived. Details of the post-mortem findings and the trial can be found in John Foot, *An appeal to the public, touching the death of Mr. George Clarke*, London, 1769.
69. Chairmen carried passengers in sedan chairs.
70. Peachey, George: "William Bromfield, 1713–1792." *Proceedings of the Royal Society of Medicine* Vol. 8, 1915, pp. 103–126.
71. Foot, *An appeal to the public*, p. 42. Also see Chirurgicus, "To the Court of Examiners of the Surgeons Company." *London Magazine*, March 1769, Vol. 38, pp. 151–2, where the author suggests the gentlemen of the court preserved the life of McQuirk.
72. The two men most closely associated with the case were the Whig statesman and prime minister, the Duke of Grafton, and the diplomat, Lord Rochford. See Thomas, Peter G. D.: *George III: King and Politicians, 1760–1770.* Manchester University Press: Manchester, 2003.
73. *The Literary Register. Or Weekly Miscellany*, Vol. 1, Newcastle, 1769, p. 83.
74. *The Literary Register*, p. 83
75. See Wall, *The History*, pp. 126–132. *The Gentleman's Magazine* Vol. 39, London, 1769 contains a series of letters regarding the case, pp. 135–140.
76. Stephens, Frederic George: *Catalogue of Prints and Drawings in the British Museum.* Chidwick Press: London, 1883, Division 1, Vol. 4, pp. 503–4. Consultation of Surgeons, 1769. An engraving of a party of surgeons grouped about a table, under the presidency of one who holds up a large bag of money in one hand, and with the other points to a scroll inscribed:—"It does not appear to us that he died—"; he says:—"This (the money) Convinces me that Cl—k did not dye of the Wound he receiv'd at Br—d" …," 503.
77. Joseph Cruttenden was an attorney-at-law and had been the company clerk since 1745. Pott was a member of the Court of Assistants from 1756 to 1783 and the Court of Examiners from 1761 until his death in 1788. He was succeeded by John Gunning (1733–98), a surgeon to St. George's Hospital.
78. Cruttenden's substantial wealth is evident in a court case at the Old Bailey in 1774. Three men (including a former servant) were indicted for breaking into Cruttenden's dwelling at the Surgeon's Hall in late October. They stole "a silver soup ladle, value thirty shillings; twelve silver table spoons, value six pounds; twelve silver tea spoons, value twenty shillings; a silver pint mug, value four pounds; two silver salvers, value twelve pounds, five silver cruet tops, value ten shillings; a silver coffee pot, value ten pounds; a silver cream pot, value ten shillings; a satin cloak, value ten shillings; a linen shirt, value five shillings; two silk handkerchiefs, value two shillings; a pair of l(e)ather breeches, value ten shillings; a

child's linen frock, value five shillings, and seventy-two halfpence." *Old Bailey Proceedings Online* (www.oldbaileyonline.org, version 7.0, 31 December 2013), December 1774, trial of William Pritchard, Peter Thane, and Edward Parker (t17741207–36).

79. Wall, *The History*, p. 169.
80. Wall, *The History*, pp. 149–52.
81. MS. 5590, "Lectures on the Practice of Surgery by Percival Pott—F.R.S. and Senior Surgeon to Bartholomew's Hospital," f. 210, *Wellcome.* This was a course of 64 lectures taken down and transcribed by an unknown student after 1765. Garrick's case is also mentioned in MS 3958, "Surgical Lectures, Vol. 2nd. Transcribed by John Grigg in 1782," *Wellcome.*
82. *The private correspondence of David Garrick: with the most celebrated persons of his time.* Boaden, James, Henry Colburn and Richard Bentley: London, 1832. Vol. 2, Mr. P. Pott to Mr. Garrick. June 14, 1776, p. 161. Pott may have treated Hannah More's sister, Sally, for vision problems. See Miss H. More to David Garrick, Bristol, July 28th, 1777, "Dear Sir The Arab [sister Sally] is grateful for your goodness to her; her eyes are vastly better, and her health almost perfectly restored; never any creature felt such great and sudden amendment: you and Mr. Pott have, I believe, a constant place in her orisons" (p. 243).
83. "An Account of the last illness" in the *Annual Register in the Year 1788*, August 2, p. 212.
84. Harvey, Diary, f. 57. As a result, Harvey was perpetually broke and had to borrow money from his brother to survive. Harvey's brother in turn spent a great deal of time trying to find a rich heiress for Ludford to marry. In 1789 an uncle left Ludford a substantial amount of money, and two years later with an income finally ensured, he married a Miss Lucy Skinner, the daughter of Alderman Skinner.
85. Cannadine, David: *Class in Britain*. Penguin Books Ltd.: London, 2000, see chapter two.
86. Pott's addresses while living with his mother were Fenchurch Street in 1737 and Bow Lane in 1740.
87. Steele, I. K.: *Atlantic Merchant Apothecary: Letters of Joseph Cruttenden, 1710–1717.* University of Toronto Press: Toronto, 1977; Steele, I. K.: "A London Trader and the Atlantic Empire: Joseph Cruttenden, Apothecary, 1710 to 1717." *The William and Mary Quarterly* Vol. 34, No. 2 1977, pp. 281–297. Also see *The Pharmaceutical Industry: A Guide to Historical Records.* Richmond, Lesley, Stevenson, Julie and Turton, Alison (eds.), Ashgate Publishing Ltd.: Farnham, 2003.
88. The South Sea Company was set up in 1711 to consolidate and reduce the national debt. In 1720 the company used bribery, deceit and obfuscation to try and increase its share capital. The price of the shares quickly rose but then crashed, and many investors lost all. See Carswell, John: *The South Sea Bubble.* Stanford University Press: Stanford, 1960 for the career of Surman. He survived the bursting of the bubble, and eventually opened his own bank. In the 1750s Surman's bank was located on Lombard Street and involved in the HEIC business.
89. On the conversion see Wilson, Walter: *History & Antiquities of the Dissenting Churches*, London, Vol. 1, 1808, pp. 208–228. The hymns can be found in Belcher, Joseph: *Historical sketches of hymns, their writers and their influence.* Lindsay and Blakiston: London, 1859, pp. 127–8. For more about Cruttenden's religious beliefs and influences, see Barry, Jonathan: *Raising Spirits: How a Conjuror's Tale Was Transmitted across the Enlightenment.* Palgrave Macmillan: New York, 2013, pp. 65–67.

90. Cruttenden, R.: *Sovereign efficacious grace! Display'd in the awakening and converting a rational, learned aged sinner. Exemplified in The experience of Robert Cruttenden, Esq. as delivered by himself to the Congregational Church, London,* 1744. Also see Porter, William: *A sermon occasioned by the death of Robert Cruttenden, Esq. (who departed this life June 23, 1763, aged 73 years) preached at Mile's-lane, on Lord's-day, August 7. To which are added, several poetical composures, by the deceased.* T. Field: London, 1763.
91. http://www.cruttenden.webspace.virginmedia.com/historical/90677.htm
92. The attack came from the Nawab of Bengal, Siraj ud-Daulah, who had objected for several years to the increasing military presence of the HEIC. It is known as the Bengal Mutiny and included what was later called the Black Hole of Calcutta incident. Edward married Elizabeth Jedderie in 1746. Their children were painted by Joshua Reynolds in c. 1760 and by Thomas Gainsborough in c. 1763. On the British who made fortunes in India, see Spear, Percival: *The Nabobs: A Study of the Social Life of the English in Eighteenth Century India.* Oxford University Press: Oxford, 1998 and Nechtman, Tillman W." *Nabobs: Empire and Identity in Eighteenth-Century Britain.* Cambridge University Press: Cambridge, 2010. Nechtman mistakenly identifies Bob Pott as William Pott (p. 75). The term "Nabob" was used for any Anglo-Indian who returned home having profited from being in South Asia.
93. The HEIC did not own its ships but chartered vessels from independent ship owners. They then a fleet to cross the seas to India.
94. P69/MRY3/A/002/MS08991, St. Mary Aldermary, Composite register, *London Metropolitan Archives.*
95. Earle, *The Chirurgical Works*, Vol. 1, p. xx. What this system entailed is discussed in the next chapter.
96. Harvey, Diary, ff. 45–6.
97. *The European Magazine*, Vol. 15, Feb. 1789, pp. 102–4, quotation from p. 103. This may have been penned by the surgeon Jessé Foot. See Foot's *The life of John Hunter*, London, 1794, p. 261 on Pott's lack of patronage.
98. John Russell, 4th Duke of Bedford (1710–1771), was the leader of the Bedford Whigs and president of the Foundling Hospital from 1739–71. James Earle performed the postmortem on Bedford's son in 1802.
99. Hastings (1732–1818) was the first Governor-General of British India. He was impeached in 1786 in the House of Commons and put on trial in 1788 on the charge of "high crimes and misdemeanours." Hastings was finally found not guilty by the House of Lords in 1795. See Dirks, Nicholas B.: *The Scandal of Empire: India and the Creation of Imperial Britain.* Harvard University Press: Cambridge, MA, 2008.
100. The Regency Crisis was a series of political maneuvers that took place in 1789 with the goal of replacing the ill George III with his son, the Prince Regent. It failed as the king recovered.
101. On the development of a cosmopolitan plutocracy (able and willing to extend patronage) in London by the mid-eighteenth century, see Rogers, Nicholas: "Money, Marriage, Mobility: The Big Bourgeoisie of Hanoverian London." *Journal of Family History* Vol. 24, No. 1, 1999, pp. 19–34. Rogers' findings are based on a survey of 247 London businessmen who held important political or commercial positions between 1740 and 1759 and were

members of parliament. All were aldermen and directors of major moneyed companies, including the Bank of England and the HEIC.

102. Thurlow never married. He had four "natural" children, a son, Charles, by the daughter of the Dean of Canterbury, and three daughters by his mistress, Polly Hervey (also known as Harvey and sometimes Humphries), the daughter of the proprietor of Nando's coffeehouse. On the history of Nando's see Lillywhite, Bryant: *The London Coffee Houses: A Reference Book of Coffee Houses of the Seventeenth, Eighteenth, and Nineteenth Centuries*. George Allen & Unwin: London, 1963, pp. 381–384.
103. From Argent, Mark: *Recollections of R.J.S. Stevens: An Organist in Georgian London*. Southern Illinois University Press: Carbondale, 1992, p. 148.
104. See Clark, Rev. Andrew: "James Marriott of Twinstead Hall, Essex." *The Essex review: An illustrated quarterly record of everything*. Vol. 15, No. 57, 1906, pp. 86–7. Clark had examined a box of papers that contained some letters of the MP James Marriott (1730–1803). In a letter dated 20th November 1790, after discussion of an operation for hemorrhoids carried out by Mr. Lucas (surgeon) at Guy's (Hospital), Marriott added, "I reflected on the fate of several of my friends and acquaintances whose lives were sacrificed to their want of resolution in a similar disorder … the present sufferings of the Bishop of Durham, who is in a most dangerous state from a long neglect of this complaint. I do not wonder to hear that his brother the Chancellor is much affected and alarmed for him; as the Chancellor himself was for a great while under the care of Pott till he died." Thomas Thurlow died in 1791, and an autopsy was carried out by John Hunter. He removed and preserved Thurlow's rectum, and it remains in the collections of the Hunterian Museum at the *Royal College of Surgeons*, London, as Object RCSHC/P 192.
105. Herbert, Lord: *Pembroke Papers (1790–94): Letters and Diaries of Henry Tenth Earl of Pembroke and His Circle*. Jonathan Cape: London, 1950, Vol. 2, p. 318. The writer of the letter was Thomas Eyre, Canon of Salisbury, Rector of Fovant and Chilmark, in Wiltshire and Chaplain to Lord Pembroke. Eyre died in 1812.
106. *Pembroke Papers*, Vol. 2, p. 319.
107. Harvey, Diary, f. 46.
108. Yorke, Philip C.: *The Diary of John Baker, Barrister of the Middle Temple, Solicitor-General of the Leeward Islands*. Hutchinson & Co.: London, 1931. John Baker's brother Thomas was a surgeon at St. Thomas's Hospital. A second brother Joseph was a surgeon in Chichester. Like Pott, John Baker had one son who entered the service of the HEIC as a writer. In 1761–2 Baker mentions outings in the Southampton area with Pott's former apprentice from Jamaica, Julian Herring, pp. 152–62.
109. Olleson, Philip: *The Journals and Letters of Susan Burney: Music and Society in Late Eighteenth-Century England*. Ashgate Publishing Ltd.: Farnham, 2012, p. 217. Susan was Fanny Burney's younger sister. In Troide, Lars E. and Cooke, Stewart J. (eds.): *Early Journals and Letters of Fanny Burney*. Oxford University Press: Oxford, 1994, Vol. 3, P. 359, there is a letter of Fanny Burney's from Brighthelmstone (Brighton) dated 10 October 1779, remarking that "all the Potts family" was in the area.
110. *The Medical Register of 1783*, London, 1783, p. 20.
111. For information on the Frye family, see Oliver, Vere Langford: *The History of the Island of Antigua, One of the Leeward Caribees in the West Indies, from the First Settlement in 1635 to the Present Time*. Mitchell and Hughes: London, 1894, pp. 284–5.

112. In 1751 the population of Montserrat was 8,853 slaves and 1,430 whites (Oliver, Preface). John Ravel Frye was a witness at James Earle's wedding to Mary, mentioned in Pott's will, and was an executor for Robert Pott. Frye was born in London at an address on Wimpole Street and reportedly died there in 1799. Sarah, his wife, pre-deceased him by 8 years.
113. *The Diary of John Baker*, p. 213.
114. *The Diary of John Baker*, p. 213.
115. *The Diary of John Baker*, p. 214.
116. *The Diary of John Baker*, p. 214.
117. He was a Whig who served as Secretary of State for thirty years and as prime minister twice.
118. To the Earl of Strafford, Strawberry Hill, August 16, 1782, from Horace Walpole, Earl of Orford. In: *Private Correspondence of Horace Walpole, Earl of Orford: Now First Collected*, Vol. 4, Rodwell and Martin: London, 1820, p. 318.
119. http://www.twickenham-museum.org.uk/detail.php?aid=113&cid=20&ctid=2
120. See L/AG/34/29/2, probate record, f. 62, IOR Bengal Administrations, *British Library.*
121. John Opie (1761–1807) was called the "Cornish Wonder." He also painted Pott's wife, Sarah, but the portrait is apparently no longer in existence. The Earle paintings are in private hands. See http://www.christies.com/lotfinder/lot/john-opie-ra-portrait-of-sir-james-2076075-details.aspx?intObjectID=2076075
122. Williams, W. R.: *The History of the Great Sessions in Wales, 1542–1830.* Edwin Davies: Welshpool, 1899, p. 186. Cox was admitted to the Inner Temple in 1775 and to Lincoln's Inn in 1781. He was Commissioner of Bankrupts from 1787–98, Second Justice of Camarthen from 1798–1804, a Master in Chancery in Ordinary (£1000 a year) from 1804–1831 and appointed Treasurer to the Foundling Hospital in 1806.
123. The marriage certificate states Percivall married Ann Belle Maria Emery (d. 1825). On what little is known of the bank he worked in, see, Price, Frederick George Hilton: *A Handbook of London Bankers.* Simpkin, Marshall, Hamilton, Kent & Company, Scribner & Welford: London, 1891. p. 201. Walpole was also MP for Great Yarmouth from 1768–90.
124. This was the same Duke of Newcastle who was the patron of Henry and Samuel Potts.
125. Charterhouse was both a school and an almshouse. It was endowed in 1611 and located in a former Carthusian monastery just behind St. Bartholomew's Hospital. Robert entered Eton College in 1765. The fee recorded as paid by his father was two guineas. See, Austen-Leigh, Richard Arthur: *The Eton College Register, 1753–1790.* Spottiswoode, Ballantine & Co. Ltd.: Eton, 1921, p. 430.
126. Add. 32968, f. 163, Newcastle Papers, Vol. CCLXXXIII, *British Library.* The letter was enclosed in one sent by a W. Pages to a Rev. T. Hurdis of Claremont in Surrey. Pages wrote that "I could not help being surprised at the contents of the inclosed which I recd. by the last post." Hurdis presumably sent Pott's and Pages' letters to the duke. If there was a reply, it has not survived. Thomas Hurdis (?–1784) was later Canon at Windsor.
127. *The Memoirs of William Hickey*, f. 742, BL G118, Private Papers, Asian Collection, *British Library.* As Hickey warns in his memoirs, there are: "Many low and indelicate anecdotes related, and many gross and filthy expressions used" (f. 1).
128. His father was Joseph Hickey, an Irish attorney in London. The poet William Cowper (1731–1800) was a law clerk for Thurlow in Ely Place, Holborn. Hickey was friends with him and they sometimes met to eat at Nando's coffeehouse.

129. Hickey, *The Memoirs*, f. 95. Four log books survive for the *Cruttenden* and they include accounts of the voyage to China and back in 1768–70, and one to Bombay, Surut, Kedgeree, and Ingelee from 1770–1772. See IOR L/MAR/A/531/A-H & 533D, *British Library.*
130. Hickey, *The Memoirs*, f. 97. Families paid the captains of the Indiamen to take their young sons and "teach them the sea." The next step was to become a midshipman, an appointment that was dependent on the captain's approval of the candidate.
131. Spencer, Alfred: *Memoirs of William Hickey*. Hurst & Blackett Ltd.: London, 1919, Vol. 1, p. 285.
132. Hickey, *The Memoirs*, f. 119.
133. Hickey, *The Memoirs*, f. 119.
134. HEIC regulations of 1765 stated that only those over 25 years of age who had performed one voyage as chief or second mate should be appointed to commands. As Jean Sutton notes, the regulations were frequently ignored. She cites Bob Pott as an example of this, in *Lords of the East: The East India Company and Its Ships*. Conway Maritime Press Ltd.: London, 1981, p. 71.
135. Hickey, *The Memoirs*, f. 127.
136. http://www.twickenham-museum.org.uk/detail.php?aid=24&cid=11&ctid=1
137. Writers' petitions, 1770–1774, IOR/J/8/428, *British Library*, contains a list of writers appointed for 1772 to the HEIC in Bengal. It includes Robert Pott, f. 430.
138. Patwardhan, R. P.: *Fort William-India House Correspondence*. Vol. 7, Government of India, Civil Lines: Delhi, 1971, p. 14. Pott was appointed a writer to the Presidency in April 1773. His father sent him £100 in 1774: "We have drawn one set of bills of exchange payable at thirty days sight and two shillings and one penny the current rupee vizt. One set for rupees nine hundred and sixty, for pounds sterling in favor of Mr. Robert Pott on order received of Mr. Percivall Pott dated the 19th December 1774," p. 90. (Rupees 960 = £100).
139. E/1/63, ff. 285–7, Bengal Miscellaneous Letters received, *British Library*. Pott asked for permission to depart for England due to ill health in a letter dated 4th September 1777 at Moorshedabad. A certificate of ill health from the surgeon he consulted is dated 24th August 1777. It states that "Pott, had in the beginning of the Year 1774 a Disorder of his Liver, which hurt his Constitution so much, that he never has recovered his former [constitution] & Strength. In December 1775 he had a severe fit of sickness which impaired his constitution still more." This was most likely malaria. In February 1778, Pott was back in India and well enough to fight a duel with James Grant. Grant was a supporter of General Clavering, first member of the Council, who opposed Governor Hastings. Pott was not surprisingly given Thurlow's patronage, described as a "staunch Hastingsite" by Hickey. See Spencer, *Memoirs*, Vol. 2, p. 154. On diseases of the liver in India see Charters, Erica: *Disease, War, and the Imperial State: The Welfare of the British Armed Forces during the Seven Year's War*. The University of Chicago Press: Chicago, 2014, pp. 155–6.
140. Robert Percival Pott, Extract of Company Letter to Bengal, 14 April 1779, IOR/H/80, ff. 1–8, *British Library.*
141. Hickey, *The Memoirs*, f. 264. Pott also told Hickey that he had paid the rent on the house 15 months in advance. This was a considerable outlay of money.
142. Harvey, Karen: "Gender, Space and Modernity in Eighteenth-Century England: A Place Called Sex." *History Workshop Journal* Vol. 51, Spring 2001, pp. 158–79, quotation from p. 174.

143. Hickey, *The Memoirs*, f. 268.
144. Hickey, *The Memoirs*, f. 268. Emily fits the definition of a courtesan according to Peakman, Julie: *Whore Biographies, 1700–1825*. Pickering & Chatto: London, 2006, Vol. 1, p. xvii. "For a courtesan, status rested on the ability to attract the wealthiest and most powerful of men … Once elevated, she needed to maintain an air of luxury and respectability while effusing sexuality; she needed her own house where possible, along with a coach and four horses, as well as a retinue of servants."
145. Hickey, *The Memoirs*, f. 269.
146. Cruickshank, Dan: *London's Sinful Secret: The Bawdy House and Very Public Passions of London's Georgian Age*. St. Martin's Press: New York, 2009, p. 214. Tim Hitchcock argues that prostitutes moved from being viewed as weak and lustful predators to the more sympathetic image of the fallen woman as victims of men. As reasons for this shift he cites the rise of the cult of seduction in the eighteenth century, changing views of sexuality, and a growing belief in the middle class origins of many prostitutes. See Hitchcock, Tim: *English Sexualities, 1700–1800*. St. Martin's Press: London, 1997, p. 99.
147. Cruikshank, p. 366. The portrait is located at Waddeson Manor (Aylsbury, Bucks, National Trust). As Phillipa Plock notes on their website, "The subject was taken from Dryden's poem, 'Alexander's Feast' which reads: 'Thaïs led the Way/To light him to his Prey/And, like another Helen, fir'd another Troy.' Thaïs was an Athenian courtesan who accompanied Alexander the Great on campaign to invade Persia. She is reputed to have persuaded him to set fire to the Palace of Persepolis in 331 BCE." http://www.waddesdon.org.uk. The 2293mm × 1448mm portrait was shown at the Royal Academy Exhibition, London, in 1781 and again at the British Institute Exhibition, London, of 1817.
148. Fanny Burney (1752–1840), saw it in Reynolds' studio and described it as "a Thaïs, for which Miss Emily, a celebrated courtesan, sat, at the desire of the Hon Charles Greville." Dobson, Austin: Frances Burney, *Diary and Letters of Madame D'Arblay*. Macmillan & Company: London, 1904, Vol. 1, p. 466. Greville quickly sold the painting to Lord Dysart as he was now keeping Emma Hart, the future Lady Hamilton. There was much mystery and confusion surrounding who was the subject of the portrait. Rumors abounded that it was Emily Pott or Warren or Bertie or Coventry. In fact these were all surnames that Emily used at different points in her life. The controversy is discussed in Waterhouse, Ellis and Blunt, Anthony: *The James A. De Rothschild Collections at Waddeson Manor: Paintings*. Fribourg, Switzerland: Office du Livre, 1967, pp. 92–94, cat. 33. Also see Hallett, Mark: *Hogarth*, Phaidon Press: London, 2000, pp. 347–350, fig. 335 and briefly in Pointon, Marcia R.: *Strategies for Showing: Women, Possession, and Representation in English Visual Culture*. Oxford University Press: Oxford, 1997, p. 213. Similar confusion surrounded the identity of the Mrs. Pott painted by George Romney in 1781. Bob Pott commissioned the portrait, and for many years it was assumed that the "Mrs Pott" was his mother. In fact the portrait, was of Mrs. Emily Pott, his mistress. Bob Pott paid Romney £21 for it in 1783, and he left it to his brother Joseph Holden in his will. See Prob. 11/1274, 102, *The National Archives*. On the portrait, see, http://www.metmuseum.org/collections/search-the-collections/437498
149. Waterhouse and Blunt, p. 364.
150. Reynolds finished the three-quarter-length portrait in 1784. It shows Pott seated in an armchair wearing a rather old-fashioned red velvet suit. There is no evidence of

him being a surgeon displayed in the painting, such as instruments or specimens. Pott is simply portrayed as a gentleman. The inscription reads, "Percivall Pott, surgeon to St. Bartholomew's Hospital. A.D. 1784, aet. 71. The gift of James, Marquis of Salisbury, and Heneage, Earl of Aylesford. A.D. 1790." It hangs today in the Great Hall at St. Bartholomew's Hospital. Pott sat for Romney and an unsigned, half-length portrait dated 1788, bought by Pott's son Joseph Holden, exists at the Royal College of Surgeons, see item RCSSC/P 193.

151. Hickey, *The Memoirs*, f. 290.
152. Hickey, *The Memoirs*, f. 290.
153. Hickey, *The Memoirs*, f. 290. Leadenhall Street was the location of East India House, the massive headquarters of the HEIC. Cheese-mongering is a slur on the trade they carried out and a reference to the supposed parsimonious nature of the directors (one of whom was of course, Bob's uncle, Edward Holden Cruttenden).
154. Hickey, *The Memoirs*, f. 290. The position of captain was permanent and conferred high status. Urmston was allowed to trade on his own account, and this included the privileges of carrying private goods for sale abroad, allocating cabin space, and setting the price of the fares for passengers. No one, however, was supposed to sail on an Indiaman without the permission of the Company and this is, perhaps, why Urmston was so worried about the discovery of Emily. See Sutton, *Lords of the East*.
155. The *Lord Mulgrave*, Ref. L/MAR/B/581A. Proceedings of the Ship Lord Mulgrave, James Urmston Commander of a Voyage to Bengall, Commencing the 10th of September 1781 and ending (no info given). Also see "letters from the court, reports the arrival of Robert Pott by the ship Lord Mulgrave, 31st May, 1781," in Gupta, Pratul Chandra: *Fort William-India House Correspondence*. Vol 13, Government of India, Civil Lines: Delhi, 1959, p. 307.
156. Hickey, *The Memoirs*, f. 374. It is quite possible that the mausoleum was never built given the architect Pott reportedly employed. Edward Tiretta was one of the mapmakers, and then Civil Architect for the HEIC. He is variously described by contemporaries as a former assistant and friend of Giacomo Casanova, a political refugee from Venice, a property speculator, and a lottery promoter. See Dutta. Krishna: *Calcutta: A Cultural History*. Interlink Publishing Ltd.: Northampton, MA, 2008, p. 82. There is evidence, however, for the existence of a column that was nicknamed "Pott's Folly" by river pilots. A photograph of it is included in *Bengal Past and Present: Journal of the Calcutta Historical Society*. Vol. 26, July–December 1923, Calcutta. Opposite p. 201.
157. Hickey, *The Memoirs*, f. 411. "Pott was appointed Resident of the Durbar and Collector of Government Customs at Moorshedabad on 31st May 1784." Saletore, B. A.: *Fort William-India House Correspondence*. Vol. 9, Government of India, Civil Lines: Delhi, 1959, p. 529.
158. Hickey, *The Memoirs*, f. 411. On the magnificence of the houses of Europeans in India, and the large number of servants, see Collingham, E. M.: *Imperial Bodies: The Physical Experience of the Raj, c. 1800–1947*. Polity Press: Cambridge, UK, 2001.
159. Add. 29165, f. 173, *British Museum*.
160. PRO 30/11/8b ff. 75–208, Cornwallis Papers, *The National Archives*, contain numerous letters from Pott to Cornwallis. Charles Cornwallis (1738–1805) was appointed

Governor-General of India and Commander-in-Chief in 1786. He returned to Britain in 1794, was reappointed Governor-General in 1805 and died in India shortly after taking up the office.

161. Pott to Cornwallis, Letter, 17th of June 1789, f. 341, Cornwallis Papers.
162. Henry Haldane to Pott, Letter, 20th of June 1789, f. 343, Cornwallis Papers.
163. This was part of *The India Act of 1786* (26 Geo. 3 c. 16).
164. Spencer, *Memoirs*, Vol. 3, p. 329. "July 24 1789, Accounts of the Weights & Measures in Moorshedabad," gives a detailed, torturous account of Pott's and Addison's accusations and counteraccusations, P/3/6 Bengal Public Council, ff. 541–723, *British Library*.
165. Letter from Moorshedabad, December 1787, Cornwallis Papers, f. 479. L/F/10/4 Bengal Civil Servants 1788–1792, Folio 19, No. 74 is an account of Pott's career in the service by the Fort William Civil Auditors Office, 30th April 1789. It records that he is now out of employ (since June 30 1788) and on a subsistence allowance amounting to 4532 rupees a year. (Approximately.£450).
166. Edward Holden Cruttenden had a daughter called Sarah, but she was alive after 1807 and married a Colonel Thomas William Ravenshaw in 1822. George Cruttenden died in 1822. He was a major in the HEIC Bengal Army. Bob Pott left him the large sum of £2000 in his will. He also left a portrait of Emily by Romney to Joseph Holden Pott, and another in ivory to a friend along with the choice of the best horse in his stable. His "Beloved wife gets everything else real and personal, 25th March 1794." Prob 11/1274, 102, The Will of Portraits mentioned:
    1) "to the Reverend Joseph Holden Pott"—"the painting of his friend Emily painted by Romney"
    2) "unto my cousin Lt. G. Cruttenden aforementioned"—"the portrait of his old friend Emily painted by Dance"
    3) "unto … Major George Russell"—"the picture of his friend Emily painted on Ivory by Sherriff" of Moorshedabad in the Province of Bengal, *The National Archives*.
167. Hickey, *The Memoirs*, f. 342.
168. On the pension see Gupta, Hira Lal: *Fort William India-House Correspondence*. Vol. 8, Governor of India Civil Lines: Delhi, 1981, pp. 241–242.
169. Sarah Pott was buried in the English Cemetery in Dacca on 18 September 1807. See Wilson, C. R.: *List of Inscriptions on Tombs or Monuments in Bengal possessing historical interest*. Office of the Superintendent of Government Printing: Calcutta, 1896, p. 206. No record of the place of burial of Bob Pott has been found.
170. Ghosh, Durba: "Decoding the Nameless: Gender, Subjectivity, and Historical Methodologies in Reading the Archives of Colonial India," pp. 297–316. In: *A New Imperial History: Culture, Identity and Modernity in Britain and the Empire, 1640–1840*. Wilson, Kathleen (ed.), Cambridge University Press: Cambridge, 2004. Ghosh examines the colonial archives for evidence of the sexual companions, domestic servants and conjugal partners of European men from 1760–1840.
171. Robert Percival Pott (Rev) to Sir Elijah Impey, 1783, f.124, Add. 16264, *British Library*.
172. For example, *Elegies, and Seimane, a Tragedy*, 1782; *Essay on Landscape-painting, with Remarks on the different Schools*, 1783; and *Testimonies of St. Paul concerning Justification*, 1846.

173. *The Gentleman's Magazine*, July 1809, p. 627.
174. See entry on Joseph Holden Pott by W. M. Jacob in the *Oxford Dictionary of National Biography*. Vol. 46, Oxford University Press: Oxford, 2004, p. 202. His possessions and valuable library were sold by auction in May 1847.
175. *The Gentleman's Magazine and Historical Chronicle*, by Sylvanus Urban, London, Vol. 68, 1798, pp. 814–5. Sylvanus Urban was the nom de plume of the chief editor and founder of the magazine, Edward Cave (1692–1754). *The Gentleman's Magazine* was launched in 1731. In 1798 it was under the editorship of the printer John Nichols (1745–1826).
176. Edward Holden Pott, 18th March 1782, Court of King's Bench: Plea Side: Affidavits of Due Execution of Articles Clerkship, Series I, II, III (KC 105–107), *The National Archives*.
177. Faye, Deirdre Le: *A Chronology of Jane Austen and Her Family: 1700–2000*. Cambridge University Press: Cambridge, 2006, p. 139.
178. When Philadelphia and her daughter returned to England, Hastings provided for them to the tune of £10,000.
179. *The London Gazette*, 2nd April 1793, Issue 8240, p. 270 and *The London Gazette*, 4th July 1797, Issue 14025, p. 633.
180. Cohen, "Liverpool's Contributions to Medicine," p. 946. Edward Holden Pott died in Liverpool.
181. *The Gentleman's Magazine*, 1798, p. 815.
182. *The Gentleman's Magazine*, 1798, p. 815.
183. Earle, *The Chirurgical Works*, Vol. 1, p. 34.
184. Prob. 11/1174, f. 354, Will of Percivall Pott of Hanover Square, *The National Archives*. Pott left his daughters Sarah and Mary £25 each for mourning rings. Elizabeth received £50. Pott left one-guinea mourning rings to the physicians, surgeons, assistant surgeons, clerk, and apothecary at St. Bartholomew's Hospital. Okey Belfour was also left 5 guineas to buy a ring. Pott at no time in his will mentions his son-in-law Samuel Potts, although his three other son-in-laws are named. Nor does he mention by name any children of Samuel Potts and Elizabeth Potts, née Pott.
185. Prob. 11/1174, f. 354.
186. Pott, Sarah: *An Address to Her Beloved Children*. Law and Gilbert: London 1811, p. 3. The address is 6 pages long.
187. Will of Sarah Pott … Widow and Relict of the late Percival Pott, Prob. 11/1519, 28, *The National Archives*. There are also records of her residing at 12 John St., off Bedford Row, in April 1793, and 5 Mortimer St., in June 1795. See MS11936/395/614328 and MS11936/400/642624, *London Metropolitan Archives*.
188. Will of Sarah Pott … Widow and Relict of the late Percival Pott, Prob. 11/1519, 28, *The National Archives*.
189. On the many meanings of politeness in Pott's lifetime see Klein, Lawrence E.: "Politeness and the Interpretation of the British Long Eighteenth-century." *Historical Journal* Vol. 454, 2002, pp. 869–898. For notions of masculinity and politeness, see Carter, Philip *Men and the Emergence of Polite Society, Britain, 1660–1800*. Pearson Education: London, 2001.
190. Earle stated that Pott had a villa in Neasden later in life, and the family spent time there in summer. Neasden, or Needsden as it was known before enclosure, was completed in

1823, was a small village consisting of six cottages, four larger houses or farms, a public house and a smithy, grouped around the green. The only clue to Pott's choice of Needsden is that there was a link to the hospital: "*St. Bartholomew's Hospital* owned a house at Church End which in 1547 was granted to the City of London; the City administered the estate on behalf of the hospital, which was still in possession in 1823. The house was still there in 1599 but had gone by 1816." http://www.british-history.ac.uk/vch/middx/vol7/pp. 216–220.

Chapter Two: "Be Firm Without Appearance of Brutality": Authority and Surgery

1. MS 00071, Box 1, Heaviside, f. 6, *Royal College of Surgeons.*
2. MS. 5590, Lectures on the Practice of Surgery by Percival Pott—F.R.S. and Senior Surgeon to Bartholomew's Hospital, 1760s–80s, f. 8. *Wellcome.*
3. Gelfand, Toby: "'Invite the philosopher, as well as the charitable': Hospital Teaching as Private Enterprise in Hunterian London," pp. 29–152. In: Bynum, W. F. and Porter, Roy (eds.), *William Hunter and the Eighteenth-Century Medical World.* Cambridge University Press: Cambridge, 1985, pp. 129–151.
4. Douglas, John: *A Syllabus of what is to be perform'd in a course on Anatomy, Chirurgical Operations and Bandages*, London, 1719, p. 1. John Douglas (d. 1743) was a Scottish surgeon and brother to Dr. James Douglas (1675–1742). He gave anatomical and surgical lectures and became surgeon-lithotomist to the Westminster Hospital.
5. See Risse, Guenther: *Hospital Life in Enlightenment Scotland: Care and Teaching at the Royal Infirmary of Edinburgh.* Edinburgh University Press: Edinburgh, 1987, pp. 140–141. A fistula is a long, narrow channel formed by discharge from an abscess or ulcer. The most common in the eighteenth century was the *fistula in ano* found in the lower part of the rectum, often caused by infections. Pott wrote on the *fistula lachrymalis*, which developed from purulent eye infections and caused a channel to form between the lachrymal sac and the skin. Following childbirth women could suffer from fistula that connected the rectum to the vagina or bladder.
6. Douglas, p. 37.
7. Douglas, p. 2.
8. Power, D'Arcy: "Nova Et Vetera." *The British Medical Journal.* Vol. 1, No. 2404, 1907, pp. 211–213.
9. Sharp (c.1700–1778) was born in Jamaica and apprenticed to William Cheselden at St. Thomas's Hospital from 1724–1731. He became a renowned surgeon at Guy's Hospital and wrote *A Treatise on the Operations of Surgery, with a description and representation of the instruments used in performing them, to which is prefix'd an introduction on the nature and treatment of wounds, abscesses and ulcers* (1739) and *A Critical Enquiry into the present state of Surgery* (1750). Sharp had spent part of his apprenticeship in France where he took a great interest in French surgery and met Voltaire.
10. See *Notes on a Course of Chyrurgical Operations performed before the Society of Navey Surgeons by Sam. Sharp of Guy's Hospital March 1746* (Incomplete) MS Hunter 216 (U.2.7.) Item 2,

Special Collections, University of Glasgow Library. The Society probably met in Covent Garden and Sharp begun the lectures in 1733. They were taken over by William Hunter in 1746.

11. Moore, Vol. 2, p. 363.
12. See *London Daily Post and General Advertiser* on 9th January and the *London Evening Post*, on 24 January 1741. The course was to begin on February 2nd. See Peachey, George: *A Memoir of William and John Hunter*. Brendan, Plymouth, 1924. In 1739 Pott lodged with his mother and half-sister on Bow Lane close to St. Bartholomew's hospital. He then moved to Fenchurch Street (1736–9), Bow Lane (1740–45), Watling street (1745–69), Lincoln's Inn Fields (1770–1777), and finally to Princes Street off Hanover Square. (1777–1788).
13. *Daily Advertiser*, Issue 3728, London, December 30, 1742.
14. *Egregious quackery display'd. Or, a narrative of the late memorable case of Seignor Capitano Masseo/Written in Spanish ... And translated into English by a faithful hand (Sarificato Sangresugeo)*. London, 1742. The two known copies of this work are in the Wellcome Library, London, and the Special Collections of the University of Cambridge. I have not discovered the identity of the author—the so-called "scourge of bloody surgery."
15. A Captain Robert Massey is listed as dying in 1748 in *The Gentleman's Magazine and Historical Chronicle*, Vol. 18, 1748, p. 428. "*Capt. Rob. Massey*, formerly in the *East India Service*, of a mortification in his arm, which was oblig'd to be cut off. He was educated in *Christ's* hospital, to which he gratefully left *500 l.*"
16. From the *Oxford English Dictionary Online*, "A person who owes his or her fortune and position, and remains subservient to, a patron; a person who is ready to do another's bidding; a puppet, a cat's paw."
17. *Egregious quackery*, p. 3.
18. *Egregious quackery*, p. 11.
19. *Egregious quackery*, p, 18. Operations could be a good source of income. Sloane 4076, f. 171, *British Library* is an undated letter to Sir Hans Sloane, signed by Nourse and five other surgeons at "your Hospitall of St. Bartholomew," requesting permission to perform the operation of lithotomy. It probably dates from the 1730s.
20. See Fischer, George: "Surgery One Hundred Years Ago." *JAMA* Vol. 28, No. 13, March 27, 1897, pp. 596–600, quotation from p. 599.
21. Quoted in Waddington, Keir: *Medical Education at St. Bartholomew's Hospital, 1123–1995*. The Boydell Press: Woodbridge, Suffolk, 2003, p. 35. The Beadles were instructed to always keep a fire burning in the room to make it habitable.
22. Jessé Foot in *The life of John Hunter*, London, 1794 praises Pott for not charging for his lectures and contrasts it with Hunter's mercenary nature: "Purchased science is of more value than that obtained, as a gratuitous book, from a surgeon of an hospital by his pupils:—thus thought John Hunter, but not so—Percivall Pott," p. 245. Foot had been examined at the Surgeon's Hall by Pott in c.1765 and greatly admired him. He disliked the Hunters intensely.
23. Bell, p. 24.
24. This is the only notice found: *St. James Chronicle or the British Evening Post*, Issue 4146. September 1, 1787.
25. Earle, *A Short Account of the*, p. xiv. 1808 edition.

26. Earle, *A Short Account of the*, p. xiv. 1808 edition.
27. Heaviside, John, "Mr. Potts Lectures taken in 1777," Introductory Lecture, f. 1, *Royal College of Surgeons.*
28. Moore, Norman: *History of St. Bartholomew's Hospital.* C. Arthur Pearson Ltd.: London, 1918. Vol. 2, p. 376. "In 1729 Saturday between 7 and 11 in the morning had been set as the time when physicians, surgeons, assistant surgeons, and the apothecary would visit all parts of the hospital in a combined group. In winter the rounds did not begin until 8 in the morning, most likely to wait for the light."
29. MS 00071 Box 1, Anon., "Mr. Potts Surgical Lectures, October 2nd, 1767." *Royal College of Surgeons.* Shand, William: "Percivall Pott, FRS (1716–1788)." *Trauma* Vol. 2, 2000, pp. 291–295, see p. 293. See Reinarz, Jonathan: "Corpus Curricula: Medical Education and the Voluntary Hospital Movement," pp. 43–52. In: Whitaker, Harry, Smith, C. U. M. and Finger, Stanley (eds.): *Brain, Mind and Medicine: Essays in Eighteenth-Century Neuroscience.* Springer Science & Business Media: London, 2007. Reinarz says that Nourse's lectures in 1734 were transferred from home to hospital, p. 48.
30. In one case Pott gave 64 lectures and these stretched into June of the following year. The same topics were covered but in greater detail. See MS 5590, *Wellcome.*
31. Pott was probably referring to Johannes Scultetus' (1595–1645) *Armamentarium chirurgicum* that was first published in 1655 and Lorenz Heister's (1683–1758) immensely popular *Chirurgie* of 1739, which went through multiple editions.
32. Heaviside, "Mr. Potts Lectures taken in 1777," f. 1.
33. His students included: Frederik Ruysch, Jan Swammerdam, Nicolaus Steno, and Reinier de Graaf. See Knoeff, Rina: *Dutch Anatomy and Clinical Medicine in 17th-Century Europe.* Published 2012-06-20, European History online, leg-ego.eu
34. *Micro-Techne; or, a methodical introduction to the art of chirurgery in which every branch thereof is handled in a most natural, compendious and perspicuous manner; and constant References are made, under each Head, to the Best Authors who have treated on that Subject more largely. Together with a Critique on the most Eminent Writers in the Art. Written in Latin by Johannes van Horne, Professor of Anatomy and Chirurgery in the University of Leyden. Translated, with additions, by Henry Banyer, surgeon.* London, 1730.
35. *Micro-Techne*, pp. xii–xiii.
36. MS B 93, The Introduction, f. 4r. *Mr. Potts Surgical Lectures Att.D. 1773 and 74, National Library of Medicine.*
37. MS B 93, f. 4r.
38. MS B 93, f. 4r.
39. MS B 93, f. 5r. This statement concurs with Earle's that Pott decided to begin with general disorders, then move to specific disorders of the head and descend "to the inferior members." Earle, *The Life of*, p. xv.
40. For example, see John Heaviside: "Lectures on Surgery by Mr. Pott, Senior Surgeon to St. Bartholomew's Hospital begun Oct. 9th 1769." *Royal College of Surgeons.* After briefly discussing "Prolapsus Vagina, Uteri; & Inversis Uterus," Pott remarks that he has only superficial knowledge, and it more properly belongs in the "Lectures on Midwifery." In 1787 Andrew Thynne a doctor of medicine of Rheims, was appointed the first lecturer in midwifery to the hospital. He died in 1814. See Moore, Vol. 2, p. 724.

41. Heaviside, 1769, Lecture 24th On Wounds of the abdomen, f. 93.
42. Heberden's description of angina pectoris was first presented to the Royal College of Physicians in 1768.
43. MS 3, "Lectures on the Practice of Surgery by Percival Pott Esq FRS and Surgeon to St. Bartholomew's Hospital," probably 1770s, f. 137, *Royal College of Surgeons.*
44. MS 3957, Lectures on Surgery by Percival Pott Esq., Given at the Theatre at Bartholomew's Hospital, First 32 lectures, c. 1770, Lect. 20 The Dropsy and the Operation call'd Paracentesis, f. 73, *Wellcome.*
45. MS 3957, f. 5.
46. MS 699, "Lectures on Surgery by Mr. Pott F. R. S & Sen. Surgeon St. Barthol-Hospital, 1775/6," f. 5, *Royal College of Physicians.* "His resolution should by no means lead him to Barbarity, he should make a difference between the senseless dead, & the Sensible & Extream [*sic*] irritable, parts of a miserable unhappy but *feeling* patient. Thus are the french [*sic*] in tracing the Spermatic Cord 5 or 6 inches up the abdomen for the removal of a Schirrous Testicle & Cord; could ye suppose they ever did it but on an inanimate Body; if otherwise that they were little less than *madmen*. How a Rational Surgeon can do this cannot be conceived yet they lay it down as a matter of fact." Also see MS 3956, The Chirurgical Lectures of Percival Pott Esq. Senior Surgeon to St. Bartholomew's hospital, Anon., first 36 lectures, c. 1770, *Wellcome.*
47. This was a condition that Pott and William Hunter disputed ownership of as its first discoverers. See chapter four.
48. MS 0071. Box 1, Anonymous, "Mr Potts Surgical Lectures, Oct. 2nd,1767." Lecture 17 on Hernias, f. 74. *Royal College of Surgeons.*
49. Heaviside, 1769, f. 81.
50. MS 5590. Lectures on the Practice of Surgery by Percival Pott—F.R.S. and Senior Surgeon to Bartholomew's Hospital. f. 131. *Wellcome.*
51. MS 5590, Lecture on Cessation of Menstruation, f. 143.
52. MS0071, Box 1, f. 19.
53. Heister, *A General System of Surgery in Three Parts*, 1743, p. 229.
54. Heister, p. 191.
55. For a review of theories and recommended operations, see Sakorafas, G. H. & Safioleas M.: "Breast Cancer Surgery: An Historical Narrative. Part II, 18th and 19th Centuries," *European Journal of Cancer Care* Vol. 19, 2010, pp. 6–29. Henri Francois Le Dran (1685–1773) argued that cancer of the breast was a local disease in its early stages and that was when an operation could be successful. Cancer spread, he believed, through the lymphatic system.
56. Gooch, Benjamin: *Cases and Remarks in Surgery. With Sketches of Machines, of Simple Construction, Easy Application and Approved Use*, London, 1758, p. 131. Gooch was apprenticed to a surgeon in Norwich and then walked the wards in London. He turned to writing about surgery when he became too ill to practice. On his life see Shaw, A. Batty: "Benjamin Gooch, Eighteenth-Century Surgeon." *Medical History* Vol. 16, 1972, pp. 40–50.
57. Gooch, *Cases*, p. 131.
58. Gooch, *Cases*, p. 131.
59. Gooch, *Cases*, p. 131.

60. Pott told his students that "the moderns" call a swelling schirrous if it "will not admit of Suppuration; these may justly be called Schirrous, or Cancerous for they are liable to be translated into cancers, by any Slight Accident as a Blow or fall, or even the Disposition of the habit." MS 699, f. 16.
61. Gooch, *Cases*, p. 131.
62. Gooch, *Cases*, p. 131.
63. Stolberg, Michael: *Experiencing Illness and the Sick Body in Early Modern Europe*. Palgrave Macmillan: Basingstoke, 2011. Stolberg makes the important point that cancer was not a hidden disease process in the past but a disease associated much more closely with images of a decaying surface. "Only those forms of cancer which were close to the body's surface and, in many cases, sooner or later destroyed it, would usually be diagnosed and experienced as cancer. Cancer was therefore experienced as a highly gender-specific disease. Aside from skin cancer, which is comparatively rare, it is largely breast and uterine (cervical) cancers that manifest themselves through palpable knots, ulcerous decay, and ugly, smelly discharge from the body." (p. 137)
64. Heister, p. 228.
65. Heister, p. 229.
66. MSS 2/0179-01, Henry Cline, *Lecture on Surgery*, last quarter 18th, College of Physicians of Philadelphia, ff. 62–66, gives a complete description of the symptoms and diagnosis of breast cancer. Cline noted that women often feel pain in their arm when they carry it backwards as tumours press on the pectoral muscle, then the woman may examine the breast and find a small lump in the Gland—"size of an hazle nut or small Walnutt, they have no pain unless they carry their arm backwards"—women sometimes noticed a small discharge from the nipple, "which stains their Shifts, and which discharge has taken place before two or three months before the Tumour has been discovered which is a sufficient proof that some alteration was at that time taking place in the structure of the breast" (f. 63)
67. Kaartinen, Marjo: *Breast Cancer in the Eighteenth Century*, Pickering & Chatto: London, 2013, pp. 65–66.
68. Churchill, Wendy D: *Female Patients in Early Modern Britain: Gender, Diagnosis, and Treatment*. Ashgate Press: Aldershot, 2012, p. 113.
69. MS 3956, f. 14, *Wellcome.*
70. MSTH/PP Whitfield, Ricardus Whitfield, *Surgical Lectures by Percivall Pott*, nd. f. 23, *King's College Archives.*
71. See Henry Fearon: *A Treatise on Cancers, with a New and Successful Method of Operating, Particularly in Cancers of the Breast and Testis*, London, 1784 and Article 38, *Observations on Cancer*, Henry Fearon, Surgeon to the Surrey Dispensary, and F.M.S., *Memoirs of the Medical Society of London*, Volume II, 1789, pp. 473–491. Fearon received the Silver Medal of the Medical Society of London. He argued that inflammation was both a proximate cause and often a fatal consequence of cancer of the breast.
72. See the case of Mrs. Elizabeth Ellis, Case IX, p. 71. Kaartinen discusses this case and others of Fearon's; see pp. 92–3.
73. Heaviside, 1769, f. 5. Similar advice is given in MS TH/PP *"Mr Pott's Practice of Surgery*, Anon., c. 1770, A Cancer in the Scrotum, f. 96, *King's.* "The greatest pain in the operation

like all others comes from dividing the skin, 'which tho I am an enemy to dexterity should be done as quick as possible."

74. Heaviside, 1769, f. 5.
75. Fearon, *A Treatise*, p. 49. Fearon quotes Pott with approval throughout and refers to him as one of the most eminent operators and authors of our age.
76. Fanny Burney, "A Mastectomy [of 30 September 1811]," Letter 595, to Esther Burney (22 March–June 1812). In: Hemlow, Joyce: *The Journals and Letters of Fanny Burney (Madame d'Arblay)*. Vol. 6, Clarendon Press: Oxford, UK, 1975, pp. 596–616. Critical commentaries include Epstein, Julia L.: "Writing the Unspeakable: Fanny Burney's Mastectomy and the Fictive Body." *Representations* Vol. 16, 1986, pp. 131–166.
77. LettersofNote.com. *Deep Sickness Seized Me*. The letter was written by Lucy Thurston, aged 60, a missionary in Hawaii to Mary her daughter. Like Burney, Thurston survived for a considerable number of years after the operation. She died 21 years later in 1876. Although chloroform was available, Mrs. Thurston's doctors advised against it as she had a previous stroke, and she wrote that in fact "I was glad they allowed me the use of my senses."
78. Heaviside, 1777, f. 72. Also see MS 5590, f. 500 where Pott stated that women must breastfeed soon after labor is over to prevent uterine discharge.
79. MS 699, f. 91. Dr. Steevens' hospital in Dublin was founded c. 1720. In all probability Pott was referring to a recipe for a caustic that an empiric named Plunkett had reportedly provided for use at the hospital. See Hughson, D.: *The New Family Receipt-book: Or Universal Repository of Domestic Economy*, London, 1817, p. 135 and the *American Medical Gazette and Journal of Health*. New York, Vol. 11, Pt. 4, 1860, pp. 530–1.
80. MS 3957, f. 62.
81. MS 3957, f. 62.
82. See Cadogan, William: *An Essay upon Nursing and the Management of Children*, London, 1748.
83. MS 0071, Box 1, f. 45.
84. Heister, *A General System*, 1753, p. 190.
85. MS D1003–1006, Anon.: *Dr. Young's Lectures on Midwifery*, Vol. I–IV, Uppsala Library. At the end of Vol. IV is the following, "Qualifications of a Manmidwife. Need a greater degree of Composure that a good Operator, because a small Oversight is attended with the worst consequence; & here you have not the assistance of your Eye in order to direct your hand."
86. MS 0071, Box 1, f. 47.
87. MS 3958, f. 54.
88. MS 3958, f. 54.
89. Pott, *A Treatise on Ruptures*, 1756, p. ix.
90. MS 0071, Box 1, f. 1.
91. *Chirurgical Works*, Vol. II, A Treatise of the Fistula in Ano, p. 213. Pott also mocked "ingenious, mechanical, or whimsical people" who had busied themselves in inventing instruments to divide the rectum, adding in a footnote: "The late Mr. Freke invented an instrument for this purpose; but it was upon trial, found to cut the operator's finger, with so much more certainty that the patient's intestine, that it has long been laid

aside," p. 212. John Freke (1688–1756) was a surgeon at St. Bartholomew's hospital and designed several new instruments, not all of which performed as badly as this one appears to have done.

92. Heaviside, 1777, f. 4. The boxes referred to contained the surgeons' instruments, bandages, and medications. They were carried by sturdy patients (who then got their meals and bed for free), and favored apprentices or dressers. Some idea of the medications at the hospital can be seen in Moore, p. 718. "On September 29, 1747, all druggists were invited to send samples of rhubarb, opium, spermaceti, gum guaiacum, aloes, manna, cantharides, ammoniacum, assafoetida, jalap, senna, gum Arabic, quicksilver, and some less important drugs, each with a price affixed. This method of selecting drugs for purchase has ever since been continued." Boxmen also had to clean, sharpen and oil instruments and then wrap them in oily muslin.
93. *Chirurgical Works*, Vol. II, An account of the Method of obtaining a Perfect or Radical Cure of the Hydrocele by Means of a Seton, p. 168. Pott was here referring to the jargon that had sprung up around diseases of the testicle.
94. Heaviside, 1777, f. 4.
95. MS TH/PP, f. 7.
96. MA 00071/6 Volume III, *Chirurgical Lectures by Percivall Pott F.R.S. and Senior Surgeon to Saint Bartholomew's Hosp.l, London*, n.d., f. 236.
97. MA 00071/6 Volume III, f. 234.
98. MS 3957, f. 104–5.
99. MS B 93, f. 1.
100. MA 00071/6 Volume III, f. 10.
101. MA 00071/6 Volume III, f. 7. Pott carried out smallpox inoculations. A letter dated the 9th of February 1776, from John Foster in London to James Baker Holroyd, mentions the inoculation of JBH's daughter, and JF's by Pott 14 days ago. See AMS5440/48, East Sussex Record Office. Foster was the first Baron Oriel (1740–1828) and Holroyd (1735–1821) was the first Earl of Sheffield.
102. Segal, Judy Z.: *Health and the Rhetoric of Medicine*. Southern Illinois University Press: Carbondale, 2008.
103. Stohlberg, p. 159.
104. Digby, Anne: *Making a Medical Living: Doctors and Patients in the English Market for Medicine, 1720–1911*. Cambridge University Press: Cambridge, 1994, p. 26.
105. Edgar, Andrew: "Professional values, aesthetic values, and the ends of trade." *Med Health Care and Philos* Vol. 4, 2011, pp. 195–201. See p. 195.
106. Edgar, p. 195.
107. Doyle, Julie: "The Spectre of the Scalpel: The Historical Role of Surgery and Anatomy in Conceptions of Embodiment." *Body & Society* Vol. 14, No. 1, March 2008, pp. 9–30. Quotation from p. 14.
108. MS 5590, f. 1.
109. MS 3957, f. 1. Also see MS B 93, f. 6.
110. MS 3956 f. 3. Also see MS TH/PP, f. 3. "in Hospital you will have frequent opportunities of this kind of knowledge, and if you omit it, the fault will be yours and you will have a great deal to answer for."

111. Heaviside, 1777, f. 1.
112. Moore, Vol. 2, p. 363 cites minutes showing that on "April 8, 1731, Barley broth is not to be sold at the Smithfield gate" and on "November 9, 1732, Apple-stalls and wheel-barrows obstructing the passage through the hospital are to be removed." But in 1746 there were still complaints that box carriers were setting up shops to sell beer and tobacco (p. 371). In 1754, April 4: "The patients called box-carriers, who carry the surgeon's box, demand a fee of 3d. or more from every patient ordered to be bled. This is an abuse, and is not to be allowed nor any other fee." (p. 369). Gibbs had been appointed a governor in 1723. He also designed St. Martin-in-the-Fields and the Radcliffe Camera at Oxford University. He died in 1754.
113. By 1734 the North Wing had been completed, and as it was to be the administrative and ceremonial heart of the hospital, the Governors searched for an artist to decorate the wing's great staircase, which led up to the Great Hall. William Hogarth put his name forward and offered to do it for no charge. Hogarth's two large paintings were installed in 1736 and 1737, and they depict the New Testament episodes of Christ's visit to the Pool of Bethesda and the Good Samaritan. Moore, Vol. 1, p. 43. Arnold, Dana: *The Spaces of the Hospital: Spatiality and Urban Change in London, 1680–1820.* Routledge: London 2013, p. 4 expresses the role of architecture in defining and constraining the patriarchal values of the elite: "The hospital gave a spatial expression to contrasting facets of urban culture articulated through the dynamic binaries of innovation/progress and restriction/containment."
114. MS 699, f. 5 and see MS 3957, f. 4, where the wording is slightly different but the sense is the same. Also see MS B 93, f. 9.
115. *Patient's Progress*, p. 69.
116. *Patient's Progress*, p. 167.
117. MS 3957, f. 5. Similar passages can be found in RCS MA 00071/6 Volume III, ff. 7–8.
118. See Payne, Lynda: *With Words and Knives: Learning Medical Dispassion in Early Modern England.* Ashgate Press: Aldershot, 2007.
119. Gladfelder, Hal: *Criminality and Narrative in Eighteenth-Century England: Beyond the Law.* Johns Hopkins University Press: Baltimore, 2001.
120. *Chirurgical Works*, A Treatise on the Hydrocele, or Watry Rupture, and other Diseases of the Testicle, 1767, Case XVIII, p. 503.
121. *Chirurgical Works*, A Treatise, Case XVIII, pp. 503–4. On the use of cicuta (an anodyne) to treat cancers, see "Observations on Cancers" by Mark Akenside, M.D. in *The Monthly Review*, Vol. 39, London, 1768, pp. 32–4. Akenside (1721–70) was a well-known poet, physician to St. Thomas Hospital and to the school of Christ's Hospital. He was a member of the Royal College of Physicians and the Royal Society, and appointed one of the physicians to Queen Charlotte in 1761. Akenside was caricatured in *The Adventures of Pergrine Pickle* (1751) by Tobias Smollett. On the use of solanum, see Gataker, Thomas: *Observations on the Internal Use of the Solanum or Nightshade*, London, 1757. Gataker was a surgeon at the Westminster Hospital, and he recommended "Garden Nightshade" for cancer among other ailments. It was prepared as a tisane and prescribed to be drunk at bedtime.
122. *Chirurgical Works*, A Treatise, Case XVIII, p. 504.

123. *Chirurgical Works*, A Treatise, Case XVIII, p. 504.
124. *Chirurgical Works*, A Treatise, Case XVIII, p. 505.
125. MS 3956, f. 3.
126. Heaviside, 1769, f. 69.
127. Heaviside, 1769, f. 103. Samuel Sharp, one of Pott's older contemporaries, always 'blooded,' or bled, his patients heavily just before a lithotomy and then sat them up, "because in this Posture [the patient] will be more liable to faint. *A Critical Enquiry Into the Present State of Surgery*, London, 1754, p. 24. Pott commented on how useful a loss of blood could be in making patients manageable to operate upon in his *A Treatise on Ruptures*, 1763, p. 63. "Children, especially very young ones, bear the loss of blood very ill, and are very apt to swoon if the quantity be at all considerable; the surgeon should embrace the opportunity which such general relaxation will afford him of reducing the rupture, especially as it gives him another advantage by preventing the child from crying, and making resistance."
128. Heaviside, 1769, f. 103.
129. Heaviside, 1769, f. 103.
130. MS3957, f. 6.
131. *Chirurgical Works*, Volume I, Observations on that Disorder of the Corner of the Eye, commonly called Fistula Lachrymalis, London, 1758, pp. 220–1.
132. Cheselden was also appointed surgeon for the stone at Westminster Infirmary, surgeon to Queen Caroline, and surgeon to St. Georges's Hospital and Chelsea Hospital. He specialized in cataract surgery as well as cutting for the stone.
133. Ellis, Harold: *A History of Bladder Stone*. Blackwell Scientific Publications: Oxford and Edinburgh, 1969 gives a comprehensive history of lithotomy operations. On Frère Jacques see pp. 12–17. The nursery rhyme does appear to be about him.
134. Stearns, Raymond Phineas: *A Journey to Paris in the Year 1698 by Martin Lister*. University of Illinois Press: Bloomington, 1967, p. 237.
135. Blackmore, Sir Richard: *Dissertation on a Dropsy, a Tympany, the Jaundice, the Stone, and a Diabetes*, London, 1727, p. 155.
136. *Public Advertiser*, London, Saturday, May 21, 1774, Issue 13029.
137. MS 3957, f. 7.
138. For example see *A treatise of lithotomy, or, Of the extraction of the stone out of the bladder written in French by Mr. Tolet ...; translated into English by A. Lovell*, London, 1683, Greenfield, John, *A Compleat Treatise of the Stone and Gravel*, London, 1710, and Douglas, James, *The history of the lateral operation, or, An account of the method of extracting a stone, by making a wound near the great protuberance of the os ischium, through the common integuments and levator ani, into the side of the bladder, without touching the urethra, prostate gland, vesiculae seminales, or any other of the urinary or seminal vessels, first attempted by Frere Jacques in France, and afterwards successfully perform'd by Professor Rau in Holland: with a postscript concerning the introduction and improvement of this method here in London*, London, 1720.
139. John Douglas had introduced the supra pubic (incision made in the lower abdomen) operation into England after he had studied in Paris, and Cheselden at first practiced this, but within two years he had switched to the lateral operation. See Ellis, p. 21.

140. Justamond, J. O.: *Surgical Tracts by the Late J. O. Justamond, FRS Surgeon to the Westminster Hospital*, 1789, p. 57. Also see *Outline of the History of Surgery collected with observations by William Houlston, Member of the Corporation of Surgeons*, London, 1789.
141. MS 3956, f. 1. Also MS 699, f. 1. The cultivation of the mystique of speed contributed to the developing image of the surgeon in the first quarter of the nineteenth century. It was exemplified by Sir Astley Paston Cooper (1768–1841), a surgeon to Guy's hospital. "You should see Sir Astley, students would say knowingly, 'he doesn't give you time to wink.'" In 1826 the Scottish surgeon John Bell (1763–1820) in *The Principles of Surgery, as they relate to wounds, ulcers, and fistulae*, compared the hospital surgeon to someone: "exhibiting on a public stage, [he] loses no occasion of charming the assemblage of spectators into an opinion of his superior skill; hence his operation is all confusion and hurry, the incisions are performed with affected dexterity, the purposes of the operation are but ill accomplished, the arteries are imperfectly secured; and in the end he huddles [hurries] up his work … to excite the plaudits of an unjudging mob."
142. *St. Bartholomew's Hospital Journal*, April 1928, p. 107. The location of this manuscript today is not known. The medical men referred to are James Earle, Edmund Pitts, Charles Blicke, William Long, Ludford Harvey, John Hunter, and Henry Cline. Moore, p. 645 gives the following information: Edmund Pitts elected assistant surgeon, Dec. 11, 1760, and surgeon Jan 22, 1784. James Earle elected asst. 1770, surgeon May 22, 1784. Resigned in 1815. William Long asst. Jan 22, 1784, surgeon 1791. Ludford Harvey elected asst. without opposition July 15, 1784, surgeon August 13, 1807. Charles Blicke succeeded Pott as senior surgeon in 1787 and was Abernethy's master. Henry Cline was surgeon to St. Thomas' hospital and an admirer of John Hunter.

Chapter Three: "He Will Talk, Until He Dies": Accidents and Violence

1. MS 3957, "Lectures in Surgery by Percivall Pott," n.d., f. 43. *Wellcome.*
2. *The Chirurgical Works of Percivall Pott*, London, 1778, Vol. I, p. 155, "Observations on the Nature and Consequences of those Injuries to Which the Head is liable from External Violence." The work was dedicated to John Darker, the treasurer of St. Bartholomew's Hospital. He died in 1785, leaving a fine library to be auctioned off with the proceeds going to the hospital. See *A catalogue of the genuine library of John Darker, Esq; deceased, late treasurer of St. Bartholomew's Hospital, and lest by will to that charity*, London, 1785. On the Jewish community in London see Endelman, Todd M.: *The Jews of Georgian England, 1714–1830: Tradition and Change in a Liberal Society*. Ann Arbor: University of Michigan, 1999.
3. MS 5590, "Lectures on the Practice of Surgery by Percival Pott." 1770s–1780s, f. 486 *Wellcome.*
4. A hydrocele testis is an accumulation of clear fluid in the tunica vaginalis, the most internal of the membranes containing a testicle. It is usually painless. A rupture or hernia is a protrusion of a tissue, structure, or part of an organ through the muscle tissue or the membrane by which it is normally contained. On works with extensive numbers of case histories by Pott see *Observations on the Nature and Consequences of those Injuries to Which*

the Head is liable from External Violence, London, printed for L. Hawes, W. Clarke, and R. Collins, Paternoster-Row, 1768; *A Treatise on Ruptures*, London, printed for C. Hitch and L. Hawes, at the Red Lion, Paternoster-Row, 1756; *Practical remarks on the hydrocele or watry rupture, and some other diseases of the testicle, its coats, and vessels; illustrated with cases; being a supplement to a general treatise on ruptures, published in the year 1756*, London, printed for C. Hitch and L. Hawes, Paternoster-Row, 1762. Quotations in this chapter are from the two-volume work of the 1778 edition of *The Chirurgical Works of Percivall Pott* unless otherwise noted.

5. See, Still, George Frederic: *The History of Paediatrics: The Progress of the Study of the Diseases of Children up to the end of the XVIIIth. Century*. Dawsons of Pall Mall: London, 1965 and Colón, A. R. and Colón, P. A.: *Nurturing Children: A History of Pediatrics*. Greenwood Press: London, 1999, especially chapter seven.
6. MS 3957, f. 6, *Wellcome*. Also see the same case briefly presented by Pott in MS. 5590, f. 118 and in MS B 93, "Mr. Pott Surgical Lectures," n.d., f. 2, *National Library of Medicine*.
7. Clare, Peter: *An Essay of the Cure of Abscesses by Caustic and on the treatment of wounds and ulcers; and a new method of curing the lues venera*, London, 1779, second edition, p. 32. Clare (1738–86) was a London surgeon who specialized in treatment for venereal diseases and especially recommended calomel being applied by friction in the mouth.
8. Wear, Andrew: "Caring for the Sick Poor in St. Bartholomew's Exchange: 1580–1676." *Medical History* Supplement No. 11, 1991, pp. 41–60, provides a good overview of the period before Pott. Also see Siena, Kevin: "Contagion, Exclusion, and the Unique Medical World of the Eighteenth-Century Workhouse," pp. 19–39. In: Reinarz, Jonathan and Schwarz, Leonard (eds.), *Medicine and the Workhouse*. University of Rochester Press: Rochester, 2013.
9. Ganz, Jeremy C. "Head Injuries in the 18th Century: The Management of the Damaged Brain." *Neurosurgery* Vol. 73, No. 1, 2013, pp. 167–75. The surgeons were Henri-François Le Dran (1685–1770) of Paris, Percivall Pott (1714–1788) of London, James Hill (1703–1776) from Dumfries, Sylvester O'Halloran (1728–1807) of Limerick in Ireland, William Dease (1750–1798) of Dublin, and John Abernethy (1764–1831) of London. Also see McCrory, P. R.: "Sir Percivall Pott—the first sports neurologist?" *British Journal of Sports Medicine* Vol. 35, 2001, pp. 278–280. McCrory claims that "Pott was the first to appreciate that the symptoms arising from a head injury are not due to the fractured skull but to injury of the brain. He also disproved the idea that extradural or subdural blood collections would inevitably become pus. This widely held concept was used to justify the enthusiastic use of trephination in many cases of head injury, even in simple concussion." 278. But as Ganz notes Le Dran had previously argued this point. In 1992 E. S. Flamm had an article titled "Percival Pott: An 18th Century neurosurgeon," published in the *Journal of Neurosurgery* Vol. 76, pp. 319–26. Jeremy Ganz responded to it in 2005 with "James Hill of Dumfries: First modern neurosurgical procedures," in the *British Journal of Neurosurgery* Vol. 29, No. 6, pp. 778–784. He specifically criticized Flamm for claiming that Pott was the first modern surgeon who performed neurosurgical procedures and argued the case for James Hill (1703–1776) instead. Hill was a surgeon-apothecary and published *Cases in surgery: particularly of cancers and disorders of the head from external violence, to which is added an account of the Sibbens*, Edinburgh, 1772. Sibbens was a contagious and chronic disease that resembled yaws.

Pott, Percivall: *Chirurgical Observations relative to the Cataract, the polypus of the nose, the cancer of the scrotum, and the mortification of the toes.* London, 1775.

Pott, Percivall: *The Chirurgical Works of Percivall Pott.* London, 1778.

Pott, Percivall: *Observations on the necessity and propriety of amputation, in certain case and under certain circumstances.* London, 1779.

Pott, Percivall: *Remarks on that kind of Palsy of the Lower Limbs, which is frequently found to accompany a Curvature of the Spine, and is supposed to be caused by it. Together with its method of cure.* London, 1779.

Pott, Percivall: *Further Remarks on the useless state of the lower limbs in consequence of a Curvature of the Spine.* London, 1782.

Sharp, Samuel: *A Treatise on the Operations of Surgery, with a description and representation of the instruments used in performing them, to which is prefix'd an introduction on the nature and treatment of wounds, abscesses and ulcers.* London, 1739.

Sharp, Samuel: *A Critical Enquiry into the present state of Surgery. London,* 1750.

Sharp, Samuel: *A Critical Enquiry Into the Present State of Surgery.* London, 1754.

Sheldrake, Jr., Timothy: *An Essay on the Various Causes and Effects of the Distorted Spine; on the improper methods usually practiced to remove that Distortion; In which that recommended by Mr. Pott is considered.* London, c. 1783.

Sinclair, G.: *Cudgel Playing Modernized and Improved; or, The Science of Defence, Exemplified in a Few Short and Easy Lessons, for the Practice of the Broad Sword or Single Stick, on Foot By Capt. G. Sinclair of the 42d Regt.* London, 1800.

Tolet, Francois: *A treatise of lithotomy, or, Of the extraction of the stone out of the bladder written in French by Mr. Tolet translated into English by A. Lovell.* London, 1683.

Wadd, William: *Nugae Chirurgicae or A Biographical Miscellany, illustrative of a Collection of Professional Portraits.* London, 1824.

Walpole, Horace: *Private Correspondence of Horace Walpole, Earl of Orford: Now First Collected.* Vol. 4, Rodwell and Martin: London, 1820.

Wilmer, B.: *Cases and Remarks in Surgery.* London, 1779.

Wilmer, B.: *Practical Observations on Herniae.* London, 1788.

Wilson, Walter: *History & Antiquities of the Dissenting Churches.* Vol. 1, 1808, pp. 208–228.

Winslow, Forbes: *Physic and Physicians: A Medical Sketch Book, exhibiting, The Public and Private Life of the Most Celebrated Medical Men of Former Days; with Memoirs of Eminent Living London Physicians and Surgeons.* Londman, Orme, Brown, and Co.: London, 1839.

Warren, Edward: *The Life of John Collins Warren, M.D., Compiled Chiefly from his Autobiography and Journals.* Ticknor and Fields: London, 1839.

Secondary Sources

Adelmann, Howard, Charles: *Percivall Pott's Role in the History of Surgery and Fracture Therapy.* Dissertation: Basel 1963.

Alberti, Fay Bound: "Bodies, Hearts, and Minds: Why Emotions Matter to Historians of Science and Medicine." *Isis* Vol. 100, No. 4, December 2009, pp. 798–810.

Kirkland, Thomas: *Observations upon Mr. Pott's General Remarks on FRACTURES, etc. IN Three LETTERS to a young SURGEON intending to settle in the Country. With a Postscript, Concerning the Cure of the Compound Dislocations; in which the usual Method of treating WOUNDS of the TENDONS and LIGAMENTS is briefly considered by Thomas Kirkland.* London, 1770.

Lagaranne M.-L. Reneaulme de: *Discours pour l'ouverture de l'École de chirurgie avec une thèse paraphrasée, sous ce titre Essay d'un traité des hernies nommées descentes, par M.-L. Reneaulme de Lagaranne.* Paris, 1726.

Lettsom, C.: *The Works of John Fothergill, MD, Member of the Royal College of Physicians and Fellow of the Royal Society of London, Fellow of the Royal College of Physicians of Edinburgh.* London, 1784.

Moore, James: *A Dissertation on the Process of Nature in the Filling up of Cavities, Healing of Wounds, and Restoring the Parts which have been Destroyed in the Human Body, which obtained the prize medal given by the Lyceum Medicum Londiense in 1789, and was ordered to be published for the use of the society.* London, 1789.

Newman, Jeremiah Whitaker: *The Lounger's Common-Place Book of 1796.* London, 1796.

Nourse, *Edward: Syllabus totam rem Anatomicam humanam complectens et praelectionibus aptatus habendis Authore E. Nourse, huic accredit syllabus chirurgicus quo exhibentur operations quarum modus peragendarum demonstrandus.* London, 1729.

Park, Henry: *An Account of a New Method of Treating Diseases of the Joints of the Knee and Elbow in a Letter to Mr. Percival.* London, 1783.

Pearson, John: *The Life of William Hey, 1758–1826.* London, 1823.

Porter, William: *A sermon occasioned by the death of Robert Cruttenden, Esq. (who departed this life June 23, 1763, aged 73 years) preached at Mile's-lane, on Lord's-day, August 7. To which are added, several poetical composures, by the deceased.* London, 1763.

Pott, Percivall: *A Treatise on Ruptures.* London, 1756.

Pott, Percivall: *An Account of a Particular Kind of Rupture, Frequently Attendant upon New-Children; and Sometimes Met with in Adult; viz. that in which the intestine, or omentum, is found in the same cavity, and in contact with the testicle.* London, 1757.

Pott, Percivall: *Observations on that disorder of the corner of the eye, commonly called fistula lachrymalis.* London, 1758.

Pott, Percivall: *Observations on the nature and consequences of those injuries to which the head is liable from external violence.* London, 1760.

Pott, Percivall: *Practical Remarks on the Hydrocele or Watery Rupture, and Some Other Diseases of the Testicle.* London, 1762.

Pott, Percivall: *Practical remarks on the hydrocele or watry rupture, and some other diseases of the testicle, its coats, and vessels; illustrated with cases; being a supplement to a general treatise on ruptures, published in the year 1756.* London, 1762.

Pott, Percivall: *Remarks on the disease, commonly called a fistula in ano.* London, 1765.

Pott, Percivall: *Treatise of the Hydrocele, or Watry Rupture and Other Diseases of the Testicle, It's Coats and Vessels.* London, 1767.

Pott, Percivall: *Observations on the Nature and Consequences of those Injuries to Which the Head is liable from External Violence.* London, 1768.

Pott, Percivall: *Remarks on the Necessity and Propriety of the Operation of Amputation.* London, 1770.

Pott, Percivall: *Some few general remarks on fractures and dislocations.* London, 1773.

10. Pott, "Observations on the Nature," in *The Chirurgical Works of Percivall Pott*, 1778, pp. 124–5. In support of Pott's statement, Le Dran is quoted in French at the bottom of 126.
11. Pott, "Observations on the Nature," p. 8.
12. An excellent article on the various overlapping theories of inflammation in the body during the eighteenth century is Christine Hallett's: "The Attempt to Understand Puerperal Fever in the Eighteenth and Early Nineteenth Centuries: The Influence of Inflammation Theory." *Medical History* Vol. 49, No. 1, 2005, pp. 1–28.
13. MS 0071, Heaviside, 1769, Lecture 8, On injuries of the scalp, f. 1, *Royal College of Surgeons*. Also see Pott, "Observations on the Nature," pp. 14–16.
14. Moore, James: *A Dissertation on the Process of Nature in the Filling up of Cavities, Healing of Wounds, and Restoring the Parts which have been Destroyed in the Human Body, which obtained the prize medal given by the Lyceum Medicum Londiense in 1789, and was ordered to be published for the use of the society*, London, 1789, p. 46. Moore was an army surgeon.
15. Pott, "Observations on the Nature," p. 156.
16. I have found no evidence of this case being referred to the authorities or going to court. The cost of proceedings would likely have been prohibitive even if a family member or a friend had chosen to pursue the case against the girl's mother. Furthermore, gender may have played a role in the decision to treat this as a domestic dispute. Gwenda Morgan and Peter Rushton have examined the casebook of a local JP in northeast England and found that even in violent assaults by women on other women, most cases were settled out of court. See "The Magistrate, the Community and the Maintenance of an Orderly Society in Eighteenth-century England." *Historical Research* Vol. 76, No. 191, pp. 54–77. On violence relating to women and girls that did come to court see Crawford, Patricia: *Parents of Poor Children in England, 1580–1800*. Oxford University Press: Oxford, 2010, especially chapter three.
17. This information has been gleaned from MJ/SP/1767/05/026, *Body Snatching Case 1767, May 21. London Metropolitan Archives*. "Voluntary confession of Joseph Pickett of the Parish of St George, Southwark in the County of Surrey, labourer, taken on oath before John Levy, one of his Majesty's Justices of the Peace for the County of Surrey. With a group of other men stole bodies at various times from burying grounds including at Brompton belonging to the Governours of St. George's Hospital (with Joseph Hoare using his mother's cart and horse.) Took the body to some place nearby in Westminster. William Francis had care of the burying ground called Mount Hill Ground belonging to the Governours of St. Bartholomew's Hospital, with Pickett stole a body and took it over London Bridge. Mark of Joseph Pickett." We know very little of how and where those who died unclaimed in St. Bartholomew's Hospital were buried.
18. MS 5590, f. 75.
19. MS 0071, ff. 30–1.
20. Greenblatt, Samuel H., Dagi T., and Epstein M. (eds.): *A History of Neurosurgery: In Its Scientific and Professional Contexts*. Thieme Medical Publications: Park Ridge, Ill., 1997, pp. 76–78 and p. 297 discuss the importance of Pott's work on head injuries in modern terms. On the frequency of skull surgery see Miles, Adrian with Connell, Brian: "New Bunhill Fields Burial Ground, Southwark, Excavations at Globe Academy, 2008." *Museum of London Archaeology*, Archaeology Series 24, 2012. In excavations at this heavily

used private burial grounds, 827 wooden coffins, 514 skeletons, 357 subadults and 157 adults were selected for full osteological analysis. The authors discovered that: "Often cut marks could be matched with the instruments used to make them … round holes seen in two of the skulls would have been made by a trephine." (p. 45)

21. Dease, William: *Observations on Wounds of the Head with a Particular Enquiry into the Parts Principally Affected, in those who die in Consequence of such Injuries*, Surgeon to the united hospitals of St. Nicholas and St. Catherine, London, re-printed for G. Robinson, Paternoster Row, 1776.
22. MS 5590, f. 61.
23. A notable exception is Thomas Rogers Forbes' long article, "Crowner's Quest" in *Transactions of the American Philosophical Society* Vol. 68, No 1 1978, pp. 1–52. In a statistical study, Forbes examined all 6351 inquests from 1788 to 1829 instigated by the City of London and Southwark, including 726 from St. Bartholomew's Hospital. Forbes concluded 3,316 were accidental deaths and classified 944 of these as occupational fatalities. Only twelve of these involved women. The most common cause of death was falls, followed by drowning, vehicle and horse accidents, and finally dangers at work such as swinging cranes. This corresponds to Pott's case histories.
24. See Porter, Roy: "Accidents in the Eighteenth Century." In: *Accidents in History: Injuries, Fatalities, and Social Relations.* Clio Medica/Wellcome Institute Series in the History of Medicine, Amsterdam: Rodopi Press, 1997, pp. 90–106, quotation from p. 91. Porter suggests that by the end of the eighteenth century, Enlightenment optimism held that hazards lay within human power. He cites the rise of the Society for the Recovery of People Apparently Drowned (1774), which changed its name to the Humane Society in 1776 and to the Royal Humane Society in 1785 (p. 97). See Kirby, Peter: *Child Labour in Britain, 1750–1870.* Palgrave Macmillan: Basingstoke, 2003 for a discussion of the large number of children involved in familial occupations.
25. Pott, "Observations on the Nature," p. 210.
26. Dodd, George: *The Food of London.* Longman, Brown & Green: London, 1856 reports that at Smithfield Market from 1740 to 1750, the average yearly sales were reported to be about 74,000 cattle and 570,000 sheep (p. 228).
27. Pott, "Observations on the Nature," p. 172.
28. I follow M. Dorothy George's definition in *London Life in the Eighteenth Century.* Academy Chicago Publishers: Chicago, 2005, that the metropolis was made up of the Cities and liberties of London and Westminster, the Borough of Southwark and parts adjacent.
29. Landers, John: *Death and the Metropolis: Studies in the Demographic History of London 1670–1830.* Cambridge University Press: Cambridge, 1993, p. 73.
30. Landers, p. 41. White, Jerry: *London in the Eighteenth Century: A Great and Monstrous Thing.* The Bodley Head: London, 2012, p. 3.
31. Landers, pp. 48–9.
32. M. Dorothy George notes that Irish women often ran lodging houses and old ruinous houses were let nightly (p. 97). On the poor and lodgings especially see, White, pp. 113–14.
33. Voth, Hans-Joachim: "Time and Work in Eighteenth-Century London." *The Journal of Economic History* Vol. 58, No. 1, 1998, pp. 29–58. Voth analyzed 2000 or so Old Bailey Sessions involving tradespeople to come up with this figure.

34. The *London Building Act of 1774* was supposed to help the situation by limiting some of the more dangerous building practices of speculators. White mentions reports of houses that suddenly collapsed on their occupants and those passing by (pp. 67–8). Numerous accidents are listed in newspapers of the day; for example, see *London Morning Penny Post*, August 2, 1751, report of a tile falling from a house in Holborn terribly fracturing the skull of a young woman. "She was immediately carried to St. Bartholomew's Hospital, where her Skull was trepann'd, but there are very little hopes of her Recovery." This was confirmed in the *Whitehall Evening Post or London Intelligencer*, August 10–13, 1751, Issue 859: "The young Woman that a few Days since had her Skull fractured, by the Fall of a Tile from a House in Holborn, is since dead in St. Bartholomew's Hospital." Also see *World and Fashionable Advertiser*, Thursday, September 20, 1787, Issue 214, "Tuesday a bricklayer's labourer fell off a scaffold near three stories high, at a new house building opposite Bridewell, in Bridge street by which he fractured his skull, and was carried to St. Bartholomew's hospital without any hope of recovery."
35. MS 3957, Lect. 11th Of Extravasation and Concussion of the Brain and the Caries of the Cranium, f. 43. Also see MS 699, "Lectures on Surgery by Mr. Pott," 1775/6, f. 60, *Royal College of Physicians*, for the same case. Christ's Hospital was founded in the sixteenth century so that poor boys could learn work skills. During Pott's lifetime, it was located in Newgate. White mentions that "Christ's Hospital licensed the drivers of 420 cars or carts to ply for hire at assigned stands and wharves," p. 225.
36. Pott, "Observations on the Nature," p. 25.
37. Pott, "Observations on the Nature," p. 32.
38. Pott, "Observations on the Nature," p. 9.
39. Pott, "Observations on the Nature," p. 90.
40. Pott, "Observations on the Nature," p. 92.
41. Williams, A. N.: "Four Candles. Original Perspectives and Insights into 18th Century Hospital Child Healthcare." *Archives of Diseases in Childhood* Vol. 92, 2007, pp. 75–79. Williams discusses two inpatient child cases (scald head and fever) and two outpatient child cases ("epileptick fits" and "asthamtick") at Northampton General Hospital in 1744–5.
42. Heaviside, 1769, f. 32.
43. Pott, "Observations on the Nature," p. 215. White gives the figure of 6,900 ships entering the docks in 1700, rising to 14,800 by 1795 (p. 167). On porters see Stern, Walter: *The Porters of London*. Longmans and Green: London, 1960.
44. Pott, "Observations on the Nature," p. 215.
45. Pott, "Observations on the Nature," p. 203. A hogshead was a large wooden barrel.
46. Pott, "Observations on the Nature," p. 204. Most goods services from London had substituted wagons for packhorses by 1750. Black, Jeremy: *Eighteenth Century Britain, 1688–1783*. Palgrave Macmillan: Basingstoke, 2008, p. 68.
47. MS B 93 f. 23.
48. See Ruisinger, Marion Maria R.: "Lorenz Heister (1683–1738) and the 'Bachmann Case': Social Setting and Medical Practice of Trepanation in Eighteenth-Century Germany," pp. 273–288. In: *Trepanation, Discovery, History, Theory*. Arnott, Robert, Finger, Stanley, and Smith, C. U. M. (eds.), Swets and Zeitlinger: Lisse: 2003 and Ruisinger, Marion Maria R.: "Lorenz Heister and the Challenge of Trepanation: A Neurosurgical Case Study From the 18th Century." *Journal of the History of Neurosciences* Vol. 11, No. 3, 2002, pp. 286–300.

49. Pott, "Observations on the Nature," p. 83–4.
50. Pott, "Observations on the Nature," p. 46.
51. Pott, "Observations on the Nature," p. 147. The Mansion House was built between 1739 and 1752 across from the Bank of England. It became the permanent residence of the lord mayor of London. Jeffery, Sally: *The Mansion House*. The History Press Ltd.: London, 1993. George Fewkes was in charge of the plastering, according to a contract signed in 1749. Intricate plastering was extensive throughout the house, and much of it remains intact today.
52. Pott, "Observations on the Nature," p. 147.
53. Pott, "Observations on the Nature," p. 151. The terms *trepan* and *trephine* appear to have been used interchangeably by Pott.
54. Pott adds that the patient took part: "In the memorable defence made by Captain Gilchrist on board as I think the Southampton man of war against the French." This case probably dated to 1757.
55. Dr. William Pitcairn (1712–91) was a physician at Saint Bartholomew's Hospital from 1750 to 1780. He was succeeded by his nephew, Dr. David Pitcairn.
56. Pott, "Observations on the Nature," p. 96.
57. Pott, "Observations on the Nature," p. 97.
58. MS 0071, f. 22.
59. Pott, "Observations on the Nature," p. 92. Hackney coaches generally operated out of inn yards and from coach stands close to the main streets of the capital. They were numbered and licensed. In 1785 there were 1,000 licensed Hackney coaches in London. See Smith, D. J.: *Discovering Horse-drawn Vehicles*. Princes Risborough: Shire Publications, 1994, p. 47.
60. Probably Daniel Brown, Surgeon, of Wellyard, Little Britain.
61. Pott, "Observations on the Nature," p. 93.
62. Pott, "Observations on the Nature," p. 137. The New Road was built between 1756 and 1757 and stretched from Edgeware Road at Paddington to the Angel Public House in Islington. The City Road opened as a toll road from Islington to Moorgate in 1761. White, p. 69.
63. Probably James Bethune (d. 1767), a surgeon in Brentford for 50 years.
64. Pott, "Observations on the Nature," pp. 93–4.
65. Pott, "Observations on the Nature," p. 142.
66. Pott, "Observations on the Nature," p. 143.
67. Pott, "Observations on the Nature," Vol. I, Cases V, XX, XXI, XXII, XXV, XXXV and XXXVI, p. 64, pp. 143–45, and pp. 205–6. Schwartz, L. D.: *London in the Age of Industrialisation: Entrepreneurs, Labour Force and Living Conditions, 1700–1850*. University of Cambridge Press: Cambridge, 1993 discusses the growing youth of the population. In 1661 the population aged below 15 was about 29%, by 1821 it was 39% (p. 26). Between the late eighteenth century and the mid nineteenth century, 17–20% of children under the age of 15 had lost one parent (p. 29).
68. Some of Pott's cases that concern injuries from playing games are transcribed in Allen, Julia: *Swimming with Dr Johnson and Mrs Thrale: Sport, Health and Exercise in Eighteenth-century England*. The Lutterworth Press: Cambridge, UK, 2012. Underdown, David: *Start of Play: Cricket and Culture in Eighteenth-Century England*. Penguin Books: London, 2000,

has an excellent chapter on "Cricket in Metropolitan Culture." On the general history of games and sport in the eighteenth century see Brailsford, Dennis: *A Taste for Diversions: Sport in Georgian England.* The Lutterworth Press: Cambridge, UK, 1999 and Tranter, Neil: *Sport, Economy and Society in Britain 1750–1914.* Cambridge University Press: Cambridge, 1998.

69. Pott, "Observations on the Nature," p. 211.
70. Underdown, p. 95. For contemporary evidence of the growing popularity of cricket, see Francis Hayman's paintings of *Cricket in the Artillery Ground* (1743) and *Cricket as Played in the Mary-le-Bone Fields* (c. 1748).
71. Pott, "Observations on the Nature," p. 66.
72. Glister or glyster was another word for a clyster or an enema administered with a clyster syringe.
73. Pott, "Observations on the Nature," p. 54.
74. See *Cudgel Playing Modernized and Improved; or, The Science of Defence, Exemplified in a Few Short and Easy Lessons, for the Practice of the Broad Sword or Single Stick, on Foot By Capt. G. Sinclair of the 42d Regt.*, London, 1800.
75. Pott, "Observations on the Nature," p. 140.
76. Pott, "Observations on the Nature," p. 141.
77. See Crawford, *Parents of Poor Children*; Turner, David M.: *Disability in Eighteenth-Century England: Imagining Physical Impairment.* Routledge: London, 2012; Borsay, Anne: *Disability and Social Policy in Britain since 1750.* Palgrave Macmillan: Basingstoke 2005; Williams, Samantha: "The Experience of Pregnancy and Childbirth for Unmarried Mothers in London, 1760–1866." *Women's History Review* Vol. 20, No. 1 2011, pp. 67–86; and Newton, Hannah: *The Sick Child in Early Modern England, 1580–1720.* Oxford University Press: Oxford, 2012. Children were believed to be more sensitive to pain.
78. Pott, "Observations on the Nature," p. 58.
79. Pott, "Observations on the Nature," p. 59.
80. Pott, "Observations on the Nature," p. 59.
81. Pott, "Observations on the Nature," p. 60.
82. Pott, "Observations on the Nature," p. 61.
83. Pott, "Observations on the Nature," p. 206. This may have been Dr. Matthew Lee (1695–1755), a physician in London and Oxford. He was also a physician to Frederick, Prince of Wales.
84. Pott, "Observations on the Nature," p. 208.
85. *Old Bailey Proceedings Online* (www.oldbaileyonline.org, version 7.0, 24 May 2012), February 1734 (17340227). The proceedings were published accounts of the trials from the sessions. On surgeons acting as witnesses in court, see Rabier, Christelle: "Defining a Profession: Surgery, Professional Conflicts and Legal Powers in Paris and London, 1760–1790," pp. 85–114. In: Christelle Rabier (ed.): *Fields of Expertise: A Comparative History of Expert Procedures in Paris and London, 1600 to Present.* Cambridge Scholars Publishing: Newcastle, UK, 2007. Pott also confirmed the evidence of Dr. Smith at the trial of Willy Sutton, a merchant, who was acquitted of the murder of Ann Bell. See *Old Bailey Proceedings Online* (www.oldbaileyonline.org, version 7.0, 05 January 2015), February 1761, trial of Willy Sutton (t17610225-18).
86. *Old Bailey Proceedings*, (17340227).

87. *Old Bailey Sessions: Sessions Papers*—Justices' Working Documents OB | PS, 5th February 1759–28th December 1759, LL ref: LMOBPS450040017. Image 17 of 71, 29th February 1759. Sessions Papers consisted of documents generated by Justices of the Peace when they dealt with various local and criminal matters.
88. In 1771 watchers were to paid 6d per night instead of 4d. Moore, Vol. 2, p. 768. See, Carré, Jacques: "Hospital Nurses in Eighteenth-Century Britain: Service without Responsibility." In: *The Invisible Woman: Aspects of Women's Work in Eighteenth-Century Britain.* Baudino, Isabelle, Carré, Jacques and Révauger, Cécile (eds.), Ashgate Press: Aldershot, 2005, pp. 89–99.
89. *Old Bailey Proceedings Online* (www.oldbaileyonline.org), December 1759 (17591205).
90. All quotations from *Old Bailey Proceedings Online* (www.oldbaileyonline.org), December 1759 (17591205).
91. MJ/SP/1767/05: f. 1. *London Metropolitan Archives.* "Information taken this Sixth day of May 1767 at the Parish of St Martin in the Fields within the Liberty of Westm.er in the County of Middlesex, on an Inquisition touching the Death of Mary Gardiner lying dead in the said Parish, Liberty and County." Earle's and Pott's depositions can be found on f. 3. Also see *Old Bailey Proceedings*, 3rd June 1767. Reference Number: 17670603, number 5, Part 1, London, published for J. Wilkie. On this case see Forbes, Thomas R.: "Percivall Pott Performs a Postmortem." *Bulletin of the New York Academy of Medicine* Vol. 51, No. 2, 1975, pp. 272–276. Coroners' inquests were required to be held within forty-eight hours of a suspicious death. The goal was to collect and record depositions from all the main witnesses and the inquest was often held in a local alehouse, a workhouse, or the place in which the death took place. The location of the inquest regarding Mary Gardiner's death was not given. See LL ref: WACWIC652070323, Image 323 of 723, 6th May 1767, City of Westminster coroners: Coroner's inquests into suspicious deaths, *Westminster Archives.*
92. MJ/SP/1767/05: f. 1. *London Metropolitan Archives.*
93. *Old Bailey Proceedings*, 3rd June 1767. Reference Number: 17670603, number 5, Part 1, London, published for J. Wilkie.
94. A mop-stick was the long thick handle of a mop. Pott, "Observations on the Nature," pp. 68–69.
95. On street sellers and entertainers see Dickie, Simon: *Cruelty and Laughter: Forgotten Comic Literature and the Unsentimental Eighteenth Century.* University of Chicago Press: Chicago, 2011, especially chapter two, and White, pp. 196–205. It is probable that as in the case of sellers of newspapers and milk, the woman would have had to purchase the rights to her "walk" or round. See M. Dorothy George, p. 98.
96. White, p. 197. Also see Hitchcock, Tim: "Begging on the Streets of Eighteenth-Century London," *Journal of British Studies* Vol. 44, July 2005, pp. 478–498.
97. Pott, "Observations on the Nature," p. 69.
98. Pott, "Observations on the Nature," p. 70.
99. Pott, "Observations on the Nature," p. 70.
100. Pott, "Observations on the Nature," p. 208.
101. Pott, "Observations on the Nature," p. 151. There is a similar case in MA 00071/6, f. 304. "Case 1st Concussion of the Brain Mr. Pott I was consulted for a young surgeon who was brought to the hospital, who had fallen from a coach, and received a blow on the left

parietal bone.' Insensible for a moment, returned home, that night violent pain to the head, convulsions, Pott opened the cranium, it bled, patient recovered his senses, bled in the arm repeatedly, high fever, uses the trephine, opened the dura mater as distended with a lancet, eighth day he died. We had no opportunity to inspect the head."

102. Pott, "Observations on the Nature," p. 154.
103. Pott, "Observations on the Nature," p. 71. A pest-house was a place where those with communicable diseases such as smallpox and tuberculosis could be forcibly quarantined. On private madhouses in this era, see Parry-Jones, William L.: *The Trade in Lunacy: A Study of Private Madhouses in England in the Eighteenth and Nineteenth Centuries*. Routledge & Kegan Paul: London, 1972, especially chapter two. "The Act of 1774 made provision for the licensing and inspection of private madhouses within the cities of London and Westminster and within a radius of seven miles thereof, by five Commissioners appointed by the College of Physicians and throughout the rest of England and Wales by justices of the peace accompanied by a medical practitioner. In addition, a medical certificate confirming the insanity was required before the confinement of non-pauper patients could take place" (p. 9). The Act was made perpetual in 1786. There were approximately 16 metropolitan licensed houses in Pott's era (p. 30).
104. Pott, "Observations on the Nature," p. 71. For context see Parry-Jones; Porter, Roy: *Mind-Forg'd Manacles: A History of Madness in England from the Restoration to the Regency*. Athlone: London, 1987; Porter, Roy: *Madmen: A Social History of Madhouses, Mad-Doctors and Lunatics*. Tempus: Stroud, 2004; Ingram, Allan: *Patterns of Madness in the Eighteenth Century: A Reader*. Liverpool University Press: Liverpool, 1998; and Andrews, Jonathan & Scull, Andrew: *Customers and Patrons of the Mad Trade: The Management of Lunacy in Eighteenth-Century London*. University of California Press: Berkeley and Los Angeles 2003.
105. Pott, "Observations on the Nature," p. 71.
106. On the wide meaning of the word "friends" in the eighteenth century, see Tadmor, Naomi: *Family & Friends in Eighteenth-Century England: Household, Kinship, and Patronage*. Cambridge University Press: Cambridge, 2007 and Houston, R. A.: "Madness and Gender in the Long Eighteenth Century." *Social History* Vol. 27, No. 3, 2002, pp. 309–326. Houston remarks that single men and women made up a large population of the mad and that suicide rates were higher for men than for women. Lunatics with families who could pay were sometimes placed in private mad houses. This appears to have been the case with this man.
107. Pott, "Observations on the Nature," p. 72.
108. Potassium carbonate, an alkali.
109. Pott, "Observations on the Nature," p. 74.
110. In the eighteenth century, a merchant generally meant someone who traded abroad.
111. Pott, "Observations on the Nature," p. 153.
112. Ennis, Daniel James: *Enter the Press Gang: Naval Impressment in Eighteenth-Century British Literature*. University of Delaware Press: Dover, 2002.
113. Watchmen were paid by the night to patrol a district of approximately 100 houses in a parish or ward. In 1755 fewer than 250 watchmen were available for the area from Whitechapel through Shoreditch, Clerkenwell, and from St. Giles to Marylebone. White, pp. 438–9.

114. Pott, "Observations on the Nature," p. 75.
115. Pott, "Observations on the Nature," p. 76.
116. Pott, "Observations on the Nature," p. 77.
117. MS 3957, f. 17.
118. A recipe for "Digestive Balsam at St. Bartholomew's Hospital" is given in Anon., *The modern practice of the London hospitals*, 1766. It consists of 12 ounces of St. John's Wort and four ounces of Arceus's liniment and is recommended for all kinds of green wounds (p. 22). Arceus's liniment generally included sheep suet, turpentine, and elemi resin from trees of the genus Icica. A soothing or anodyne cataplasm was often a mixture of linseed oil and powdered opium smeared on a plaster (then known as a cataplasm). It was applied to try and draw a wound together and to dry up ulcers. On bandages see Bishop, W. J.: *A History of Surgical Dressings*. Robinson and Sons Ltd.: Chesterfield, 1959. Women provided many fine and coarse pounds of lint to the hospitals in London every year. Lint was made from scraping fine, p. 34.
119. See, for example, MS 5590, f. 19.
120. Moore, *A Dissertation*, p. 33.
121. Pott may have also attended the following case, given that John Abernethy worked with him. See MSS 1020 D 2/1, Transcript of a Course of Lecture on the Theory and Practice of Surgery as Delivered in the Theatre of St. Bartholomew's Hospital by J. Abernethy F.R.S., Lecturer on Anatomy & Surgery & Assist. Surgeon to that Institution. Collated from Notes taken by Wm. Robarts Anno 1810, *Clendening Library*. "At the time of the Riots in 1780—a Boy was brought into this hospital [Bartholomews] who was wounded in the heel by a soldier, with a sabre while standing on a little hut in Fleetmarket—Tetanus came on—& he took Opium till increased to xi every hour & 1 drachm at bedtime—& then it was left off & the spasms diminished & the boy recovered—." f. 29. One drachm was 20 grains or 4 grams or one teaspoonful. See Crellin, John K.: "How Shall I Take My Medicine? Dosages and Other Matters in Eighteenth-Century Medicine." *Caduceus: A Humanities Journal for Medicine and the Health Sciences* Vol. 13, No. 1, 1997, pp. 39–50. See also Simmons, Anna: "Medicines, Monopolies and Mortars: the Chemical Laboratory and Pharmaceutical Trade at the Society of Apothecaries in the Eighteenth Century." *Ambix* Vol. 53, No. 3, 2006, pp. 221–236. It is not clear if doses in the eighteenth century were prescribed for just waking hours or for a 24-hour day.
122. See Haywood, Ian and Seed, John (eds.): *The Gordon Riots: Politics, Culture and Insurrection in Late Eighteenth-Century Britain*. Cambridge University Press: Cambridge, 2012; Hibbert, Christopher: *King Mob: The London Riots of 1780*. Dorset Press: New York, 1958; Shoemaker, Robert: *London Mob: Violence and Disorder in Eighteenth-Century England*. Hambledon Continuum: London, 2007. White, p. 541 gives the following figures for "Black Wednesday": 210 rioters shot dead in the street, with 75 dying in hospitals, and an unknown number dead from drinking neat liquor at Langdale's. I have not been able to find the original source for the citation concerning the number of patients in the hospitals, but it probably came from a report by the military. Historians now estimate 700–850 people were wounded or killed by the military. Sixty-two were condemned to death and 5 women were executed; see Gatrell, Vic: *The First Bohemians: Life and Art in London's Golden Age*. Allen Lane: London, 2013, p. 353.

123. Hibbert, p. 113. Bob Pott, Emily and William Hickey are discussed in chapter one. Also see Green, Dominic: "George Gordon: A Biographical Reassessment," pp. 245–264, In: *The Gordon Riots*, p. 247 on Hickey's acquaintance with Gordon.
124. MS 4337, f. 62. Jesuit's Bark was Cinchona bark, and according to Patrick Wallis it made up 40 percent of all direct American drug imports into early modern England. See "Exotic Drugs and English Medicine: England's Drug Trade, c. 1550–c. 1800." *Social History of Medicine* Vol. 25, No. 1, 2011, pp. 20–46, especially p. 33. Cinchona bark acts against malarial parasites.
125. MS 4337, "Medical Notes Taken at St. Bartholomew's Hospital, 1778–81," *Wellcome*. The manuscript consists of a casebook with clinical notes taken by one of the house physicians on cases in the Hospital. Hannah Stewart's case is dated 12 June 1780, although she was admitted five days earlier, f. 59. She may have been shot by the militia which, led by the Sheriff of London, fired for several minutes on rioters surrounding the Bank of England on the 7th.
126. MS 4337, f. 59.
127. See the following for a discussion of why hospital patients consented to or refused amputations. Herault, Pascal: "Les pauvres et l'amputation a la maison—dieu de Montmorillon (En Poitou) aux xviie et xviiie siècles."*Bulletin de la Société française d'histoire des hôpitaux* Vol. 69, 1993, pp. 23–33.
128. Pott may have been on his way to the Southwark Outhouse in what is now known as the Old Kent Rd. It was a Lock hospital for male venereal patients and run by St. Bartholomew's Hospital. There is a possibility that Pott was a guide (a surgeon who received a daily salary) to the Southwark Outhouse. See, Lloyd, G. Marner: "The Life and Works of Percivall Pott, 1714–1789, Wix Prize Essay 1933."*Saint Bartholomew's Hospital Reports* Vol. 46, 1933, pp. 291–336, p. 302. On Lock hospitals see Siena, Kevin: *Venereal Disease, Hospitals and the Urban Poor: London's "Foul Wards," 1600–1800.* Routledge: New York and London, 2004, particularly chapter four. The outhouses (Lock and Kingsland) were closed in 1760 for financial reasons. Male patients were then admitted to St. Bartholomew's hospital to the aptly named Job and Lazarus wards, and female patients to the Hope and Charity wards (p. 123).
129. Earle, *The Chirurgical Works*, Vol. 1, 1808, xiii.
130. Earle, *The Chirurgical Works*, Vol. 1, 1808, xiv.
131. Clare, Peter: *A New and Easy Method of Curing the Lues Venerea: By the Introduction of Mercury into the System through the Orifices of the absorbent Vessels on the inside of the Mouth, With the Remarks of Dr. Hunter and Mr. Cruikshank in favour of this Practice. Also An Essay on Abscesses and other Observations in Surgery*, London, Third Edition, 1780. "Previous to his own accident, Mr. *Pott* had treated cases of this kind in the hospital with great success; amongst which was that of a boy of eight or ten years of age, who had a fracture of the radius, which protruded through the skin. It was bound up as a simple fracture, and the wound was healed in a fortnight" (p. 25).
132. Few accounts have been located of what amputation of a limb felt like to the patient before general anesthesia was developed. See Heath, Christophe: "A Lecture on a Century of Surgery, Delivered in University College Hospital on January 8th, 1900. *The British Medical Journal* Vol. 1, No. 2037, Jan. 13, 1900, pp. 61–65. "I had an opportunity once of talking to a patient who had had his thigh amputated before the days of anaesthesia, and I asked him

to tell what it was like. "Well," he said, you know what a bad burn is." I said, "yes, I do." He said, "Well, it was exactly like that; when the knife went through the flesh of my thigh it was exactly as if I was burned as severely as possible." One can easily understand that that [*sic*] does represent very fairly the feeling which would be induced by the transfixion of the living tissues of the limb by a long knife carried rapidly through it," p. 61.

133. Heaviside, 1769, f. 19.
134. Heaviside, 1769, f. 21.
135. Heaviside, 1769, f. 21.
136. Earle. *The Chirurgical Works*, 1808, Vol. I, p. xv.
137. MS 5590, f. 486.
138. Aitkin, John: *Thoughts on Hospitals*, London, 1771, p. 25. Aitkin attended hospital lectures in London, spent two years at the University of Edinburgh from 1774 to 1776, and finally earned his M.D. from the University of Leyden in 1784. Aitkin was the first pupil of the noted Unitarian Phillip Doddridge at the Kibworth Academy. Doddridge was a friend of Pott's father-in-law who became a Unitarian in 1742. See chapter one.
139. Heaviside, 1777, f. 22.
140. Heaviside, 1777, f. 22.
141. On the history of amputations see Sachs, Michael, Bojunka, Jörg, and Encke, Albrecht: "Historical Evolution of Limb Amputation." *World Journal of Surgery* Vol. 23, 1999, pp. 1088–1093; Kirkup, John, R.: *A History of Limb Amputation*. Springer-Verlag: London, 2007; Kocher, Mininder S.: "Early Limb Salvage: Open Tibia Fractures of Ambrose Paré (1510–1590) and Percivall Pott (1714–1789)" *World Journal of Surgery* Vol. 21, 1007, pp. 116–122.
142. Heaviside, 1769, f. 22.
143. MA 00071/6, f. 288.
144. On Bilguer see Kirkup, *A History of Limb Amputation*, pp. 76–77.
145. Bilguer, Johann Ulrich: A *dissertation on the inutility of the amputation of limbs*. London, 1764, p. 13.
146. MS 3957, f. 27.
147. MS 3957, f. 28.
148. Heaviside, 1781, f. 125.
149. Heaviside, 1781, f. 125.
150. Pott: "Observations on the necessity and propriety of amputation, in certain cases, and under certain circumstances." In: *Chirurgical Works*, Vol. II, 1779, p. 308.
151. Pott, "Observations on the necessity," p. 308.
152. A web of cells—cells being the spaces of the web. See Forrester, J. M.: "The Homoeomerous Parts and Their Replacement by Bichat's Tissues." *Medical History* Vol. 38, No. 4, 1994, pp. 444–458, particularly, p. 452.
153. Pott, "Observations on the necessity," p. 311.
154. Pott, "Observations on the necessity," p. 315.
155. Pott, "Observations on the necessity," p. 319.
156. Pott, "Observations on the necessity," p. 323.
157. 1787, 12 September, OBP t17870912-96. oldbaileyonline.org. James Weston, Coroner's depositions, *London Metropolitan Archives*, LSP/1787/Jul. Tried for manslaughter.

158. OBP t17870912-96.
159. OBP t17870912-96.
160. OBP t17870912-96.

Chapter Four: "A Poor Man Came to St. Bartholomew's": Chronic Conditions

1. "Observations and Cases Relative to Ruptures, etc." In: *The Chirurgical Works of Percivall Pott,* London, 1778, Vol. II, p. 424.
2. *London Magazine*, May 1771: Issue 40, p. 275.
3. The terms hernia and rupture were interchangeable in the early modern period. On hernias see Mills, Philip R.: "Privates on Parade: Soldiers, Medicine and the Treatment of Inguinal Hernias in Georgian England." In: Hudson, Geoffrey L., *British Military and Naval Medicine, 1600–1830,* pp. 149–182. Rodopi: Amsterdam, 2007.
   Also, Smith, Lisa Wynne: "The Body Embarrassed? Rethinking the Leaky Male Body in Eighteenth-Century England and France." *Gender & History* Vol. 23, No. 1, 2010, pp. 26–46.
4. On quacks see Porter, Roy: *Quacks: Fakers & Charlatans in English Medicine.* Tempus: Stroud, 2000.
5. "A Treatise on the Hydrocele, or Watry Rupture and Other Diseases of the Testicle, It's [*sic*] Coats and Vessels." In: *The Chirurgical Works*, Vol. II, 1778, p. 13.
6. MS 3958, "These Lectures were written down in time of Lecture by Mr. J. Grigg Surgeon & were carefully corrected at his apartments at St. Bartholomew's Hospital, 1782, London," f. 32. *Wellcome.* Not much is known about Grigg except he practiced as a surgeon in Bath.
7. MS 3958, f. 32. On the pox in the eighteenth century, see Siena, Kevin: *Venereal Disease, Hospitals and the Urban Poor: London's "Foul Wards," 1600–1800.* Routledge: New York and London, 2004.
8. The claret probably came from the tavern where the operation took place. A surgeon's mate was an apprentice to a ship's surgeon.
9. "A Treatise on the Hydrocele." Vol. II, pp. 15–16.
10. "A Treatise on the Hydrocele." Vol. I, p. 493. (The Treatise begins in Volume I and continues in Volume II of *The Chirurgical Works*, London, 1778.)
11. MS 3958, f. 13.
12. MS 3958, f. 7.
13. MS 0071, Heaviside, 1780 & 1781, f. 118. *Royal College of Surgeons.*
14. Hitchcock, Tim: *Down and Out in Eighteenth-Century London.* Bloomsbury Press: London, 2004. p. 110.
15. "A Treatise on the Hydrocele." Vol. 1, pp. 434–5. Jesuit drops were similar to Friar's Balsam.
16. "A Treatise on the Hydrocele." Vol. II, pp. 14–15.
17. White, Jerry: *London in the Eighteenth Century: A Great and Monstrous Thing.* The Bodley Head: London, 2012, p. 92. White, p. 192.
18. "A Treatise on the Hydrocele." Vol. II, pp. 14–15.

19. "A Treatise on the Hydrocele." Vol. II, 14–15. The epididymis is a curved structure behind the testicle. Eighteenth-century specimens survive today. See Hirsh, A. V.: "The anatomical preparations of the human testis and epididymis in the Glasgow Hunterian Anatomical Collection." *Human Reproduction Update* Vol. 11, No. 5, 1995, pp. 515–521.
20. "Observations and Cases Relative to Ruptures, etc.," was included in the two-volume collected works of Pott in 1778. All quotations are from this edition. As discussed in chapter three, Pott first published a *Treatise on Ruptures* in 1756 when he was recovering from a horse accident. He continued to expand his theories and cases. Subsequent editions of the *Treatise* appeared in 1763, 1769, and 1775. Pott wrote two additional monographs related to hernias: *An Account of a Particular Kind of Rupture, Frequently Attendant upon New-Children; and Sometimes Met with in Adults* (1757) and *Practical Remarks on the Hydrocele or Watery Rupture, and Some Other Diseases of the Testicle* (1762).
21. Dickie, Simon: *Cruelty and Laughter: Forgotten Comic Literature and the Unsentimental Eighteenth Century*. University of Chicago Press: Chicago, 2011, p. 92. Dickie uses Margaret Pelling's groundbreaking works on early modern Norwich to suggest that around 25% of poor men and women were severely disabled by the age of sixty, and that the probability of disability increased exponentially every year beyond that age. See p. 93.
22. Dickie, p. 93. See Turner, David M. and Withey, Alun: "Technologies of the Body: Polite Consumption and the Correction of Deformity in Eighteenth-Century England." *History: The Journal of the Historical Association* Vol. 454, 2002, pp. 775–796.
23. Dickie, Simon: "Hilarity and Pitilessness in the Mid-Eighteenth Century: English Jestbook Humor." *Eighteenth-Century Studies* Vol. 37, No. 1, Fall, 2003, pp. 1–22. On physical discrimination, see, Dawson, Mark S.: "First Impressions: Newspaper Advertisements and Early Modern English Body Imaging, 1651–1750." *Journal of British Studies* Vol. 50, April 2011, pp. 277–306.
24. "Observations and Cases Relative to Ruptures, etc." Vol. II, p. 416. A journey-man was someone who had completed an apprenticeship but was not yet a master of a trade as he had not taken the required exams.
25. "Observations and Cases Relative to Ruptures, etc." Vol. II, p. 416.
26. "Observations and Cases Relative to Ruptures, etc." Vol. II, p. 416.
27. "Observations and Cases Relative to Ruptures, etc." Vol. II, p. 416.
28. "A Treatise on Ruptures." In: *The Chirurgical Works*. Vol. I, 1778, p. 339.
29. "A Treatise on the Hydrocele." Vol. I, p. 437. *The London Chronicle* from Saturday March 6, to Tuesday March 9, 1762, reports "Saturday died Mr. Hollingsworth, surgeon, in Cowcross," p. 225.
30. "A Treatise on the Hydrocele." Vol. I, p. 437.
31. "A Treatise on the Hydrocele." Vol. I, p. 437.
32. An escharotic is a corrosive salve to burn away the skin and thus draw the cancer out. The thick dry scab that develops on the skin is called an eschar and hence the name escharotic. In MS 699, Lectures on Surgery by Mr. Pott, 1775/79, Pott revealed to his pupils that the "Boasted Secret" of the Quack's caustic is "The Meadow crow-foot, Dogfennel, Sulph. Vivum & Arsenic made into a paste with a yoke of Egg," f. 91. *Royal College of Surgeons.*

33. "A Treatise on the Hydrocele." Vol. I, p. 437. Pott and Hollingsworth examined the man after death and found that he had a diseased cancerous testicle lying in the groin.
34. "A Treatise on Ruptures." Vol. I, p. 407.
35. "A Treatise on the Hydrocele." Vol. I, p. 56.
36. John Freke (1688–1756) became an assistant surgeon at St. Bartholomew's hospital in 1726 and was elected a senior surgeon in 1729. He became Master of the Company of Surgeons in 1746 and remained a senior hospital surgeon until 1755. He appears to have also been the first curator of the hospital museum, and from around 1727 couched for cataracts and took care of the poor with diseases of the eye. Hospital minutes record that Freke would charge "six shillings and eight pence for each person so couched as is paid on other operations." See *Dictionary of National Biography* Vol. 20, 1885–1900.
37. "A Treatise on the Hydrocele." Vol. I, p. 56.
38. "A Treatise on the Hydrocele." Vol. II, 142.
39. MS TH/PP, f. 88. *Kings College Archives.*
40. Heaviside, 1769, f. 75. *Royal College of Surgeons.*
41. "A Treatise on the Hydrocele." Vol. I, p. 435.
42. "A Treatise on the Hydrocele." Vol. I, p. 436.
43. "A Treatise on the Hydrocele." Vol. I, p. 462. This was Mr. William Sharp (1729–1810) who, from 1755 to 1779, was a surgeon to St. Bartholomew's hospital. His brother was Granville Sharp, an advocate for the abolition of slavery.
44. "A Treatise on the Hydrocele." Vol. I, p. 464.
45. A Winchester pint is roughly equal to two Imperial quarts, or 2.25 liters.
46. "A Treatise on the Hydrocele." Vol. I, p. 464.
47. "Observations and Cases Relative to Ruptures, etc." Vol. II, p. 471.
48. "A Treatise on Ruptures." Vol. I, p. 340.
49. "Observations and Cases Relative to Ruptures, etc." Vol. II, p. 472.
50. "Observations and Cases Relative to Ruptures, etc." Vol. II, p. 472.
51. Redford, Bruce: *The Letters of Samuel Johnson*. Princeton University Press: Princeton, NJ, 1992.
52. *The Letters.* Vol. 4, p. 201. John Taylor (1711–88) was a school friend of Johnson's.
53. *The Letters.* Vol. 4, p. 218. To Mrs. Thrale at Bath, Monday Sept. 22, 1783.
54. *The Letters.* Vol. 4, p. 220. To Mrs. Thrale on October 9, 1783.
55. Johnson repeats the story to Mudge on October 9th. "Mr. Pot, seeing at his return, so great an alteration, thought it proper to suspend all violence, and as Nature has so far favoured us, to wait the process. This he thinks more reasonable, if I understood him rightly, because the diseased part is totally free from all scirrosity, and he therefore thinks the spermatick cord in no danger. The disorder, he says is purely local, and indicates no depravity of the constitution." *The Letters.* Vol. 4, p. 223. Johnson was obviously concerned that the illness was systemic or one of habit.
56. *The Letters.* Vol. 4, pp. 223–4. See McDonald, Stuart W.: "William Cruikshank (1745–1800), Anatomist and Surgeon, and His Illustrious Patient, Samuel Johnson." *Clinical Anatomy* Vol. 28, 2015, pp. 836–843.
57. *The Letters.* Vol. 4, p. 233.
58. *The Letters.* Vol. 4, p. 235. To Bowles on Wed. Jan. 14, 1784.

59. See, Wiltshire, J.: *Samuel Johnson in the Medical World: The Doctor and the Patient.* Press Syndicate of the University of Cambridge: Cambridge, 1991, on Johnson's testicle and Pott diagnosis and treatment of it.
60. *The Letters.* Vol. 4, p. 223.
61. "Wit" meaning mental faculties or intellect. Mrs. Thrale was to bury eight of her twelve children between October 1765 and April 1783. She also lost her mother in June 1773 and her first husband in April 1781. John Gay (1685–1732) poet, dramatist, and author of *The Beggar's Opera* (1728) had his Fables published in 1727. Fable III, "The Mother, the Nurse and the Fairy," is the story of a boy stolen from his bed and replaced with a changeling (a shocking, awkward creature, a fool in ev'ry feature). The mother is blind to the condition of the changling and cries, "I see wit sparkle in his eyes." *Gay's Fables in one volume complete.* London, 1808, p. 14. On Gay see Lewis, Jayne Elizabeth: *Literary Culture, 1651–1740.* Cambridge University Press: Cambridge, 1996. On Pott and the Thrales see, Hyde, Mary: *The Thrales of Streatham Park.* Harvard University Press: Cambridge, 1977, p. 85: "The true state of Ralph's clinical condition was to be revealed rather brutally to the Thrales by the revered physician, Dr Percival Pott of St Bartholomew's Hospital." Also see McIntyre, Ian: *Hester: The Remarkable Life of Dr Johnson's 'Dear Mistress.'* Constable: London, 2008, p. 109 also Morgan, Lee: *Dr. Johnson's "own Dear Master," The Life of Henry Thrale.* University Press of America, Inc.: Lanham, Maryland, 1998, p 136 and finally, James, R. M.: "The effect on family life during the late Georgian period of indisposition, medication, treatments and the resultant outcomes." PhD thesis. Oxford Brookes University, 2010.
62. Hyde, p. 105.
63. Hyde, p. 110. Dr. Daniel Sutton (c. 1735–1819) provided a remedy of antimony, mercury and calomel to reduce the danger of live inoculation. The Sutton family (father and three sons) carried out thousands of inoculations with live smallpox.
64. Hyde, p. 115.
65. Hyde, p. 116.
66. Porter, Roy: *Bodies Politic: Disease, Death, and Doctors in Britain, 1650–1900.* Cornell University Press: Ithaca, NY, 2001, p. 173.
67. An idiot was someone with impaired mental ability (Johnson's definition in his *Dictionary* is "A fool; a natural; a changeling; one without the powers of reason.")
68. Hydranencephaly, or hydroanencephaly, is a congenital condition in which the brain's cerebral hemispheres are absent to varying degrees and the resulting empty cranial cavity is filled with cerebrospinal fluid. See Hubble, Douglas: "Mrs Thrale Keeping Notes." *The British Medical Journal* Vol. 1, No. 6116, Apr. 1, 1978, pp. 832–833. Dr. Lucas Pepys (1742–1830) was a physician to the Middlesex.
69. Hyde, p. 122.
70. Between 1769 and 1776 Pott treated Boswell 11 times for gonorrheal urethritis. See Ober, William B.: *Boswell's Clap and Other Essays.* Southern Illinois University Press: Carbondale, 1979, p. 19.
71. Ober, p. 17.
72. Ober, p. 22 and p. 24.
73. *The Cullen Project*, http://cullenproject.ac.uk [ID: 2228] From: Mr J. Spens/To: Dr William Cullen (Professor Cullen)/Regarding: Mr J. Spens (Patient)/6 June 1782/(Incoming). Spens has not been identified.

74. They were invented and patented in 1747 by the physician Robert James (1703–1776), a close friend of Samuel Johnson's. The powders were prescribed for many disorders in humans and cattle. The primary ingredients were antimony and phosphate of lime.
75. The X referred to this note on page 11 of the long letter: "X this Mr. Hunter told me was not His Common practice. but my mentioning the effect of Mr Potts Pill. He thought perhaps that might best answer my Constitution."
76. *The Cullen Project*, [ID: 2228] 14. Spens gives the recipe at the end of his letter as {illeg} ounces of Gum Arabic Mucilage, half an ounce of Balsam of Capivi, eight ounces of Clear Cinnamon Water, one ounce of Nutmeg and one ounce of Simple Syrup [M Capt.: Cocj iiij Man Sero?]
77. *The Cullen Project*, [ID: 2228] p. 3.
78. *The Cullen Project*, [ID: 2228] p. 5.
79. *The Cullen Project*, [ID: 579] p. 1. From: Dr William Cullen (Professor Cullen)/To: Mr J. Spens/Regarding: Mr J. Spens (Patient)/19 June 1782/(Outgoing)
80. *The Cullen Project*, [ID: 579] p. 1.
81. *The Cullen Project*, [ID: 579] p. 2.
82. *The Cullen Project*, [ID: 628] From: Dr William Cullen (Professor Cullen)/To: Mr J. Spens/Regarding: Mr J. Spens (Patient)/26 August 1782/(Outgoing). "In the present irritable state of your urethra I am not fond of your using any of my Balsamic medicines but the time may come when you can abstain from the use of bougies that the balsamics may be again usefull to you. They are the medicines I would chiefly depend upon for Strengthening the urethra and was you more free of Spasms I should not be so much afraid of stopping your gleet as Mr Pott is" (pp. 2–3). It is possible that Pott also advised in the following, *The Cullen Project*, [ID: 2898] From: Dr Ralph Irving/To: Dr William Cullen (Professor Cullen)/Regarding: Governor George Johnstone (Johnston) (Patient)/5 October 1786/Incoming. George Johnstone (1730–1787) was a Royal Naval Officer, MP, Director of the EIC, and the first Governor of West Florida from 1763–1767. He suffered from chronic venereal complaints.
83. MS 3957, Lect. 30 Deseases of the Urethra continue, f. 110, *Wellcome*. MS 699 has the same case but the address is given as Canon St, f. 185, *Royal College of Surgeons*.
84. MS 3957, f. 112.
85. MS 3957, f. 116. And no doubt it was very alarming to the patient too.
86. Plaut, G: "Dr. John Fothergill and Eighteenth-century Medicine." *Journal of Medical Biography* Vol. 7, No. 4, 1999, pp. 192–6. Also see Lettsom, C.: *The Works of John Fothergill, MD, Member of the Royal College of Physicians and Fellow of the Royal Society of London, Fellow of the Royal College of Physicians of Edinburgh.* London, 1784.
87. MS 4337, "Medical Notes taken at Barts 1778–1781." *Wellcome*. These are clinical notes taken by one of the house physicians on cases in the hospital. There is an index of diseases at the back. The "Operation for strangulated femoral artery by Mr. Pott with p.m. (post mortem) Pit (Dr. William Pitcairn)," is the first entry, f. 1.
88. MS 4337, f. 2. *Wellcome*.
89. MS 4337, f. 2. *Wellcome*.
90. See additional case histories at the back of MA 00071/6 Volume III, *Royal College of Surgeons*. For example, Case 11th Retention of Urine, ff. 323–5. Here Pott diagnosed a

patient as having a distended bladder that pushed out to the anus, so he perforated it and made an artificial passage for the patient to use.

91. In a femoral hernia, part of the intestines push the membrane that lines the abdomen (peritoneum) downward through the opening where the femoral artery and vein pass into the thigh (femoral canal). They are more common in women then men.
92. MA 00071/6 Volume III, f. 326, *Royal College of Surgeons.*
93. MA 00071/6 Volume III, f. 329, *Royal College of Surgeons.*
94. "A Treatise on Ruptures." Vol. I, p. 285.
95. "Observations and Cases Relative to Ruptures, etc." Vol. II, p. 443. On trusses, see Rabier, Christelle & Pérez, Liliane: "Self-Machinery? Steel Trusses and the Management of Ruptures in Eighteenth-Century Europe." *Technology and Culture* Vol. 54, No. 3, pp. 460–502. http://doi.org/10.1353/tech.2013.0096
96. "A Treatise on Ruptures." Vol. I, p. 320.
97. Medicinal use of tobacco in the eighteenth century is touched upon in Stewart, Grace G.: "A History of the Medicinal Uses of Tobacco, 1492–1860." *Medical History* Vol. 11, 1967, pp. 228–268.
98. "Observations and Cases Relative to Ruptures, etc." Vol. I, p. 441 and p. 445.
99. "Observations and Cases Relative to Ruptures, etc." Vol. I, p. 442. This case is dated September 1767.
100. Clare, Peter: *A New and Easy Method of Curing the Lues Venerea: By the Introduction of Mercury into the System through the Orifices of the absorbent Vessels on the inside of the Mouth … Also An Essay on Abscesses and other Observations in Surgery.* London, Third Edition, 1780, "On Hernias," p. 115. This description is provided in a footnote.
101. MS 5590, f. 180. *Wellcome.*
102. MS 5590, f. 181. *Wellcome.*
103. "A Treatise of Ruptures." Vol. I, p. 333.
104. "Observations and Cases Relative to Ruptures, etc." Vol. II, p. 474.
105. "Observations and Cases Relative to Ruptures, etc." Vol. II, p. 478.
106. "Observations and Cases Relative to Ruptures, etc." Vol. II, p. 479.
107. "Observations and Cases Relative to Ruptures, etc." Vol. II, p. 479.
108. MS TH/PP, f. 255. *Kings College Archives.*
109. "An Account of the Method of obtaining a perfect or radical Cure of the Hydrocele or Watery Rupture, by Means of a Seton." In: *The Chirurgical Works.* 1778, Vol. II, p. 174.
110. London magazine, May 1771: 40, p. 275, Of New Publications, XIV. *An Account of the Method of obtaining a perfect or radical Cure of the Hydrocele or Watery Rupture, by Means of a Seton*, by Percivall Pott, F.R.S.
111. "An Account of the Method of obtaining a perfect or radical Cure of the Hydrocele or Watery Rupture, by Means of a Seton." In: *The Chirurgical Works.* 1778, Vol. II, p. 171.
112. Gregory, George: *Elements of the Theory and Practice of Medicine designed for the Use of Students.* London, 1820. Discusses "scrophulous incurvation to which infants and children are liable … This disorder, from having been very accurately described in the works of Mr. Pott, has received the name of Pott's Palsy" (p. 375). Gregory (1790–1853) trained at Barts in medicine.

113. Pott, Percivall: *Remarks on that kind of Palsy of the Lower Limbs which is frequently found to accompany Curvature of the Spine, and is supposed to be caused by it. Together with its method of cure*. London, 1771, p. 9.
114. *Remarks on that kind of Palsy*, p. 10.
115. *Remarks on that kind of Palsy*, p. 10.
116. *Remarks on that kind of Palsy*, p. 15.
117. Sorge-English, Lynn: *Stays and Body Image in London: The Staymaking Trade, 1680–1810*. Pickering and Chatto: London, 2011, p. 128.
118. In 1762 they advertised as workmen to St. Bartholomew's, St. Thomas's, Guy's, St. George's, the Middlesex and Foundling Hospitals, and the London Infirmary. Billheads that survive from 1773 show that Christ's, London, had been added but the Middlesex removed. The same year they received a lucrative contract to provide trusses to the Royal Navy. Sorge-English, p. 128.
119. *Remarks on that kind of Palsy*, p. 15. See the response to Pott's condemnation of the inutility of machines in Sheldrake, Jr., Timothy, *An Essay on the Various Causes and Effects of the Distorted Spine; on the improper methods usually practiced to remove that Distortion; In which that recommended by Mr. Pott is considered*. London, c. 1783. Sheldrake advocated the use of Vacher's machine and new elastic trusses with flexible pads to correct the deformity of the spine after treatment with issues. He praised Pott for being the "only gentleman who has written on the causes, as well as the effects and methods of treating the disease," but criticized him for being seemingly content to stop at offering a cure for the disorder, and "rather too hastily said, that the deformity occasioned by it must always remain …" (p. 47). Vacher was Francois Guillaume Levacher de la Feutrie (1732–1816) who introduced the first mechanical bed in France in 1764. Sheldrake was truss maker to the HEIC and to the Westminster hospital. He died in 1806.
120. *Remarks on that kind of Palsy*, p. 17.
121. *Remarks on that kind of Palsy*, p. 17. The predecessor was spinal tuberculosis, which led quickly to the neurological condition of paraplegia, caused by the pressure of pus, granulated and necrotic tissue. Sometimes the vertebrae would crumble and collapse too. Draining fluid from around the initial area of infection through an artificial abscess cum issue may have helped relieve the numbness in the legs in some cases but in all probability it was the enforced rest that helped them the most. See Power, D'Arcy: "Pott's Disease of the Spine." *The British Journal of Surgery*. Vol. 11, No. 41, July 1923, pp. 1–6. See Evans, Jonathan: "Barts and the London's Medical Museum Collections," pp. 115–137. In: *Anatomical Dissection in Enlightenment England and Beyond: Autopsy, Pathology and Display*. Mitchell, Piers (ed.), Ashgate Press: Aldershot, 2012. Other specimens collected by Pott included three preparations demonstrating tuberculosis of the spine (Pott's disease) dating from c. 1780 (C57, C58, T232). The specimens illustrate angular curvature of the spine resulting from partial destruction of vertebra with compression of the spinal cord that resulted in paraplegia" (p. 118).
122. *Remarks on that kind of Palsy*. p. 18. Sorge-English, p. 98. "Stays were made up of four layers of fabric, often a layer of paper and/or buckram, whalebone and lining." Also see Schillace, Brandy Lain: "Reproducing Custom: Mechanical Habits and Female Machines in Augustan Women's Education." *Feminist Formations* Vol. 25, 2013, pp. 111–137.

123. Sorge-English, p. 113.
124. Kirkup, John R.: "Nicolas Andry and 250 Years of Orthopaedy." *The Journal of Bone and Joint Surgery* Vol. 73, No. 8, 1991, pp. 361–362.
125. Cadogan, William: *An Essay upon Nursing and the Management of Children*. London, 1748, pp. 14–15. Cadogan's essay went through nine reprintings.
126. *Remarks on that kind of Palsy*. p. 21.
127. Dr. Thomas Cameron (1704–1777) was a Scottish physician who set up practice in 1727 and helped found the Worcester Infirmary in 1747.
128. Henry Vaughan Jeffreys (1722–1803), a surgeon to the Infirmary from 1747.
129. *Remarks on that kind of Palsy*, p. 24. Pott got permission to dissect the infant.
130. *Remarks on that kind of Palsy*, p. 24.
131. *Remarks on that kind of Palsy*, p. 26.
132. The plant *Symphytum officinale* was also widely known as "Knitbone."
133. Isinglass was made from the dried air bladders of sturgeon, perch or cod, and other freshwater fish. It was used to congeal liquids.
134. *Remarks on that kind of Palsy*, p. 26.
135. *Remarks on that kind of Palsy*, p. 27.
136. *Remarks on that kind of Palsy*, p. 28.
137. *Remarks on that kind of Palsy*, p. 30.
138. Page, Anthony: *John Jebb and the Enlightenment Origins of British Radicalism*. Praeger Publishers: Westport, CT, 2003.
139. Jebb, John: *Select Cases of the Disorder commonly termed the Paralysis of the Lower Extremities*. London, 1782, p. 5.
140. Jebb, *Select Cases*, p. 6.
141. Jebb, *Select Cases*, p. 9.
142. Jebb, *Select Cases*, p. 9.
143. Jebb, *Select Cases*, p. 13.
144. Jebb, *Select Cases*, p. 14. MS 4337, *Wellcome* includes the sad case of Mary Burton admitted to Martha Ward, who was treated by Jebb, James Earle, William Cruikshank, and William Hunter, ff. 130–134. The account of her illness was written in the book on May 19, 1778. Burton was described as middle-aged, used to hard work, and she had drunk freely according to her friends. She thought the violent pain in her loins and the swelling of her legs were due to her being four months pregnant, but after the midwives (described as ignorant), Earle, Jebb and Hunter examined her and thought she was not with child but had perhaps a tumour and/or a retroverted uterus. Both her pulse and inspirations a minute were recorded. Burton died on the 31st of May screaming in pain, and her body was dissected, but the uterus was found to be sound.
145. Jebb, *Select Cases*, p. 18.
146. MS 4337, f. 218. *Wellcome*. A note in front of the book states that this was a case of spinal caries.
147. Jebb, *Select Cases*, pp. 8–20.
148. Jebb, *Select Cases*, p. 22.
149. Jebb, *Select Cases*, p. 49.
150. Jebb, *Select Cases*, p. 50.

151. Jebb, *Select Cases*, p. 37.
152. Jebb, *Select Cases*, p. 40.
153. Belloni, L.: "Percivall Pott's Disease of the Spine, Discussed in Two Letters of J. Hunczovsky from London, 1779, to G. A. Brambilla in Vienna." *Medical History* Vol. 16, No. 1, 1972, pp. 78–80.
154. Belloni, p. 80.
155. Pott, "Farther Remarks on the useless State of the Lower Limbs, in consequence of a Curvature of the Spine." In: *Chirurgical Works*, 1790, Vol. III, p. 449.
156. "Farther Remarks," p. 457.
157. "Farther Remarks," p. 449.
158. "Farther Remarks," p. 449.
159. "Farther Remarks," p. 484.
160. Gelfand, Toby: "'Invite the philosopher, as well as the charitable': Hospital Teaching as Private Enterprise in Hunterian London," pp. 29–152. In: Bynum, W. F. and Porter, Roy (eds.), *William Hunter and the Eighteenth-Century Medical World.* Cambridge University Press: Cambridge, 1985, p. 39. "The writings of Percivall Pott, in particular, were avidly translated into French. A second edition came out in 1776. It was also translated into German in 1770, Dutch in 1779, and Italian in 1801."
161. Gonzalès, Jacques: "Le mal de Pott avant les antituberculeux: de Pott à Ménard." *Histoire des Sciences Médicales*, Tome 39: 3, 2005, pp. 291–301.
162. MA 00071/6 Volume III, Case 8th Curvature of the Spine, f. 317. *Royal College of Surgeons.*
163. MA 00071/6 Volume III, f. 318.
164. MA 00071/6 Volume III, f. 318
165. MA 00071/6 Volume III, f. 320
166. MA 00071/6 Volume III, f. 320
167. MA 00071/6 Volume III, Case 7th Paralysis, January 1786, f. 316.
168. MA 00071/6 Volume III, f. 316.
169. Ravitch, Mark M.: "Invective in Surgery: William Hunter Versus Monro Primus, Monro Secundus, and Percival Pott." *Bulletin of the New York Academy of Medicine* Vol. 50, No. 7, 1974, pp. 797–816 and Beekman, Fenwick: "'The Hernia Congenita' and an Account of the Controversy It Provoked between William Hunter and Percivall Pott." *Bulletin of the NY Academy of Medicine* Vol. 22, No. 9, 1946, pp. 486–500.
170. Porter, Roy: William Hunter: A Surgeon and a Gentleman," pp. 7–34. In: Bynum, W. F. and Porter, Roy (eds.), *William Hunter and the Eighteenth-Century Medical World.* Cambridge University Press: Cambridge, 1985.
171. Pott, Percivall: *A Treatise on Ruptures*. London, 1763, p. 138.
172. *A Treatise on Ruptures*, p. 138.
173. *A Treatise on Ruptures*, p. 140.
174. *A Treatise on Ruptures*, p. 140.
175. *A Treatise on Ruptures*, p. 140.
176. Sultan, Georg: *Atlas and Epitome of Abdominal Hernias*. W. B. Saunders & Co.: Philadelphia and London, 1902, p. 51. Lagaranne M.-L. Reneaulme de: *Discours pour l'ouverture de l'École de chirurgie avec une thèse paraphrasée, sous ce titre Essay d'un traité des hernies nommées descentes, par M.-L. Reneaulme de Lagaranne*. Paris, 1726.

177. *A Treatise on Ruptures*, p. 140.
178. *A Treatise on Ruptures*, p. 144.
179. *A Treatise on Ruptures*, p. 145.
180. *A Treatise on Ruptures*, p. 145.
181. *A Treatise on Ruptures*, p. 146.
182. *A Treatise on Ruptures*, pp. 159 and 161.
183. *A Treatise on Ruptures*, p. 148.
184. *The Critical Review*, March 1757, 3, 284–5. From 1756 to 1817 the editor was Tobias George Smollett (baptized 1721–1771). Samuel Johnson and John Hunter both wrote reviews for the periodical.
185. *The Critical Review*, p. 284.
186. *The Critical Review*, p. 284.
187. The *Monthly Review*, May 1757, 16, p. 464. Ralph Griffith (1749–1845), a non-conformist bookseller, founded the *Monthly Review*. It was the first periodical to offer reviews.
188. *The Critical Review*, December 1763, 16, pp. 464–5. Quotation from p. 464.
189. *The Critical Review*, July 1764, 18, pp. 47–49.
190. *The Critical Review*, July 1764, pp. 47.
191. *The Critical Review*, July 1764, pp. 48.
192. *The Critical Review*, July 1764, pp. 49.
193. *Monthly Review*, Feb 1765, 42, pp. 109–110.
194. *Monthly Review*, Feb. 1765, pp. 110–112.
195. *Monthly Review*, Feb. 1765, p. 110.
196. *Monthly Review*, Feb. 1765, p. 112.
197. Brand, T.: *Strictures in Vindication of some of the doctrines misrepresented by Mr. Foot in his two pamphlets entitled, Observations upon the New Opinions of John Hunter in his late treatise on the venereal disease; including Mr. Pott's plagiarisms and misinformation on the subject of pus or matter in his Observations on that disorder … commonly called fistula lachrymalis*, London, 1774. Thomas Brand (d. 1820) was surgeon to the Royal Hospital Greenwich and to the Soho Square Dispensary for the Relief of the Infant Poor. He had studied with the Hunters. See a review of the pamphlet "The Case of a Boy who had been mistaken for a girl," by TB surgeon, London, 1787 in *The English Review*, Vol. 11, Art. 29, 1788, pp. 69–70 and Warren, Carol A. B.: "Gender Reassignment Surgery in the Eighteenth Century." *Sexualities* Vol. 17, No. 7, 2014, pp. 872–884. Jessé Foot was surgeon to the Middlesex. In *The Life of John Hunter*, London, 1794 he takes Pott's side and praises Haller's work on the congenial hernia.
198. *The Monthly Review*, Vol. 77, July–December inclusive, 1787, p. 241 condemned Brand's *Strictures in Vindication* with "As a pupil of Mr. Hunter, it was laudable in our Author to defend the tenets of his master; but he is very unequal to the task. Independent of his censures on Mr. Foot, this heated writer attacks Sharpe, Gataker, and Pott,—men who have been ornaments to their profession, and whose acknowledged veracity and integrity would not suffer them on any account to insert what Mr. B. calls a falsehood, in their useful publications … It is too great arrogance and presumption to attribute every improvement in anatomy and surgery to one man."

Epilogue: Pott's Legacy: Then and Now

1. Cooper, Samuel: *A Dictionary of Practical Surgery: containing a complete exhibition of the present state of theprinciples and practice of surgery, collected from the best and most original sources of information and illustrated by critical remark.* London, 1809, p. 882. This description has been wrongly ascribed to the surgeon Edward Alanson of Liverpool in several secondary sources on Pott. The mistake appears to go back to a biography of Alanson that quoted Cooper from 1809 as if it was Alanson. See Murray, R. W.: *Edward Alanson and his Times*. Samuel Hill & Sons: Liverpool, 1914.
2. Blizard, William: *The Hunterian oration: delivered in the theatre of the Royal College of Surgeons, on the 14th Day of February*. Rivington's, London, 1815, p. 53.
3. Canter, David: "Cancer." In: Bynum, W. F. and Porter, Roy (eds.), Roy. *Companion Encyclopedia of the History of Medicine*. Routledge: London, 1993. p. 556.
4. *The European Magazine*, February 1789, 15, pp. 102–4.
5. *The European Magazine*, pp. 102–3.
6. *The Gentlemen's Magazine*, November 1794, pp. 64–5, pp. 1017–1023 and p. 1018. "The three disputes abovementioned were carried on in the Critical review; and the system of that undertaking was in great measure broken in upon to be made subservient to the purposes of the Hunters, who had obtained that ascendancy over the editor as to command his services in the promotion of any cause that their views or ambition suggested. All the attacks and all the replies of the Hunters were revised, corrected, and published, under the immediate eye, influence, and direction, of Smollett," p. 1018.
7. *The Gentlemen's Magazine*, p. 103.
8. *The Gentlemen's Magazine*, p. 103.
9. *The Gentlemen's Magazine*, p. 104.
10. *Critical Review*, August 1791, 2, pp. 361–368
11. *Critical Review*, p. 361.
12. *Critical Review*, p. 361.
13. *Critical Review*, p. 361.
14. Newman, Jeremiah Whitaker: *The Lounger's Common-Place Book of 1796*. London, 1796, Vol. II, pp. 94–96.
15. *The Lounger's*, p. 95.
16. *The Lounger's*, p. 95.
17. Jane Stanhope, Countess of Harrington (1755–1824), was a society hostess and rich heiress.
18. *The Lounger's*, p. 96.
19. MSS/ADDITIONAL/33107. James Earle, 1801 Letter to Lady Holdernesse, f. 420. *British Library*. Mary Doublet was the widow of the fourth. Earl of Holdernesse. She died in late 1801 from breast cancer.
20. Earle, *Chirurgical operations*, Vol. I, p. 10.
21. Hey, William, *Practical Observations in Surgery, Illustrated with Cases*. London, 1803, p. 1.
22. Hey, p. 1.
23. Hey, p. 122.

24. Hey, p. 195.
25. Hey, p. 119.
26. Hey, p. 120.
27. The president at this time used to sit in "Mr. Pott's old chair." Moore, Norman: *History of St. Bartholomew's Hospital.* C. Arthur Pearson Ltd.: London, Vol. 2, 1918, p. 827. It was renamed The Abernethian Society in 1832.
28. MSS 1020 D/21, "Transcript of a Course of Lectures on the Theory and Practice of Surgery as Delivered in the Theatre of St. Bartholomew's Hospital by J. Abernethy F.R.S., Lecturer on Anatomy & Surgery & Assist. Surgeon to that Institution, collated from Notes taken by Wm. Robarts Anno 1810," f. 80. *Clendening Library.*
29. Abernethy, John, *Surgical Observations on the Injuries of the Head and on Miscellaneous Subjects.* London, 1815. See pp. 140, 142 and 159.
30. Abernethy, p. 154.
31. Abernethy, p. 154. In Lloyd G. Marner: The Life and Works of Percivall Pott, 1714–1789, Wix Prize Essay, 1933, *Saint Bartholomew's Hospital Reports,* Vol. XLVI, London: John Murray, 1933, pp. 291–336 uncited stories were included such as Pott having removing nasal polyps from himself with bone adhering to some of them and Abernethy remarking that he disagreed with Pott's cranial surgery, saying about Pott's treatment of wounds of the longitudinal sinus, "Though I do not believe it killed the patients, yet there always a dripping of blood till they died." See pp. 307 and 310.
32. Cooper, Samuel: *A Dictionary of Practical Surgery: containing a complete exhibition of the present state of the principles and practice of surgery, collected from the best and most original sources of information and illustrated by critical remarks.* London, 1809, p. 882. Cooper (1781–1848) trained at St. Bartholomew's hospital in 1800 and became a surgeon's mate in 1801. By 1805 he had established a surgical practice in Golden Square, London. Cooper was a prodigious writer. In 1809 the first edition of his great surgical dictionary for the use of students appeared. It was instantly successful in Britain, Europe and America, and as *Cooper's Surgical Dictionary* it continued to be revised and issued until 1838.
33. Cooper, *A Dictionary,* p. 883.
34. Blizard, p. 49. He added that the authors referred to in the Works of Percival Pott are Albucasis; Ambrose Parè [*sic*]; Andreas a Crucè [*sic*]; Archigenes; Bertapal; Berengarius Carpensis; Bilguer; Brunus; Celsus; Cheselden; De la Faye; Dionis; Du Verney; Fabritius [*sic*] Hildanus; Fabritius ab Aquapendente; Faget; Fallopius; Galen; Garengeot; Guido; Gulielmus de Saliceto; Heister; Hippocrates; Lanfranc; Le Dran; Lowe; Monro; Morgagni; Mukreen; Munnicks; Muys; Oribasius; Paulus Aegineta; Petrus e Marcheti; Petrus Paaw; Platner; Rhazes; Richter; Rolandus; Ruysch; Severinus; Schenkius; Siculus; Theodorus; Tissot; Turner; Van Swieten; Verduc; Wirtz; and Wiseman (pp. 48–49).
35. Blizard, p. 51.
36. Blizard, p. 52.
37. Blizard, p. 52.
38. For example see Winslow, Forbes, *Physic and Physicians: A Medical Sketch Book, exhibiting, The Public and Private Life of the Most Celebrated Medical Men of Former Days; with Memoirs of Eminent Living London Physicians and Surgeons.* London: Londman, Orme, Brown,

and Co., 1839, Vol. II, pp. 116–9. Winslow includes stories that I have not found elsewhere concerning Pott, such as, "On one occasion he had performed a complicated and dangerous operation. He had seen the patient three times during the day; and during the following night he dreamed that the assistant at the hospital had forgotten to administer a particular medicine that he had ordered, and from which he had anticipated much good effect. He could not remain easy whilst this impression was on his mind. He rose from his bed, dressed himself, and in the middle of the night without disturbing any of the family, went to the hospital, gained admission, had the house-surgeon summoned to his side, in order to satisfy himself that his instructions had been punctually obeyed. To his great astonishment he found that the medicine had not been exhibited! Pott always declared that his dream had saved his patient's life" (p. 118).

39. See, biographies of John Hunter such as Ottley, Drewery: *The Life of John Hunter*. Longman, Rees, Orman, Brown, Green and Longman: London, 1853; Kobler, John: *The Reluctant Surgeon: a Biography of John Hunter.* Heinemann: London, 1960; and most recently, Moore, Wendy: *The Knife Man: The Extraordinary Life and Times of John Hunter, Father of Modern Surgery*. Bantam: London, 2005.
40. Macilwain, George: *Memoirs of John Abernethy*. Hurst and Blackett: London, 1853, p. 361. Italics in original text.
41. Paget, Sir James: *The Hunterian Oration of 1877*. Longmans, Green and Co.: London, 1877, p. 54.
42. Paget, p. 29.
43. Owen, Edmund: "Remarks on Hernia—Particularly in Children." *British Medical Journal* Vol. 1, No. 2422, June 1, 1907, pp. 1285–9.
44. Robinson, James O.: "The Royal and Ancient History of St. Bartholomew (founded 1123)," *Journal of Medical Biography*, Vol. 1: 1, 1993, pp. 23–30. See p. 28.
45. *Critical Review*, August 1791, 2, pp. 361–368, quotation from p. 362.
46. See Kipling, M. D. and Waldron, H. A.: "Percivall Pott and Cancer Scroti." *British Journal of Industrial Medicine* Vol. 32, No. 3, 1975, pp. 244–50; also Brown, John R. and Thornton, John L.: "Percivall Pott (1714–1788) and Chimney Sweepers' Cancer of the Scrotum." *British Journal of Industrial Medicine* Vol. 14, No. 1, 1957, pp. 68–70; and Denkler, Keith: "Sir Percivall Pott, Sir James Paget, and Soot Cancer of the Hand." *Lancet*, Vol. 364, August 14, 2004, pp. 555–636.
47. The 1788 *The Act for the Better Regulation of Chimney Sweeps and their Apprentices* was poorly applied. It required no boy under the age of eight to be apprenticed to a sweep. 1803 the *Society for Superseding the Necessity of Climbing Boys, by Encouraging a New Method of Sweeping Chimneys and for Improving the Condition of Children and Others Employed by Chimney Sweepers* was formed and advocated for replacing chimney boys with mechanical sweeping devices. It was largely unsuccessful. In 1834 the apprenticeship age was raised to ten, and further acts raised it to sixteen. Finally in 1875 sweeps were required to be licensed. A notable exception to the argument that Pott's essay was a prelude to reform is that of Niels van Manen. He gave a paper, titled Skin Politics: Scrotal Cancer and the Regulation of Child Labour in Chimney Sweeping in Britain, c. 1773–1840, that partly discussed this claim at The History of the Skin Conference at the University of Birmingham, UK, October 28–30, 2010. van Manen particularly noted that in the early to

mid-nineteenth century, surgeons debated before Parliamentary hearings on child labor and in their own works whether this as in fact an adult disease, perhaps a hereditary one, or secondary to another disorder. I am grateful that I heard his paper.

48. Pott, Percivall: "Chirurgical observations relative to the cataract, the polypus of the nose, the cancer of the scrotum, the different kinds of rupture etc." In: *Chirurgical Works*, London, 1778, p. 64.
49. Jonas Hanway (1715–1786) had published *Observations on the Causes of Dissoluteness which Reigns among the Lower Classes of the People ... Likewise a Plan for Preventing the Extraordinary Mortality of the Children of the Labouring Poor in London and Westminster* (1772) and *A Sentimental History of Chimney Sweepers, in London and Westminster, Shewing the Necessity of Putting Them Under Regulation, To Prevent the Grossest Inhumanity to the Climbing Boys, With a Letter to a London Clergyman on Sunday Schools Calculated to the Preservation of the Children of the Poor* (1785). He was a governor and then vice president of the Foundling hospital, a merchant, traveler and philanthropist.
50. Pott, "Chirurgical observations," p. 65. On chimney sweeps see Phythian-Adams Charles: "Milk and Soot: The Changing Vocabulary of a Popular Ritual in Stuart and Hanoverian London," in *The Pursuit of Urban History*, edited by Fraser, Derek and Sutcliffe, Anthony (eds.), London: Edward Arnold Publishers Ltd., 1983, pp. 83–104. Judge, Roy: *The Jack-in-the-Green: A May Day Custom.* Cambridge, UK: D. S. Brewer Ltd. and Rowman and Littlefield for the Folklore Society, 1979. Holden, Robert: *Orphans of History: The Forgotten Children of the First Fleet.* The Text Book Publishing Company: Melbourne 1999. Phillips, George Lewis: *England's Climbing Boys: A History of the Long Struggle to Abolish Child Labor in Chimney-sweeping.* Baker Library, Harvard Graduate School of Business Administration: Boston, MA, 1949.
51. Pott, "Chirurgical observations," p. 67.
52. Pott, "Chirurgical observations," p. 67.
53. Pott, "Chirurgical observations," p. 68.
54. *The London Review*, Number 1175, April 1775, pp. 268–70. Quotation from p. 269.

Bibliography

Primary Sources

Archives Consulted

Barts and The London NHS Archives
British Library
Clendening History of Medicine Library
College of Physicians of Philadelphia
Ebling Library for the Health Sciences, University of Wisconsin
Kings College Archives
London Metropolitan Archives
The National Archives (UK)
United States National Library of Medicine
Royal College of Surgeons of London
Royal College of Physicians of London
University of Uppsala Library, Special Collections
Wellcome Library

Electronic Resources Used

Old Bailey Proceedings Online

Ancestry.com UK, Register of Duties Paid for Apprentices' Indentures, 1710–1811 [database on-line]. Provo, UT, USA: Ancestry.com Operations, Inc., Board of Stamps: Apprenticeship Books, Series IR 1; The National Archives of the UK (TNA), Kew, Surrey, England.

The Cullen Project: The Consultation Letters of Dr William Cullen (1710–1790) at the Royal College of Physicians of Edinburgh.

Periodicals Consulted

Annual Register

The Boston Medical and Surgical Journal

The Critical Review

The European Magazine

The Gentlemen's Magazine

The Gentleman's Magazine and Historical Chronicle

Hibernian Magazine

The Literary Register. Or Weekly Miscellany

The London Chronicle

London Magazine

London Morning Penny Post

The London Review

The Monthly Review

St. James Chronicle or the British Evening Post

The Universal Magazine

The Westminster Magazine

Whitehall Evening Post or London Intelligencer

World and Fashionable Advertiser

Abernethy, John: *Surgical Observations on the Injuries of the Head and on Miscellaneous Subjects.* London, 1815.

Abernethy, John: *Surgical and Physiological Essays.* London, 1793.

Aitkin, John: *Thoughts on Hospitals.* London, 1771.

Alanson, Edward: *Practical Observations on Amputation and the After Treatment.* London, 1782.

Andry, Nicolas: *Orthopaedia, or the art of correcting and preventing deformities in children. Translated from the French of M. Andry.* London, 1743.

Anon.: *The modern practice of the London hospitals.* 1766.

Anon.: *Egregious quackery display'd. Or, a narrative of the late memorable case of Seignor Capitano Masseo/Written in Spanish … And translated into English by a faithful hand (Sarificato Sangresugeo).* London, 1742.

Bell, Benjamin: *A Treatise on the Theory and Management of Ulcers.* 1778.

Bell, John: *The Principles of Surgery, as they relate to wounds, ulcers, and fistulae.* Edinburgh, 1826.

Bilguer, Johann Ulrich: *A dissertation on the inutility of the amputation of limbs*. London, 1764.

Blackmore, Sir Richard: *Dissertation on a Dropsy, a Tympany, the Jaundice, the Stone, and a Diabetes*. London, 1727.

Blicke, Charles: *An Essay on the Bilious of Yellow Fever of Jamaica Collected from the Manuscript of a Late Surgeon*. London, 1791.

Blizard, William: *Suggestions for the Improvement of Hospitals and other Charitable Institutions*. London, 1796.

Blizard, William: *The Hunterian oration: delivered in the theatre of the Royal College of Surgeons, on the 14th Day of February*. Rivington's, London, 1815.

Brand, T.: *Strictures in Vindication of some of the doctrines misrepresented by Mr. Foot in his two pamphlets entitled, Observations upon the New Opinions of John Hunter in his late treatise on the venereal disease; including Mr. Pott's plagiarisms and misinformation on the subject of pus or matter in his Observations on that disorder commonly called fistula lachrymalis*. London, 1774.

Cadogan, William: *An Essay upon Nursing and the Management of Children*. London, 1748.

Clare, Peter: *An Essay of the Cure of Abscesses by Caustic and on the treatment of wounds and ulcers; and a new method of curing the lues venera*. London, 1779.

Clare, Peter: *A New and Easy Method of Curing the Lues Venerea: By the Introduction of Mercury into the System through the Orifices of the absorbent Vessels on the inside of the Mouth, With the Remarks of Dr. Hunter and Mr. Cruikshank in favour of this Practice. Also An Essay on Abscesses and other Observations in Surgery*. London, 1780.

Cooper, Samuel: *A Dictionary of Practical Surgery: containing a complete exhibition of the present state of the principles and practice of surgery, collected from the best and most original sources of information and illustrated by critical remark*. London, 1809.

Cruttenden, R.: *Sovereign efficacious grace! Display'd in the awakening and converting a rational, learned aged sinner. Exemplified in The experience of Robert Cruttenden, Esq. as delivered by himself to the Congregational Church*. London, 1744.

Dease, William: *Observations on the different methods made use of for the radical cure of the hydrocele, or watry rupture, and on other diseases of the testicle: to which is added a comparative view of the different methods of cutting for the stone*. Dublin, 1782.

Douglas, James: *The history of the lateral operation, or, An account of the method of extracting a stone, by making a wound near the great protuberance of the os ischium, through the common integuments and levator ani, into the side of the bladder, without touching the urethra, prostate gland, vesiculae seminales, or any other of the urinary or seminal vessels, first attempted by Frère Jacques in France, and afterwards successfully perform'd by Professor Rau in Holland: with a postscript concerning the introduction and improvement of this method here in London*. London, 1720.

Douglas, John: *A Syllabus of what is to be perform'd in a course on Anatomy, Chirurgical Operations and Bandages*. London, 1719.

Earle, James: *The Chirurgical Works of Percival Pott, F.R.S. a new Edition, with his Last Corrections. To which are added A Short Account of the Life of the Author, a Method of curing the Hydrocele by Injection, and occasional Notes and Observations*. London, 1790.

Earle, James: The Chirurgical Works of Percivall Pott, F.R.S. London, 1789.

Earle, James: *A Treatise on the Hydrocele*. London, 1791.

Earle, James: *Practical Observations on the Operation for the Stone*. London, 1793.

Earle, James: *An appendix to a Treatise on the Hydrocele*. London, 1793.

Earle, James: *An Appendix to a Treatise on the operation for the stone*. London, 1796.

Earle, James: *Observations on the cure of the curved spine and the means of lessening the effects of fire on the human body*. London, 1799.

Earle, James: *Observations on Hemorrhoidal Excresences*. London, 1799.

Else, Joseph: *An Essay on the cure of the hydrocele of the tunica vaginalis*. London, 1770.

Fearon, Henry: *A Treatise on Cancers, with a New and Successful Method of Operating, Particularly in Cancers of the Breast and Testis*. London, 1784.

Fearon, Henry: "*Observations on Cancer*." *Memoirs of the Medical Society of London*, Volume II, Article 38, London, 1789.

Foot, John: *An appeal to the public, touching the death of Mr. George Clarke*. London, 1769.

Foot, Jessé: *The Life of John Hunter*. London, 1794.

Gataker, Thomas: *Observations on the Internal Use of the Solanum or Nightshade*. London, 1757.

Gay, John: *Gay's Fables in one volume complete*. London, 1808.

Gooch, Benjamin: *Cases and Remarks in Surgery. With Sketches of Machines, of Simple Construction, Easy Application and Approved Use*. London, 1758.

Greenfield, John: *A Compleat Treatise of the Stone and Gravel*. London, 1710.

Gregory, George: *Elements of the Theory and Practice of Medicine designed for the Use of Students*. London, 1820.

Hanway, Jonas: *Observations on the Causes of Dissoluteness which Reigns among the Lower Classes of the People … Likewise a Plan for Preventing the Extraordinary Mortality of the Children of the Labouring Poor in London and Westminster*. London, 1772.

Hanway, Jonas: *A Sentimental History of Chimney Sweepers, in London and Westminster, Shewing the Necessity of Putting Them Under Regulation, To Prevent the Grossest Inhumanity to the Climbing Boys, With a Letter to a London Clergyman on Sunday Schools Calculated to the Preservation of the Children of the Poor*. London, 1785.

Heister, Lorenz: *A General System of Surgery in Three Parts*. London, 1743.

Hey, William: *Practical Observations in Surgery, Illustrated with Cases*. London, 1803.

Houlston, William: *Outline of the History of Surgery collected with observations by William Member of the Corporation of Surgeons*. London, 1789.

Howship, John: *Practical observations on the symptoms, discrimination and treatment, of some of the most important diseases of the lower intestines and anus*. London, 1820.

Hughson, D.: *The New Family Receipt-book: Or Universal Repository of Domestic Economy*. London, 1817.

Jackson, William: *Cautions and advice to the public, respecting some abuses in medicine*. London, 1787.

Jebb, John: *Select Cases of the Disorder commonly termed the Paralysis of the Lower Extremities*. London, 1782.

Jebb, John: *Select Cases of a Disorder commonly termed the Paralysis of the Lower Extremities to which is added a Case of Catalepsy*. London, 1783.

Jones, John: *Plain, concise, practical remarks on the treatment of wounds and fractures*. John Holt: New York, 1776.

Justamond, J. O.: *Surgical Tracts By the Late J.O. Justamond, F.R.S., Surgeon to the Westminster Hospital, London, 1789. Part One is Outlines of the History of Surgery, collected with observations by William Houlston, Member of the Corporation of Surgeons*. London, 1789

Allen, Julia: *Swimming with Dr Johnson and Mrs Thrale: Sport, Health and Exercise in Eighteenth-century England.* The Lutterworth Press: Cambridge, UK, 2012.

Amussen, Susan Dwyer: "'Being Stirred to Much Unquietness': Violence and Domestic Violence in Early Modern England." *Journal of Women's History* Vol. 6, No. 2, 1994, pp. 70–89.

Andrews, Jonathan and Scull, Andrew: *Customers and Patrons of the Mad Trade: The Management of Lunacy in Eighteenth-Century London.* University of California Press: Berkeley and Los Angeles, 2003.

Androutsos, G.: "The Outstanding British Surgeon Percivall Pott (1714–1789) and the First Description of an Occupational Cancer." *Journal of BUON* Vol. 11, 2006, pp. 533–39.

Anning, S. T.: "The General Infirmary at Leeds. Vol. 1, the First Hundred Years, 1767–1869." S T, Livingstone: Edinburgh, 1963.

Anon.: *American Medical Gazette and Journal of Health.* Vol. 11, Pt. 4 1860, pp. 530–1.

Anon.: *Bengal Past and Present, The Journal of the Calcutta Historical Society* Vol. 26, Parts I and II, July–December 1923.

Anon.: Written by a Pupil of St. *Bartholomew's Hospital on the Resignation of Mr. Pott." St. Bartholomew's Hospital Journal* April 1928, p. 107.

Argent, Mark: *Recollections of R.J.S. Stevens: An Organist in Georgian London.* Southern Illinois University Press: Carbondale, 1992.

Arnold, Dana: *The Spaces of the Hospital: Spatiality and Urban Change in London, 1680–1820.* Routledge: London 2013.

Austen-Leigh, Richard Arthur: *The Eton College Register, 1753–1790.* Spottiswoode, Ballantine & Co. Ltd.: Eton, 1921.

Bailey, Joanne: "Reassessing Parenting in Eighteenth-Century England." In: Berry, H. and Foster, E. (eds.), *The Family in Early Modern England.* Cambridge University Press: Cambridge, 2007, pp. 209–232.

Bailey, Joanne: "'I dye [*sic*] by Inches': Locating Wife Beating in the Concept of a Privatization of Marriage and Violence in Eighteenth-century England." *Social History* Vol. 31, No. 3, 2006, pp. 273–294.

Bailey, Joanne: *Unquiet Lives: Marriage and Marriage Breakdown in England, 1660–1800.* Cambridge University Press: Cambridge, 2003.

Barry, Jonathan: *Raising Spirits: How a Conjuror's Tale Was Transmitted across the Enlightenment.* Palgrave Macmillan: New York, 2013.

Beekman, Fenwick: "The 'Hernia Congenita' and an Account of the Controversy It Provoked between William Hunter and Percivall Pott." *Bulletin of the NY Academy of Medicine* Vol. 22, No. 9, 1946, pp. 486–500.

Belcher, Joseph: *Historical sketches of hymns, their writers and their influence.* Lindsay and Blakiston: London, 1859.

Bell, Whitfield, J.: "James Hutchinson (1752–1793): Letters from an American Student in London." *Transactions & Studies of the College of Physicians of Philadelphia* Vol. 34, No. 1, 1966, pp. 20–25.

Belloni, L.: "Percivall Pott's Disease of the Spine, Discussed in Two Letters of J. Hunczovsky from London, 1779, to G. A. Brambilla in Vienna." *Medical History* Vol. 16, No. 1, 1972, pp. 78–80.

Bennion, Elisabeth: *Antique Medical Instruments*. University of California Press: Berkeley, 1979.

Bishop, W. J.: *A History of Surgical Dressings*. Robinson and Sons Ltd.: Chesterfield, 1959.

Black, Jeremy: *Eighteenth Century Britain, 1688–1783*. Palgrave Macmillan: Basingstoke, 2008.

Bloom, H. T. G., Richardson, W. W., and Harries, E. J.: "Natural History of Untreated Breast Cancer (1805–1933): Comparison of Untreated and Treated Cases According to Histological Grade of Malignancy." *The British Medical Journal* Vol. 2, No. 5299, 1962, pp. 213–221.

Borsay, Anne: *Disability and Social Policy in Britain since 1750*. Palgrave Macmillan: Basingstoke, 2005.

Brailsford, Dennis: *A Taste for Diversions: Sport in Georgian England*. The Lutterworth Press: Cambridge, 1999.

Brock, Claire: *The Feminization of Fame, 1750–1830*. Palgrave Macmillan: Basingstoke, 2006.

Brock, Helen: "The Many Facets of William Hunter (1718–83)". *History of Science* Vol. 32, 1994, pp. 387–404.

Brown, John R. and Thornton, John L.: "Percivall Pott (1714–1788) and Chimney Sweepers' Cancer of the Scrotum." *British Journal of Industrial Medicine* Vol. 14, No. 1, 1957, pp. 68–70.

Brown, Michael: *Performing Medicine: Medical Culture and Identity in Provincial England, c. 1760–1850*. Manchester University Press: Manchester, 2011.

Buchan, James: *Capital of the Mind: How Edinburgh Changed the World*. John Murray Publishers: London, 2004.

Bucholz, Robert O. and Ward, Joseph P.: *London: A Social and Cultural History, 1550–1750*. Cambridge University Press: Cambridge, 2012.

Bynum, William F.: "Physicians, Hospitals, and Career Structures in Eighteenth-Century London." In: Bynum, W. F. and Porter, Roy (eds.), *William Hunter and the Eighteenth-Century Medical World*. Cambridge University Press: Cambridge, 1985, pp. 105–28.

Callahan, Charles W.: "Construction Crew Discovers Grave of 'Tiny Tim'." *The Journal of Infectious Diseases* Vol. 176, No. 6, 1997, pp. 1653–1654.

Cannadine, David: *Class in Britain*. Penguin Books Ltd.: London, 2000.

Cantor, David: "Cancer." In: Bynum, W. F. and Porter, Roy (eds.), *Companion Encyclopedia of the History of Medicine*. Vol. 1. Routledge: London, 1993, pp. 537–561.

Carré, Jacques: "Hospital Nurses in Eighteenth-Century Britain: Service without Responsibility." In: Baudino, Isabelle, Carré, Jacques and Révauger, Cécile (eds.), *The Invisible Woman: Aspects of Women's Work in Eighteenth-Century Britain*. Ashgate Press: Aldershot, 2005, pp. 89–99.

Carswell, John: *The South Sea Bubble*. Stanford University Press: Stanford, 1960.

Carter, Philip: *Men and the Emergence of Polite Society, Britain, 1660–1800*. Pearson Education: London, 2001.

Cash, Arthur: *John Wilkes: The Scandalous Father of Civil Liberty*. Yale University Press: New Haven, 2006.

Caton, Donald: *What a Blessing She Had Chloroform: The Medical and Social Response to the Pain of Childbirth from 1800 to the Present*. Yale University Press: New Haven, 1999.

Chakrabarti, Pratik: *Materials and Medicine: Trade, Conquest and Therapeutics in the Eighteenth Century*. Manchester University Press: Manchester, 2010.

Chaplin, Arnold: *Medicine in England during the Reign of George III.* Henry Klimpton: London, 1919.

Chaplin, Simon: "Nature Dissected, or Dissection Naturalized? The Case of John Hunter's Museum." *Museum and Society,* Vol. 6, No. 2, Jul. 2008, pp. 135–151.

Chaplin, Simon David John: "John Hunter and the 'museum economy', 1750–1800." Unpublished dissertation, University of London, May 2009.

Charters, Erica: *Disease, War, and the Imperial State: The Welfare of the British Armed Forces during the Seven Year's War.* The University of Chicago Press: Chicago, 2014.

Churchill, Wendy D: *Female Patients in Early Modern Britain: Gender, Diagnosis, and Treatment.* Ashgate Press: Aldershot, 2012.

Clarke, J. F.: *Autobiographical recollections of the medical profession.* J. & A. Churchill: London, 1874.

Clark, Rev. Andrew: "James Marriott of Twinstead Hall, Essex." *The Essex Review: An Illustrated Quarterly Record of Everything.* Vol. 15, No. 57, 1906, pp. 86–7.

Cockayne, Emily: *Hubbub: Filth, Noise and Stench in England.* Yale University Press: New Haven, 2007.

Cody, Lisa Forman: "Living and Dying in Georgian London's Lying-In Hospitals." *Bulletin of the History of Medicine.* Vol. 78, No. 2, 2004, pp. 309–48.

Cohen, Lord: "Liverpool's Contributions to Medicine." *The British Medical Journal,* Vol. 1, No. 5440, 1965, pp. 945–948.

Collingham, E. M.: *Imperial Bodies: The Physical Experience of the Raj, c. 1800–1947.* Polity Press: Cambridge, UK, 2001.

Colón, A. R. and Colón, P. A.: *Nurturing Children: A History of Pediatrics.* Greenwood Press: London, 1999.

Cook, Harold: *The Decline of the Old Medical Regime in Stuart London.* Ithaca, NY: Cornell University Press, 1986.

Cooper, David K. C.: "John Collins Warren (1778–1856): An American Surgeon in London." *British Medical Journal* Vol. 345, No. 7888, 2012, pp. 42–43.

Cope, Zachary: *The History of the Royal College of Surgeons of England.* Anthony Blond: London, 1959.

Costa, Palmira Fontes Da: *The Singular and the Making of Knowledge at the Royal Society of London in the Eighteenth Century.* Cambridge Scholars Publishing: Newcastle upon Tyne, 2009.

Cozens-Hardy, Basil: *The Diary of Sylas Neville, 1767–1788.* Oxford University Press: Oxford, 1950.

Crawford, Catherine: "Patients' Rights and the Law of Contract in Eighteenth-Century England." *Social History of Medicine* Vol. 13, No. 3, 2000, pp. 381–410.

Crawford, Patricia: *Parents of Poor Children in England, 1580–1800.* Oxford University Press: Oxford, 2010.

Crellin, John K.: "How Shall I Take My Medicine? Dosages and Other Matters in Eighteenth-Century Medicine." *Caduceus: A Humanities Journal for Medicine and the Health Sciences* Vol. 13, No. 1 1997, pp. 39–50.

Crimmin, Pat: "The Shortage of Surgeons and Surgeons' Mates, c.1740–1806: 'An Evil of a Serious Nature to the Service.'" *Transactions of the Naval Dockyards Society Publications* Vol. 6, 2010, pp. 49–55.

Cristancho, S. M., Apramian, T., Vanstone, M., Lingard, L., Ott, M., Novick, R. J.: Understanding Clinical Uncertainty: What Is Going on When Experienced Surgeons Are Not Sure What To Do?" *Academic Medicine* Vol. 88, No. 10, October 2013, pp. 1–5.

Croxson, Bronwyn: "The Price of Charity to the Middlesex Hospital, 1750–1830." In: Gorsky, Martin and Sheard, Sally (eds.), *Financing Medicine: The British Experience since 1750.* Routledge: London and New York, 2006, pp. 23–39.

Cruickshank, Dan: *London's Sinful Secret: The Bawdy House and Very Public Passions of London's Georgian Age*. St. Martin's Press: New York, 2009.

Curl, James Stevens: *Spas, Wells, & Pleasure Gardens of London*. Historical Publications Ltd.: London, 2010.

Dacome, Lucia: "'To what purpose does it think?': Dreams, Sick bodies and Confused minds in the Age of Reason." *History of Psychiatry* Vol. 15, No. 4, 2004, pp. 395–416.

Dawson, Mark S.: "First Impressions: Newspaper Advertisements and Early Modern English Body Imaging, 1651–1750." *Journal of British Studies* Vol. 50, April 2011, pp. 277–306.

Denkler, Keith: "Sir Percivall Pott, Sir James Paget, and Soot Cancer of the Hand." *Lancet*, Vol. 364, August 14, 2004, pp. 555–636.

Dickie, Simon: *Cruelty and Laughter: Forgotten Comic Literature and the Unsentimental Eighteenth Century*. Chicago: University of Chicago Press, 2011.

Dickie, Simon: "Hilarity and Pitilessness in the Mid-Eighteenth Century: English Jestbook Humor." *Eighteenth-Century Studies* Vol. 37, No. 1, Fall, 2003, pp. 1–22.

Digby, Anne: *Making a Medical Living: Doctors and Patients in the English Market for Medicine, 1720–1911*. Cambridge University Press: Cambridge, 1994.

Dillon, Patrick: *Gin: The Much-lamented Death of Madam Geneva: The Eighteenth-Century Gin Craze.* Justin, Charles & Co.: Boston, 2003.

Dirks, Nicholas B.: *The Scandal of Empire: India and the Creation of Imperial Britain*. Harvard University Press: Cambridge, MA, 2008.

Dobson, Austin: Frances Burney, *Diary and Letters of Madame D'Arblay.* Macmillan & Company: London, 1904.

Dobson, Jesse: "Percivall Pott." *Annuals of the Royal College of Surgeons of England* Vol. 50, 1972, pp. 54–65.

Dodd, George: *The Food of London*. Longman, Brown & Green: London, 1856.

Doyle, Julie: "The Spectre of the Scalpel: The Historical Role of Surgery and Anatomy in Conceptions of Embodiment." *Body & Society* Vol. 14, No. 1, March 2008, pp. 9–30.

Dutta, Krishna: *Calcutta: A Cultural History*. Interlink Publishing Ltd.: Northampton, MA, 2008.

Edgar, Andrew: "Professional Values, Aesthetic Values, and the Ends of Trade." *Med Health Care and Philos* Vol. 4, 2011, pp. 195–201.

Eigen, Joel Peter: *Witnessing Insanity: Madness and Mad-Doctors in the English Court*. Yale University Press: New Haven, CT, 1995.

Ellis, Harold: *A History of Bladder Stone*. Blackwell Scientific Publications: Oxford and Edinburgh, 1969.

Ennis, Daniel James: *Enter the Press Gang: Naval Impressment in Eighteenth-Century British Literature*. University of Delaware Press: Dover, 2002.

Endelman, Todd M.: *The Jews of Georgian England 1714–1830: Tradition and Change in a Liberal Society*. University of Michigan Press: Ann Arbor, 1999.

Epstein, Julia L.: "Writing the Unspeakable: Fanny Burney's Mastectomy and the Fictive Body." *Representations* Vol. 16, 1986, pp. 131–166.

Evans, Jennifer: "'It is caused of the womans part or of the mans part': The Role of Gender in the Diagnosis and Treatment of Sexual Dysfunction in Early Modern England." *Women's History Review* Vol. 20, No. 3, July 2011, pp. 439–457.

Evans, Jonathan: "Barts and the London's Medical Museum Collections." In: Mitchell, Piers (ed.), *Anatomical Dissection in Enlightenment England and Beyond: Autopsy, Pathology and Display*. Ashgate Press: Aldershot, 2012, pp. 115–137.

Faye, Deirdre Le: *A Chronology of Jane Austen and Her Family: 1700–2000*. Cambridge University Press: Cambridge, 2006.

Fischer, George: "Surgery One Hundred Years Ago." *JAMA* Vol. 28, No. 13, March 27, 1897, pp. 596–600.

Fissell, Mary, *Patients, Power and the Poor in Eighteenth-Century Bristol*. Cambridge University Press: Cambridge, 2002.

Flamm, E. S.: "Percival Pott: An 18th Century Neurosurgeon." *Journal of Neurosurgery* Vol. 76, 1992, pp. 319–26.

Flavell, Julie: *When London Was Capital of America*. Yale University Press: New Haven, CT, 2010.

Forbes, Thomas Rogers: "Crowner's Quest." *Transactions of the American Philosophical Society* Vol. 68, No. 1, 1978, pp. 1–52.

Forbes, Thomas R.: "Percivall Pott Performs a Postmortem." *Bulletin of the New York Academy of Medicine*, Vol. 51, No. 2, Feb 1975, pp. 272–276.

Forrester, J. M.: "The Homoeomerous Parts and Their Replacement by Bichat's Tissues." *Medical History* Vol. 38, No. 4, 1994, pp. 444–458.

Foyster, Elizabeth: *Marital Violence: An English Family History, 1660–1857*. Cambridge University Press: Cambridge, 2005.

Foyster, Elizabeth: "Male Honour, Social Control and Wife Beating in Late Stuart England." *Transactions of the Royal Historical Society* Vol. 6, 1996, pp. 215–24.

Freidson, Eliot: *Profession of Medicine: A Study of the Sociology of Applied Knowledge*. The University of Chicago Press: Chicago, 1988.

Fu, Louis Kuo-Tai: "Notable Names in the History of Surgery: Percivall Pott (1714–1788)." *Annals of the College of Surgeons of Hong Kong* Vol. 4, 2000, pp. 110–122.

Ganz, Jeremy C.: "Head injuries in the 18th Century: The Management of the Damaged Brain." *Neurosurgery* Vol. 73, No. 1, 2013, pp. 167–75.

Ganz, Jeremy C.: "James Hill of Dumfries: First Modern Neurosurgical Procedures" *British Journal of Neurosurgery* Vol. 29, No. 6, 2005, pp. 778–784.

Ganz, Jeremy C.: "Hippocrates, Celsus and Galen: Head Injury, the Brain, and the Bone." *Istoriya meditsiny History of Medicine*. Vol. 2. No. 1, 2000, pp. 92–103.

Garrick, David: *The private correspondence of David Garrick: with the most celebrated persons of his time*. James Boaden, Henry Colburn and Richard Bentley Publishers: London, 1832.

Gask, George E.: "Percivall Pott." In: Power, D'Arcy (ed.), *British Masters of Medicine.* Books for Libraries Press: Freeport, New York, 1969.

Gatrell, Vic: *City of Laughter: Sex and Satire in 18th Century London.* Bloomsbury Publishing: New York, 2007.

George, M. Dorothy: *London Life in the Eighteenth Century.* Academy Chicago Publishers: Chicago, 2005.

Geyer-Kordesch, Johanna and MacDonald, Fiona: *The History of the Royal College of Physicians and Surgeons of Glasgow 1599–1858.* The Hambledon Press: London, 1999.

Ghosh, Durba: "Decoding the Nameless: Gender, Subjectivity, and Historical Methodologies in Reading the Archives of Colonial India." In: Wilson, Kathleen (ed.), *A New Imperial History: Culture, Identity and Modernity in Britain and the Empire, 1640–1840.* Cambridge University Press: Cambridge, 2004, pp. 297–316.

Gladfelder, Hal: *Criminality and Narrative in Eighteenth-Century England: Beyond the Law.* Johns Hopkins University Press: Baltimore, 2001.

Godfrey, Walter H. and Marcham, W. McB. (eds.): *Survey of London.* London County Council: London, Vol. 24, 1952.

Gonzalès, Jacques: "Le mal de Pott avant les antituberculeux: de Pott à Ménard." *Histoire des Sciences Médicales,* Tome 39: 3, 2005, pp. 291–301.

Granshaw, Lindsay: "The Rise of the Modern Hospital in Britain." In: Wear, Andrew (ed.), *Medicine in Society: Historical Essays.* The Press Syndicate of the University of Cambridge: Cambridge, 1992, pp. 197–218.

Gray, Drew D.: *Crime, Prosecution and Social Relations: The Summary Courts of the City of London in the Late Eighteenth Century.* Palgrave Macmillan: Basingstoke, 2009.

Green, Dominic: "George Gordon: a biographical Reassessment." In: Haywood, Ian and Seed, John (eds.), *The Gordon Riots: Politics, Culture and Insurrection in Late Eighteenth-Century Britain.* Cambridge University Press: Cambridge, 2012, pp. 245–264.

Greenblatt, Samuel H., Dagi T., and Epstein M. (eds.): *A History of Neurosurgery: In Its Scientific and Professional Contexts.* Thieme Medical Publications: Park Ridge, IL., 1997.

Gupta, Hira Lal: *Fort William India-House Correspondence.* Vol. 8, Government of India, Civil Lines: Delhi, 1981.

Gupta, Pratul Chandra: *Fort William-India House Correspondence.* Vol. 13, Government of India, Civil Lines: Delhi, 1959.

Hakulinen, E.: "Mannen Bakom Syndrome: Percivall Pott." *Läkartidningen* Vol. 82, No. 34, 1985, pp. 2784–5.

Hallett, Christine: "The Attempt to Understand Puerperal Fever in the Eighteenth and Early Nineteenth Centuries: The Influence of Inflammation Theory." *Medical History* Vol. 49, No. 1, 2005, pp. 1–28.

Hallett, Mark: *Hogarth.* Phaidon Press: London, 2000.

Hamilton, Bernice: "The Medical Professions in the Eighteenth Century." *The Economic History Review* Vol. 4, No. 2, 1951, pp. 147–162.

Hargreaves, A. S.: *White as Whales Bone: Dental Services in Early Modern England.* Northern Universities Press: Leeds, 1998.

Harland, Kathleen: "Royal Naval Surgeons Afloat and Ashore, 1700–1750." *Transactions of the Naval Dockyards Society Publications* Vol. 6, 2010, pp. 9–30.
Harvey, Karen: "Gender, Space and Modernity in Eighteenth-Century England: A Place Called Sex." *History Workshop Journal* Vol. 51, Spring 2001, pp. 158–79.
Haslam, Fiona: *From Hogarth to Rowlandson: Medicine in Art in Eighteenth Century Britain.* Liverpool University Press: Liverpool, 1996.
Haywood, Ian and Seed, John (eds.): *The Gordon Riots: Politics, Culture and Insurrection in Late Eighteenth-Century Britain.* Cambridge University Press: Cambridge, 2012.
Heath, Christopher: "A Lecture on a Century of Surgery, Delivered in University College Hospital on January 8th 1900." *British Medical Journal* Vol. 1, No. 2037, 1900, pp. 61–65.
Hee, R. Van: "Surgeons and the Collegium Medicum Antverpiense: Professionalisation of Surgical Practice in 17th Century Antwerp." *Acta Chirurgica Belgica*, Vol. 3, 2011, pp. 184–91.
Helm, Jürgen and Wilson, Renate (eds.): *Medical Theory and Therapeutic Practice in the Eighteenth Century: A Transatlantic Perspective.* Franz Steiner Verlag: Stuttgart, 2008.
Hemlow, Joyce: *The Journals and Letters of Fanny Burney (Madame d'Arblay).* Vol. 6, Clarendon Press: Oxford, UK, 1975.
Herault, Pascal: "Les pauvres et l'amputation a la maison–dieu de Montmorillon (En Poitou) aux xviie et xviiie siècles." *Bulletin de la Société française d'histoire des hôpitaux* Vol. 69, 1993, pp. 23–33.
Herbert, Lord: *Pembroke Papers (1790–94): Letters and Diaries of Henry, Tenth Earl of Pembroke, and His Circle.* Jonathan Cape: London, 1950.
Hibbert, Christopher: *King Mob: The London Riots of 1780.* Dorset Press: New York, 1958.
Hirsh, A. V.: "The Anatomical Preparations of the Human Testis and Epididymis in the Glasgow Hunterian Anatomical Collection." *Human Reproduction Update* Vol. 11, No. 5, 1995, pp. 515–521.
Hitchcock, Tim: "Begging on the Streets of Eighteenth-Century London" *Journal of British Studies* Vol. 44, July 2005, pp. 478–498.
Hitchcock, Tim: *Down and Out in Eighteenth-Century London.* Bloomsbury Press: London, 2004.
Hitchcock, Tim: *English Sexualities, 1700–1800.* St. Martin's Press: London, 1997.
Hitchcock, Tim, King, Peter and Sharpe, Pamela (eds.): *Chronicling Poverty: The Voices and Strategies of the English Poor, 1640–1840.* St. Martin's Press Inc.: New York, 1997.
Holden, Robert: *Orphans of History: The Forgotten Children of the First Fleet.* The Text Book Publishing Company: Melbourne, 1999.
Hoppit, Julian: *Risk and Failure in English Business, 1700–1800.* Cambridge University Press: Cambridge, 1987.
Horder, Thomas J.: "The Life and Works of Percivall Pott. Being the Wix Prize Essay for the year 1894." *Saint Bartholomew's Hospital Reports* Vol. 30, 1894, pp. 163–187.
Houblon, Lady Alice Archer: *The Houblon Family: Its Story and Times.* Archibald, Constable and Company Ltd.: London, 1907.
Houston, R. A.: "Explanations for Death by Suicide in Northern Britain during the Long Eighteenth Century." *History of Psychiatry* Vol. 23, No. 1, 2011, pp. 53–64.
Houston, R. A.: *Punishing the Dead: Suicide, Lordship, and Community in Britain, 1500–1830.* Oxford University Press: Oxford, 2010.

Houston, R. A.: "Madness and Gender in the Long Eighteenth Century." *Social History* Vol. 27, No. 3, 2002, pp. 309–326.

Hubble, Douglas: "Mrs Thrale Keeping Notes." *The British Medical Journal* Vol. 1, No. 6116 Apr. 1, 1978, pp. 832–833.

Hunt, Margaret R.: *The Middling Sort: Commerce, Gender, and the Family in England, 1680–1780.* University of California Press: Berkeley, CA, 1996.

Hunt, Margaret R.: "Wife Beating, Domesticity and Women's Independence in Eighteenth-Century London." *Gender and History.* Vol. 4, No. 1, 1992, pp. 10–33.

Hurl-Eamon, Jennine: "The Fiction of Female Dependence and the Makeshift Economy of Soldiers, and Their Wives in Eighteenth-century London." *Labor History* Vol. 49, No. 4, November 2008, pp. 481–501.

Hyde, Mary: *The Thrales of Streatham Park.* Harvard University Press: Cambridge, MA, 1977.

Ingram, Allan: *Patterns of Madness in the Eighteenth Century: A Reader.* Liverpool University Press: Liverpool, 1998.

Jackson, Graham, and Ludlow, Cate: *A Grim Almanac of Georgian London.* The History Press: Stroud, 2011.

Jacob, W. M.: *Oxford Dictionary of National Biography.* Vol. 46, Oxford University Press, 2004, p. 202.

James, R. M.: "The Effect on Family Life During the Late Georgian Period of Indisposition, Medication, Treatments and the Resultant Outcomes." PhD thesis. Oxford Brookes University, 2010.

Jeffery, Sally: *The Mansion House.* The History Press Ltd.: London, 1993.

Jenner, Mark S. R. and Wallis, Patrick (eds.): *Medicine and the Market in England and Its Colonies, c.1450–c.1850.* Palgrave Macmillan: Basingstoke, 2007.

Jewson, Nicholas D.: "Medical Knowledge and the Patronage System in 18th Century England." Sociology Vol. 8, 1974, pp. 369–383.

Judge, Roy: *The Jack-in-the-Green: A May Day Custom.* D. S. Brewer Ltd. and Rowman and Littlefield for the Folklore Society: Cambridge, UK, 1979.

Kaartinen, Marjo: *Breast Cancer in the Eighteenth Century.* Pickering & Chatto: London, 2013.

Kelly, Ian: *Mr Foote's Other Leg: Comedy, Tragedy and Murder in Georgian London.* Picador: London, 2012.

Keynes, M.: "The Miserable Health of Dr. Samuel Johnson." *Journal of Medical Biography* Vol. 3, No. 3 1995, pp. 161–9.

Kipling, M. D. and Waldron, H. A.: "Percivall Pott and Cancer Scroti." *British Journal of Industrial Medicine* Vol. 32, No. 3, 1975, pp. 244–50.

Kirby, Peter: *Child Labour in Britain, 1750–1870.* Palgrave Macmillan: Basingstoke, 2003.

Kirkup, John R.: "Nicolas Andry and 250 Years of Orthopaedy." *The Journal of Bone and Joint Surgery* Vol. 73, No. 8, 1991, pp. 361–362.

Kirkup, John, R.: *A History of Limb Amputation.* Springer-Verlag: London, 2007.

Klein, Lawrence E.: "Politeness and the Interpretation of the British Long Eighteenth-century." *Historical Journal* Vol. 454, 2002, pp. 869–898.

Knoeff, Rina: *Dutch Anatomy and Clinical Medicine in 17th-Century Europe.* Published 2012–06–20, European History online, leg-ego.eu

Kobler, John: *The Reluctant Surgeon: A Biography of John Hunter.* Heinemann: London, 1960.

Kocher, Mininder S.: "Early Limb Salvage: Open Tibia Fractures of Ambrose Paré (1510–1590) and Percivall Pott (1714–1789)." *World Journal of Surgery* Vol. 21, 1007, pp. 116–122.

Labianca, Dominick A. and Reeves, William J.: "Science Literacy at Brooklyn College." *College Teaching*. Vol. 37, No. 4, 1989, pp. 135–137.

Landers, John: *Death and the Metropolis: Studies in the Demographic History of London, 1670–1830.* Cambridge University Press: Cambridge, 1993.

Lane, Joan: *A social history of medicine: Health, healing and disease in England, 1750–1950*, Routlege: London, 2001.

Lane, Joan: "Eighteenth-Century Medical Practice: A Case Study of Bradford Wilmer, Surgeon of Coventry, 1737–1813." *Social History of Medicine* Vol. 3, No. 3, 1990, pp. 369–86.

Lane, Joan: "The Role of Apprenticeship in Eighteenth-Century Medical Education in England." In: Bynum, William and Porter, Roy (eds.), *William Hunter and the Eighteenth-Century Medical World.* Cambridge University Press: Cambridge, 1985, pp. 57–104.

Lawrence, Christopher: "Medical Minds, Surgical Bodies: Corporeality and the Doctors." In: Lawrence, Christopher and Shapin, Steven (eds.), Science Incarnate: *Historical Embodiments of Natural Knowledge*. University of Chicago Press: Chicago, 1998, pp. 156–201.

Lawrence, Christopher: *Medicine in the Making of Modern Britain 1700–1920.* Routledge: London, 1994.

Lawrence, Christopher: "'Democratic, Divine and Heroic': The History and Historiography of Surgery." In: Lawrence, Christopher (ed.), *Medical Theory, Surgical Practice: Studies in the History of Surgery*, Routledge: London, 1992, pp. 1–47.

Lawrence, Susan C.: *Charitable Knowledge: Hospital Pupils and Practitioners in Eighteenth-century London*. Cambridge University Press: Cambridge, 1996.

Lawrence, Susan C.: "Educating the Senses: Students, Teachers and Medical Rhetoric in Eighteenth-Century London." In: Bynum W. F. and Porter, Roy (eds.), *Medicine and the Five Senses.* Cambridge University Press, Cambridge, 1993, pp. 154–178.

Lawrence, Susan C: "Desirous of Improvements in Medicine, Barts, 1795–1815." *Bulletin of the History of Medicine* Vol. 59, 1985, pp. 89–104.

Leong, E.: "Making medicines in the early modern household." *Bulletin of the History of Medicine* Vol. 82, 2008, pp. 145–168.

Leunig, Tim, Minns, Chris and Wallis, Patrick: "Networks in the Premodern Economy: The Market for London Apprenticeships, 1600–1749." *Journal of Economic History* Vol. 71, No. 2, 2011, pp. 413–443.

Levene, Alysa: *The Childhood of the Poor: Welfare in Eighteenth-Century London*. Palgrave Macmillan: Basingstoke, 2012.

Levene, Alysa: "Parish Apprenticeship and the Old Poor Law in London." *Economic History Review* Vol. 63, No. 4, 2010, pp. 915–41.

Levene, Alysa: "'Honesty, sobriety and diligence': Master-apprentice Relations in Eighteenth- and Nineteenth-century England." *Social History* Vol. 33, No. 2, 2008, pp. 183–200.

Levene, Alysa: *Childcare, Health and Mortality at the London Foundling Hospital, 1741–1800.* Manchester University Press: Manchester, 2007.

Lewis, Jayne Elizabeth: *Literary Culture, 1651–1740.* Cambridge University Press: Cambridge, 1996.

Lillywhite, Bryant: *The London Coffee Houses: A Reference Book of Coffee Houses of the Seventeenth, Eighteenth, and Nineteenth Centuries.* George Allen & Unwin: London, 1963.

Lloyd, G. Marner: "The Life and Works of Percivall Pott, 1714–1789, Wix Prize Essay 1933." *Saint Bartholomew's Hospital Reports* Vol. 46, 1933, pp. 291–336.

Lloyd, Sarah: *Charity and Poverty in England, c.1680–1820: Wild and Visionary Schemes.* Manchester University Press: Manchester, 2009.

Longstaffe-Gowan, Todd: *The London Square.* Yale University Press: New Haven, CT, 2012.

Loudon, Irvine: "Medical Practitioners 1750–1850 and the Period of Medical Reform in Britain." In: *Medicine in Society*: Historical Essays. Wear, Andrew, Cambridge University Press: Cambridge, 1992, pp. 219–247.

Macilwain, George: *Memoirs of John Abernethy* Hurst and Blackett: London, 1853.

Macleish, D. G.: "Pott, Pedantry and Precision." *Aust. NZ Surg.* Vol. 67, 1997, pp. 520–23.

Martin S.: *A Calculus of Suffering: Pain, Professionalism, and Anesthesia in Nineteenth-Century America.* Columbia Press: New York, 1985.

McCrory, P. R.: "Sir Percivall Pott—the First Sports Neurologist?" *British Journal of Sports Medicine* Vol. 35, 2001, pp. 278–280.

McDonald, Stuart W.: "William Cruikshank (1745–1800), Anatomist and Surgeon, and His Illustrious Patient, Samuel Johnson." *Clinical Anatomy* Vol. 28, 2015, pp. 836–843.

McIntyre, Ian: *Hester: The Remarkable Life of Dr Johnson's 'Dear Mistress.'* Constable: London, 2008.

McKenzie, Andrea: *Tyburn's Martyrs: Execution in England, 1675–1775*, Continuum Books: London, 2007.

Melicow, Meyer M. "Percivall Pott (1713–1788): 200th Anniversary of First Report of Occupation-Induced Cancer of Scrotum in Chimney Sweepers." *Urology* Vol. 6, No. 6, 1975, pp. 745–49.

Mellick, S. A.: "Abernethy and the Golden Age of Surgical Teaching." *Aust. N.Z. J. Surg.* Vol. 67, 1997, pp. 528–33.

Miles, Adrian with Connell, Brian: "New Bunhill Fields Burial Ground, Southwark, Excavations at Globe Academy, 2008." *Museum of London Archaeology,* Archaeology Series 24, 2012.

Miller, Elizabeth C. and Miller James A.: "Milestones in Chemical Carcinogenesis." *Oncology* Vol. 6, No. 4, 1979, pp. 445–56.

Mills, Philip R.: "Privates on Parade: Soldiers, Medicine and the Treatment of Inguinal Hernias in Georgian England." In: Geoffrey L. Hudson (ed.), *British Military and Naval Medicine, 1600–1830.* Rodopi: Amsterdam, 2007, pp. 149–182.

Milne I. A., Passmore, R., Doig, A., and Ferguson J. P. S.: *William Cullen and the Eighteenth Century Medical World: A Bicentenary Exhibition and Symposium Arranged by the Royal College of Physicians of Edinburgh.* Edinburgh University Press: Edinburgh, 1993.

Minns, Chris and Wallis, Patrick: "Rules and Reality: Quantifying the Practice of Apprenticeship in Early Modern England." *Economic History Review* Vol. 65, No. 2. 2012, pp. 556–579.

Minns, Chris and Wallis, Patrick: "The Price of Human Capital in a Pre-industrial Economy: Premiums and Apprenticeship Contracts in 18th Century England." *Explorations in Economic History* Vol. 50, 2013, pp. 333–350.

Moore, Norman: *History of St. Bartholomew's Hospital.* C. Arthur Pearson Ltd.: London, 1918.

Moore, Wendy: *The Knife Man: The Extraordinary Life and Times of John Hunter, Father of Modern Surgery.* Bantam: London, 2005.

Morgan, Sir Clifford Naunton: "Surgery and Surgeons in 18th-Century London." *Annals of the Royal College of Surgeons of England.* Vol. 42, 1968, pp. 1–37.

Morgan, Gwenda and Rushton, Peter: "The Magistrate, the Community and the Maintenance of an Orderly Society in Eighteenth-century England." *Historical Research* Vol. 76, No. 191 2003, pp. 54–77.

Morgan, Lee: *Dr. Johnson's "own Dear Master," The Life of Henry Thrale.* University Press of America, Inc.: Lanham, MD, 1998.

Moulin, D. De: "The Treatment of Compound Fractures in the Eighteenth Century." *The Netherlands Journal of Surgery.* Vol. 37, No. 2, 1985, pp. 54–59.

Mumford, James Gregory: *Surgical Memoirs: and Other Essays*, Moffat, Yard and Company: New York, 1908.

Murdoch, Tessa and Vigne, Randolph: *The French Hospital in England: Its Huguenot History and Collections.* Adamson: Cambridge, UK, 2009.

Murray, R. W.: *Edward Alanson and His Times.* Samuel Hill & Sons: Liverpool, 1914.

Nechtman, Tillman W.: *Nabobs: Empire and Identity in Eighteenth-Century Britain.* Cambridge University Press: Cambridge, 2010.

Neve, M.: "Orthodoxy and Fringe: Medicine in Late Georgian Bristol." In: Bynum, W. F. and Porter, Roy (eds.), *Medical Fringe & Medical Orthodoxy, 1750–1850.* Croom Helm: Beckenham, 1987, pp. 40–55.

Newton, Hannah: *The Sick Child in Early Modern England, 1580–1720.* Oxford University Press: Oxford, 2012.

Newton, Hannah: "Children's Physic: Medical Perceptions and Treatment of Sick Children in Early Modern England, c. 1580–1720." *Social History of Medicine* Vol. 23, No. 3, 2010, pp. 456–474.

Ober, William B.: *Boswell's Clap and Other Essays.* Southern Illinois University Press: Carbondale, 1979.

Oliver, Vere Langford: *The History of the Island of Antigua, One of the Leeward Caribees in the West Indies, from the First Settlement in 1635 to the Present Time.* Mitchell and Hughes: London, 1894.

Olleson, Philip: *The Journals and Letters of Susan Burney: Music and Society in Late Eighteenth-Century England.* Ashgate Publishing Ltd.: Farnham, 2012.

Ottaway, S. R.: *The Decline of Life: Old Age in Eighteenth-century England.* The Press Syndicate of the University of Cambridge: Cambridge, 2004.

Ottley, Drewery: *The Life of John Hunter.* Longman, Rees, Orman, Brown, Green and Longman: London, 1853.

Owen, Edmund: "The Huntarian Oration on John Hunter and His Museum, Delivered at the Royal College of Surgeons of England." *The British Medical Journal* Vol. 1, No. 2616, 1911, pp. 341–347.

Owen, Edmund: "Remarks on Hernia—Particularly in Children." *The British Medical Journal* Vol. 1, No. 2422, 1907, pp. 128–9.

Page, Anthony: *John Jebb and the Enlightenment Origins of British Radicalism*. Praeger Publishers: Westport, CT, 2003.

Paget, Sir James: *The Hunterian Oration of 1877*. Longmans, Green and Co.: London, 1877.

Paley, Ruth: *Justice in 18th-Century Hackney: The Justicing Notebook of Henry Norris and the Hackney Petty Sessions Book*. London Record Society: London, 1991.

Parry-Jones, William L.: *The Trade in Lunacy: A Study of Private Madhouses in England in the Eighteenth and Nineteenth Centuries*. Routledge & Kegan Paul: London, 1972.

Patwardhan, R. P.: *Fort William-India House Correspondence*. Vol. 7, Government of India, Civil Lines: Delhi, 1971.

Peachey, George: *John Heaviside*. St. Martin's Press: London, 1931.

Peachey, George: *A Memoir of William and John Hunter*. Brendan, Plymouth, 1924.

Peachey, George: "William Bromfield, 1713–1792," *Proceedings of the Royal Society of Medicine*. Vol. 8, 1915, pp. 103–126.

Peakman, Julie: *Laviscious Bodies. A Sexual History of the Eighteenth Century*. Atlantic: London, 2004.

Peakman, Julie: *Whore Biographies 1700–1825*. Pickering & Chatto: London, 2006.

Pelling, Margaret: "Corporatism or Individualism: Parliament, the Navy, and the Splitting of the London Barber-Surgeons' Company in 1745." In: Gadd, Ian and Wallis, Patrick (eds.): *Guilds and Associations in Europe, 900–1900*. Centre for Metropolitan History: London, 2006, pp. 57–82.

Peltier, Leonard F.: "Percivall Pott and Pott's Fracture." *Surgery* Vol. 51, No. 2, 1962, pp. 280–286.

Pernick, Martin S.: *A Calculus of Suffering: Pain, Professionalism, and Anesthesia in Nineteenth-Century America*, Columbia Press, 1985.

Phythian-Adams, Charles: "Milk and Soot: The Changing Vocabulary of a Popular Ritual in Stuart and Hanoverian London." In: Fraser, Derek and Sutcliffe, Anthony (eds.): *The Pursuit of Urban History*. Edward Arnold Publishers Ltd.: London, 1983, pp. 83–104.

Plaut, G: "Dr. John Fothergill and Eighteenth-century Medicine." *Journal of Medical Biography* Vol. 7, No. 4 1999, pp. 192–6.

Pointon, Marcia R.: *Strategies for Showing: Women, Possession, and Representation in English Visual Culture*. Oxford University Press: Oxford, 1997.

Porter, Dorothy and Porter, Roy: *Patient's Progress: Doctors and Doctoring in Eighteenth-Century England*. Polity Press: Cambridge, UK, 1989.

Porter, Roy: *Madmen: A Social History of Madhouses, Mad-Doctors and Lunatics*. Tempus: Stroud, 2004.

Porter, Roy: *Bodies Politic: Disease, Death, and Doctors in Britain, 1650–1900*. Cornell University Press: Ithaca, NY, 2001.

Porter, Roy: *Quacks: Fakers & Charlatans in English Medicine*. Tempus: Stroud, 2000.

Porter, Roy: "Accidents in the Eighteenth Century." In: Roger Cooter (ed.), *Accidents in History: Injuries, Fatalities, and Social Relations*. Clio Medica/Wellcome Institute Series in the History of Medicine. Rodopi Press: Amsterdam, 1997, pp. 90–106.

Porter, Roy: "Medical Lecturing in Georgian London." *The British Journal for the History of Science* Vol. 28, No. 1, 1995, pp. 91–99.

Porter, Roy: "'Expressing Yourself Ill': The Language of Sickness in Georgian England." In: Burke, P. and Porter, Roy (eds.), *Language, Self and Society: A Social History of Language*. Polity Press: Cambridge, 1991, pp. 276–299.

Porter, Roy: *Health for Sale: Quackery in England, 1660–1850*. Manchester University Press: Manchester, 1989.

Porter, Roy: *Mind-Forg'd Manacles: A History of Madness in England from the Restoration to the Regency*. Athlone: London, 1987.

Porter, Roy: "William Hunter: A Surgeon and a Gentleman." In: Bynum, W. F. and Porter, Roy (eds.), *William Hunter and the Eighteenth-Century Medical World*. Cambridge University Press: Cambridge, 1985, pp. 7–34.

Power, D'Arcy: "Two Liverpool Surgeons." *The British Journal of Surgery* Vol. 24, No. 94, 1936, pp. 205–207.

Power, D'Arcy: Pott's Disease of the Spine." *The British Journal of Surgery*. Vol. 11, No. 41, July 1923, pp. 1–6.

Power, D'Arcy: "Nova Et Vetera." *The British Medical Journal*, Vol. 1, No. 2404, 1907, pp. 211–213.

Power, D'Arcy: *Memorials of the Craft of Surgery in England compiled by John Flint South*. Cassell & Company: London, 1886.

Powers D. Arcy: *The Dictionary of National Biography*. Vol. 46, London: Smith, Elder & Co. 1885–1900, pp. 207–211.

Price, Frederick George Hilton: *A Handbook of London Bankers*. Simpkin, Marshall, Hamilton, Kent & Company, Scribner & Welford: London, 1891.

Rabier, Christelle & Hilaire-Pérez, Liliane: "Self-Machinery? Steel Trusses and the Management of Ruptures in Eighteenth-Century Europe." *Technology and Culture* Vol. 54, No. 3, pp. 460–502. http://doi.org/10.1353/tech.2013.0096

Rabier, Christelle: "Defining a Profession: Surgery, Professional Conflicts and Legal Powers in Paris and London, 1760–1790." In: Rabier, Christelle (ed.), *Fields of Expertise: A Comparative History of Expert Procedures in Paris and London, 1600 to Present*. Cambridge Scholars Publishing: Newcastle, 2007, pp. 85–114.

Ravitch, Mark M.: "Invective in Surgery: William Hunter Versus Monro Primus, Monro Secundus, and Percival Pott." *Bulletin of the New York Academy of Medicine* Vol. 50, No. 7, 1974, pp. 797–816.

Redford, Bruce: *The Letters of Samuel Johnson*. Princeton University Press: Princeton, NJ, 1992.

Reinarz, Jonathan: "Corpus Curricula: Medical Education and the Voluntary Hospital Movement." In: Harry Whitaker, C.U.M. Smith, Stanley Finger, Lesley Richmond, Julie Stevenson, Alison Turton (eds.), *The Pharmaceutical Industry: A Guide to Historical Records*. Ashgate Publishing Ltd.: Farnham, 2003, pp. 43–52.

Richardson, Ruth: *Death, Dissection and the Destitute*. University of Chicago Press: Chicago, 2000.

Richmond, Lesley, Stevenson, Julie and Turton, Alison (eds.): *The Pharmaceutical Industry: A Guide to Historical Records*. Ashgate Publishing Ltd.: Farnham, 2003.

Risse, Guenther: *Mending Bodies—Saving Souls: A History of Hospitals*. Oxford University Press: New York, 1999.

Risse, Guenther: *Hospital Life in Enlightenment Scotland: Care and Teaching at the Royal Infirmary of Edinburgh*. Cambridge University Press, New York, 1986.

Roberts, Lissa: "Science Becomes Electric: Dutch Interaction with the Electrical Machine during the Eighteenth Century." *Isis* Vol. 90, No. 4, 1999, pp. 680–714.

Robinson, James O.: "The Royal and Ancient History of St. Bartholomew (founded 1123)." *Journal of Medical Biography* Vol. 1, No. 1, 1993, pp. 23–30.

Rogers, John Jope: *Opie and His Works: Being a Catalogue of 760 Pictures by John Opie, R. A.* Paul and Dominic Connaught: London, 1878.

Rogers, Nicholas: "Money, Marriage, Mobility: The Big Bourgeoisie of Hanoverian London." *Journal of Family History* Vol. 24, No. 1, 1999, pp. 19–34.

Rosenthal, Laura J.: *Nightwalkers: Prostitute Narratives from the Eighteenth Century*, Broadview Press: Toronto, 2008.

Ross, John A., "Percivall Pott, 1714–1788." *Paraplegia* Vol. 24, 1986, pp. 287–292.

Rubenhold, Hallie: *The Covent Garden Ladies: Pimp General Jack & the Extraordinary Story of Harris's List*. Tempus Publishing: Stroud, 2006.

Ruisinger, Marion Maria R.: "Lorenz Heister (1683–1738) and the 'Bachmann Case': Social Setting and Medical Practice of Trepanation in Eighteenth-Century Germany." In: Arnott, Robert, Finger, Stanley, and Smith, C. U. M. (eds.): *Trepanation, Discovery, History, Theory*. Swets and Zeitlinger: Lisse, 2003, pp. 273–288.

Ruisinger, Marion Maria R.: "Lorenz Heister and the Challenge of Trepanation: A Neurosurgical Case Study From the 18th Century." *Journal of the History of Neurosciences* Vol. 11, No. 3, 2002, pp. 286–300.

Ruston, Sharon: "One of the 'modern sceptics': Reappraising Shelley's Medical Education." *Romanticism* Vol. 9, No. 1, 2003, pp. 1–20.

Sachs, Michael, Bojunka, Jörg, and Encke, Albrecht: "Historical Evolution of Limb Amputation." *World Journal of Surgery* Vol. 23, 1999, pp. 1088–1093,

Sakorafas, G. H. & Safioleas, M.: "Breast Cancer Surgery: An Historical Narrative. Part II, 18th and 19th centuries." *European Journal of Cancer Care* Vol. 19, 2010, pp. 6–29.

Saletore, B. A.: *Fort William-India House Correspondence*. Vol. 9, Government of India, Civil Lines: Delhi, 1959.

Salzman, L. F.: *A History of the County of Sussex*. Vol. 4, Victoria County History: London, 1953.

Schlich, Thomas: "'The Days of Brilliancy are Past': Skill, Styles and the Changing Rules of Surgical Performance, ca. 1820–1920." *Medical History* Vol. 59, No. 3, 2015 July, pp. 379–403.

Schlich, Thomas: *The Origins of Organ Transplantation: Surgery and Laboratory Science, 1880–1930*. University of Rochester Press: Rochester, 2012.

Schlich, Thomas: "The Emergence of Modern Surgery," In: Brunton, D. (ed.), *Medicine Transformed: Health, Disease and Society in Europe, 1800–1930*. Manchester University Press: Manchester, 2004, pp. 61–91.

Schillace, Brandy Lain: "Reproducing Custom: Mechanical Habits and Female Machines in Augustan Women's Education." *Feminist Formations* Vol. 25, 2013, pp. 111–137.

Schwartz, L. D.: *London in the Age of Industrialisation: Entrepreneurs, Labour Force and Living Conditions, 1700–1850*. University of Cambridge: Cambridge, 1993.

Segal, Judy Z.: *Health and the Rhetoric of Medicine*. Southern Illinois University Press: Carbondale, 2008.

Shand, William: "Percivall Pott, FRS (1716–1788)." *Trauma* Vol. 2, 2000, pp. 291–295.

Shaw, A. Batty: "Benjamin Gooch, Eighteenth-Century Surgeon." *Medical History* Vol. 16, 1972, pp. 40–50.

Shesgreen, Sean: *Images of the Outcast: The Urban Poor in the Cries of London*. Manchester University Press: Manchester, 2002.

Shoemaker, Robert: *London Mob: Violence and Disorder in Eighteenth-Century England*. Hambledon Continuum: London, 2007.

Siena, Kevin: *Venereal Disease, Hospitals and the Urban Poor: London's "Foul Wards," 1600–1800*. Routledge: New York and London, 2004.

Siena, Kevin: "Hospitals for the Excluded or Convalescent Homes? Workhouses, Medicalization and the Poor Law in Long Eighteenth-Century London and Pre-Confederation Toronto." *CBMH/BCHM* Vol. 27, No. 2010, pp. 5–25.

Siena, Kevin: "Suicide as an Illness Strategy in the Long Eighteenth Century." In: Weaver, John and Wright, David (eds.), *Histories of Suicide: International Perspectives on Self-Destruction in the Modern World*. University of Toronto: Toronto, 2009, pp. 53–72.

Siena, Kevin: "Stage-Managing a Hospital in the Eighteenth-Century: Visitation at the London Lock Hospital." In: Graham Mooney and Jonathan Reinarz (eds.). *Permeable Walls: Historical Perspectives on Hospital and Asylum Visiting*. Editions Rodopi: Amsterdam, 2009, pp. 175–198.

Siena, Kevin: "Contagion, Exclusion, and the Unique Medical World of the Eighteenth-Century Workhouse." In: Reinarz, Jonathan and Schwarz, Leonard (eds.), *Medicine and the Workhouse*. University of Rochester Press: Rochester, 2013, pp. 19–39.

Simmons, Anna: "Medicines, Monopolies and Mortars: The Chemical Laboratory and Pharmaceutical Trade at the Society of Apothecaries in the Eighteenth Century." *Ambix* Vol. 53, No. 3, 2006, pp. 221–236.

Smith, D. J.: *Discovering Horse-drawn Vehicles*. Princes Risborough: Shire Publications, 1994.

Smith, Greg T.: "Expanding the Compass of Domestic Violence in the Hanoverian Metropolis." *Journal of Social History* Vol. 41, No. 1, 2007, pp. 31–54.

Smith, Lisa Wynne: "The Body Embarrassed? Rethinking the Leaky Male Body in Eighteenth-Century England and France." *Gender & History* Vol. 23, No. 1, 2010, pp. 26–46.

Smith, L. W.: "Reassessing the Role of the Family: Women's Medical Care in Eighteenth-century England." *Social History of Medicine* Vol. 16, No. 3, 2003, pp. 327–342.

Snow, Stephanie J.: *Blessed Days of Anesthesia: How Anaesthetics Changed the World.* Oxford University Press: Oxford, 2008.

Sorge-English, Lynn: *Stays and Body Image in London: The Staymaking Trade, 1680–1810.* Pickering and Chatto: London, 2011.

South, John Flint: *Memorials of the Craft of Surgery in England.* Cassell and Co.: London, 1886.

Spear, Percival: *The Nabobs: A Study of the Social Life of the English in Eighteenth Century India.* Oxford University Press: Oxford, 1998.

Spencer, Alfred: *Memoirs of William Hickey.* Hurst & Blackett Ltd.: London, 1919.

Stanley, Peter: *For Fear of Pain. British Surgery, 1790–1850.* Amsterdam: Rodopi Press, 2003.

Stearns, Raymond Phineas: *A Journey to Paris in the Year 1698 by Martin Lister.* University of Illinois Press: Bloomington, 1967.

Steele, I. K.: "A London Trader and the Atlantic Empire: Joseph Cruttenden, Apothecary, 1710 to 1717." *The William and Mary Quarterly* Vol. 34, No. 2, 1977, pp. 281–297.

Steele, I. K.: *Atlantic Merchant Apothecary: Letters of Joseph Cruttenden, 1710–1717.* University of Toronto Press: Toronto, 1977.

Stephens, Frederic George: *Catalogue of Prints and Drawings in the British Museum.* Chidwick Press: London, 1883.

Stern, Walter: *The Porters of London.* Longmans and Green: London, 1960.

Sternbach, G.: "Percivall Pott: Tuberculous Spondylitis." *The Journal of Emergency Medicine* Vol. 14, No. 1, 1996, pp. 79–83.

Stewart, Grace G.: "A History of the Medicinal Uses of Tobacco, 1492–1860." *Medical History* Vol. 11, 1967, pp. 228–268.

Still, George Frederic: *The History of Paediatrics: The Progress of the Study of the Diseases of Children up to the End of the XVIIIth Century.* Dawsons of Pall Mall: London, 1965.

Stookes, Alexander: "Obstetrics: Past, Present, and Future." *British Medical Journal* Vol. 2, No. 3074, 1919, pp. 701–703.

Stolberg, Michael: *Experiencing Illness and the Sick Body in Early Modern Europe.* Palgrave Macmillan: Basingstoke, 2011.

Stone J. L. & Hockley A. D.: "Percivall Pott and the Miners of Cornwall." *British Journal of Neurosurgery* Vol. 16, No. 5, 2002, pp. 501–6.

Straub, Kristina: *Domestic Affairs: Intimacy, Eroticism, and Violence between Servants and Masters in Eighteenth-Century Britain.* Johns Hopkins University Press: Baltimore, 2008.

Sultan, Georg: *Atlas and Epitome of Abdominal Hernias.* W. B. Saunders & Co.: Philadelphia and London, 1902.

Sutton, Jean: *Lords of the East: The East India Company and Its Ships.* Conway Maritime Press Ltd.: London, 1981.

Tadmor, Naomi: *Family & Friends in Eighteenth-Century England: Household, Kinship, and Patronage.* Cambridge University Press: Cambridge, 2007.

Thomas, Peter G. D.: *George III: King and Politicians, 1760–1770.* Manchester University Press: Manchester, 2003.

Thornton, John L.: *John Abernethy: A Biography.* Simpkin Marshall Ltd.: London, 1953.

Towner, Elizabeth & Towner, John: "Developing the History of Unintentional Injury: The Use of Coroners' Records in Early Modern England." *Injury Prevention* Vol. 6, 2000, pp. 102–105.

Tranter, Neil: *Sport, Economy and Society in Britain 1750–1914*. Cambridge University Press: Cambridge, 1998.

Troide, Lars E. and Cooke, Stewart J. (eds.): *Early Journals and Letters of Fanny Burney*. Oxford University Press: Oxford, 1994.

Turner, David M.: *Disability in Eighteenth-Century England: Imagining Physical Impairment*. Routledge: London, 2012.

Turner, David M. and Withey, Alun: "Technologies of the Body: Polite Consumption and the Correction of Deformity in Eighteenth-Century England." *History: The Journal of the Historical Association* Vol. 454, 2002, pp. 775–796.

Underdown, David: *Start of Play: Cricket and Culture in Eighteenth-Century England*. Penguin Books: London, 2000.

Vickery, Amanda: "An Englishman's Home Is His Castle? Thresholds, Boundaries and Privacies in the Eighteenth-Century London House." *Past & Present* Vol. 199, 2008, pp. 147–173.

Voth, Hans-Joachim: "Time and Work in Eighteenth-Century London." *The Journal of Economic History* Vol. 58, No. 1 1998, pp. 29–58.

Waddington, Keir: *Medical Education at St. Bartholomew's Hospital, 1123–1995*. The Boydell Press: Woodbridge, Suffolk, 2003.

Walfpord, Edward: *Old and New London*, Vol. 6. Cassell, Petter & Galpin: London, 1878, pp. 29–44.

Wall, Cecil: *The History of the Surgeon's Company, 1745–1800*. Hutchinson's Scientific & Technical Publications: London, 1937.

Wall, Cecil, Cameron, H. Charles, and Underwood, E. Ashford: *A History of the Worshipful Society of Apothecaries of London*, Vol. I, 1617–1815. Oxford University Press: London, 1963.

Wallis, Patrick: "Apprenticeship and Training in Premodern England." *Journal of Economic History* Vol. 68, No. 3, 2008, pp. 832–861.

Wallis, Patrick: "Exotic Drugs and English Medicine: England's Drug Trade, c.1550–c.1800." *Social History of Medicine* Vol. 25, No. 1, 2011, pp. 20–46.

Wallis, P. J. and Wallis, R. V.: *Eighteenth Century Medics*. P. J. Phibb: P. J., 1988.

Wangensteen, Owen H. and Wangensteen, Sarah D.: *The Rise of Surgery: From Empiric Craft to Scientific Discipline*. Dawson: Folkestone, 1978.

Ward, Candace: *Desire and Disorder: Fevers, Fictions, and Feelings in English Georgian Culture*. Bucknell University Press: Lewisburg, 2007.

Warner, Jessica: *Craze: Gin and Debauchery in the Age of Reason*. Four Walls Eight Windows: New York, 2002.

Warner, John Harley: *The Therapeutic Perspective: Medical Practice, Knowledge, and Identity in America, 1820–1885*. Princeton University Press: Princeton, NJ, 2014.

Warren, Carol A. B.: "Gender Reassignment Surgery in the Eighteenth Century." *Sexualities*, Vol. 17, No. 7, 2014, pp. 872–884.

Waterhouse, Ellis and Blunt, Anthony: *The James A. De Rothschild Collections at Waddeson Manor: Paintings*. Fribourg, Switzerland: Office du Livre, 1967.

Wear, Andrew: *Knowledge and Practice in English Medicine, 1550–1680*. Cambridge University Press: Cambridge, 2000.

Wear, Andrew: "Caring for the Sick Poor in St. Bartholomew's Exchange: 1580–1676." *Medical History* Supplement No. 11, 1991, pp. 41–60.

Weiner, M-F., and Silver, J. R.: "The Contribution to Our Understanding of Spinal Disorders by the Great Windmill Street School of Anatomy." *Spinal Cord* Vol. 49, 2011, pp. 323–332.

Whitaker, Harry, Smith, C.U.M., and Finger, Stanley (eds.): *Brain, Mind and Medicine: Essays in Eighteenth-Century Neuroscience.* Springer Science & Business Media: London, 2007.

White, Jerry: *London in the Eighteenth Century: A Great and Monstrous Thing.* The Bodley Head: London, 2012.

Wild, W.: *Medicine-by-post: The Changing Voice of Illness in Eighteenth-century British Consultation Letters and Literature.* Editions Rodopi: Amsterdam, 2006.

Wiltshire, J.: *Samuel Johnson in the Medical World: The Doctor and the Patient.* Press Syndicate of the University of Cambridge: Cambridge, 1991.

Williams, A. N.: "Four Candles. Original Perspectives and Insights into 18th Century Hospital Child Healthcare." *Archives of Diseases in Childhood* Vol. 92, 2007, pp. 75–79.

Williams, Samantha: "The Experience of Pregnancy and Childbirth for Unmarried Mothers in London, 1760–1866." *Women's History Review* Vol. 20, No. 1, 2011, pp. 67–86.

Williams, W. R.: *The History of the Great Sessions in Wales, 1542–1830.* Edwin Davies: Welshpool, 1899.

Wilson, C. R.: *List of Inscriptions on Tombs or Monuments in Bengal possessing historical interest.* Office of the Superintendent of Government Printing: Calcutta, 1896.

Wilson, P.: "An Enlightenment Science? Surgery and the Royal Society." In: Porter, Roy (ed.), *Medicine in the Enlightenment.* Clio Medica, Rodopi: Amsterdam, 1995, pp. 360–286.

Wilson, William James Erasmus: *The History of Middlesex Hospital During the First Century of Its Existence.* John Churchill: London, 1865.

Winslow, Forbes: *Physic and Physicians: A Medical Sketch Book, exhibiting, The Public and Private Life of the Most Celebrated Medical Men of Former Days; with Memoirs of Eminent Living London Physicians and Surgeons.* Londman, Orme, Brown, and Co.: London, 1839.

Wrightson, Keith: *Earthly Necessities: Economic Lives in Early Modern Britain.* Yale University Press: New Haven, CT, 2000.

Yorke, Philip C.: *The Diary of John Baker, Barrister of the Middle Temple, Solicitor-General of the Leeward Islands.* Hutchinson & Co.: London, 1931.

Zigarovich, Jolene: "Preserved Remains: Embalming Practices in Eighteenth-Century England." *Eighteenth-Century Life* Vol. 33, Fall 2009, pp. 65–104.

Index

Note: Page numbers in italic indicate figures.

A

B

C

D

E

F

G

H

I

J

K

L

M

N

O

P

Q

R

S